Musculoskeletal Examination

Musculoskeletal Examination

Chief Author and Editor

Vivek Pandey MBBS MS (Orthopedics)
Associate Professor
Trauma, Joint Replacement, Sports Medicine, and
Arthroscopy Division
Department of Orthopedic Surgery
Kasturba Medical College
Manipal Academy of Higher Education
Manipal, Karnataka, India

Co-Author

Hitesh Shah MBBS MS
Associate Professor
Pediatric Orthopedic Division
Department of Orthopedic Surgery
Kasturba Medical College
Manipal Academy of Higher Education
Manipal, Karnataka, India

Forewords

M Shantharam Shetty MS
Mandeep S Dhillon MS
W Jaap Willems MD PhD

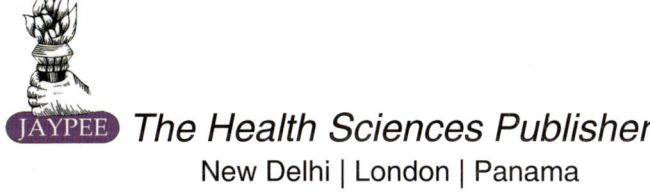

JAYPEE *The Health Sciences Publisher*
New Delhi | London | Panama

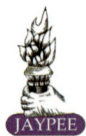

Jaypee Brothers Medical Publishers (P) Ltd

Headquarters

Jaypee Brothers Medical Publishers (P) Ltd.
4838/24, Ansari Road, Daryaganj
New Delhi 110 002, India
Phone: +91-11-43574357
Fax: +91-11-43574314
E-mail: jaypee@jaypeebrothers.com

Overseas Offices

JP Medical Ltd.
83, Victoria Street, London
SW1H 0HW (UK)
Phone: +44-20 3170 8910
Fax: +44(0)20 3008 6180
E-mail: info@jpmedpub.com

Jaypee-Highlights Medical Publishers Inc
City of Knowledge, Bld. 235, 2nd Floor, Clayton
Panama City, Panama
Phone: +1 507-301-0496
Fax: +1 507-301-0499
Email: cservice@jphmedical.com

Jaypee Brothers Medical Publishers (P) Ltd.
17/1-B, Babar Road, Block-B, Shyamoli
Mohammadpur, Dhaka-1207
Bangladesh
Mobile: +08801912003485
E-mail: jaypeedhaka@gmail.com

Jaypee Brothers Medical Publishers (P) Ltd.
Bhotahity, Kathmandu, Nepal
Phone: +977-9741283608
E-mail: kathmandu@jaypeebrothers.com

Website: www.jaypeebrothers.com
Website: www.jaypeedigital.com

© 2018, Jaypee Brothers Medical Publishers

Inquiries for bulk sales may be solicited at: jaypee@jaypeebrothers.com

Musculoskeletal Examination

First Edition: **2018**

ISBN: 978-93-5270-329-6

Printed at: Samrat Offset Pvt. Ltd.

Dedicated to

My Parents; Kuldip Narain Pandey and Manju Pandey
My wife Deeksha and son Krish
My brother and his family; Abhishek, Susanne, Demira and Maya
My Teachers and Students!

Contributors and Reviewers

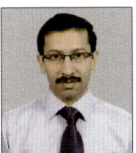

Ashwath Acharya MS ortho FNB (Hand Surgery)
Associate Professor
Department of Orthopedics
Kasturba Medical College
Manipal, Karnataka, India

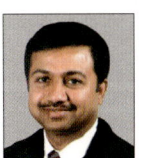

BC Navadgi
MS (Orth) MRCS MSc MCh (Orth) FRCS (T&O)
Consultant Orthopedic Surgeon
Great Western Hospital
Swindon, UK

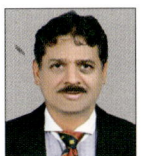

KR Prathap Kumar
MBBS FRCS (Tr&Orth) FRCS (Gen) D'Orth
Senior Consultant and Head
Shoulder and Upper Limb Unit
Sunrise Hospital
Kochi, Kerala, India

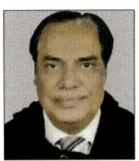

KN Pandey MS
Consultant Surgeon
BCM Hospital
Sitapur, Uttar Pradesh, India

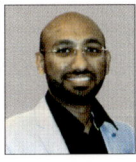

Darshan Jain MS ortho
Assistant Professor
Department of Orthopedics
MS Ramaiah Medical College
Bengaluru, Karnataka, India

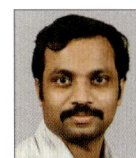

Raghuraj K MS ortho
Assistant Professor
Department of Orthopedics
Kasturba Medical College
Manipal, Karnataka, India

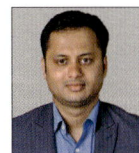

Nishanth A MS ortho
Assistant Professor
Department of Orthopedics
Kasturba Medical College
Manipal, Karnataka, India

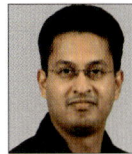

Sandesh M MS Ortho
Assistant Professor
Department of Orthopedics
Kasturba Medical College
Manipal, Karnataka, India

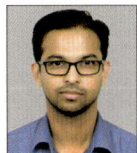

Sujayendra DM MS ortho
Senior Resident
Department of Orthopedics
St John's Medical College
Bengaluru, Karnataka, India

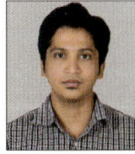

Naveen Mathai MS ortho
Senior Resident
Department of Orthopedics
Kasturba Medical College
Manipal, Karnataka, India

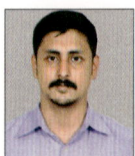

Jayakrishnan KN MS ortho
Senior Resident
Department of Orthopedics
Kasturba Medical College
Manipal, Karnataka, India

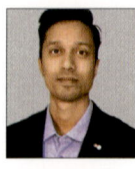

Sameer Qureshi DNB Ortho
Assistant Professor
Amaltas Institute of Medical Sciences
Dewas, Madhya Pradesh, India

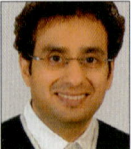

Krishnaprasad PR MS D'Ortho
Assistant Professor
Foot and Ankle Specialty Clinic
Department of Orthopedics
Kasturba Medical College
Manipal, Karnataka, India

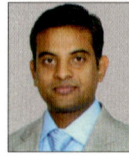

Kishore Reddy MS ortho
Consultant Musculoskeletal
Oncologist
Omni Hospital
Hyderabad, Telangana, India

Foreword

I feel it is indeed a pleasure for me for having been requested to scribe the foreword to Dr Vivek Pandey's book on *Musculoskeletal Examination*. To me a sound clinical examination is paramount in the diagnosis and management of patients with variable presentations.

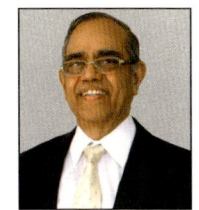

In this era of unparalleled bio-technological developments where a clinician and even an orthopedic trainee are forgetting the art and science of a sound clinical examination, this book emphasized on the fundamentals of clinical diagnosis. It is sad that many a times, an elaborate investigation is ordered before a clinical assessment.

Dr Vivek has indeed burnt many midnight lamps to bring out this outstanding treatise on clinical examination. He as a teacher, surgeon, examiner and a clinician has understood the importance of a shabbily done clinical examination, which can have a bad impact on the daily life of our patients who come to us with so much of faith and hope.

In his well-illustrated book of 15 chapters, Dr Pandey has gone into the fundamentals and at the same time, the depth of most of the commonly faced musculoskeletal injuries and disorders. His book is comprehensive, well structured and made easy to arrive at a clinical diagnosis. I am sure this book will be a landmark amongst the large number of books which have come out on clinical examination. It is so different from others and it is bound to stand out from others because of the excellent flow of thoughts, clear photographic illustrations and more than all the passion with which this book has been written.

I should really compliment Dr Vivek Pandey for realizing his dreams and for his tenacity of purpose for this monumental work. I am sure all of us from senior most surgeons to the junior residents, postgraduate to undergraduate students will greatly be benefitted by going through this book. It shall definitely adorn the shelves of all our libraries as a ready reference book.

I would like to end my foreword by quoting these famous words from Upanishad:

ॐ असतो मा सद् गमय । तमसो मा ज्योतिर्गमय । मृत्योर्माऽमृतम् गमय ।।

This book has indeed brought in light from darkness, from ignorance to enlightenments and from death to the very essence of life.

M Shantharam Shetty
Pro-Chancellor, NITTE University
Mangaluru, Karnataka, India
Past President – Indian Orthopedic Association
Past AO Trustee & AO Trauma India Council Chairman

Foreword

It is with great pleasure that I write this brief foreword for this interesting book *Musculoskeletal Examination*, written specifically for young surgeons and surgeons in training. A much overdue tome for the Asian population, the aim of this book is to bring about clarity in the understanding of orthopedic examination by surgeons in training, which it does in a very structured and pictorial format. Focused both on undergraduate students who are only beginning to grasp medicine, and postgraduate students who are attempting to grasp Orthopedics, this is a timely effort, as there is no appropriate modern orthopedic examination book available for both segments of the medical trainee population.

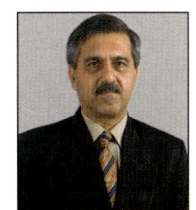

With 15 chapters, starting from the basics of orthopedic examination, including tips and know hows, the book advances to cover joint examinations in detail, covering some aspects of anatomy and function, followed by history taking and examination. The key element of note is the numerous pictures that illustrate the text, which go on to enhance the understanding of these problems in the minds of these young students struggling for comprehension of complex orthopedic situations.

The structure and format of all the chapters is similar for easier understanding. An added feature is that each chapter has a proforma, which emphasizes key points, which are helpful to remember for medical examination. Each chapter then ends with some basic information about common diseases affecting the joint, allowing some sort of overview of the situation, albeit for the student levels.

I compliment Dr Vivek Pandey for this excellent book, and I hope that it becomes the standard references for medical and orthopedic students

Mandeep S Dhillon MBBS MS (Orth) FAMS FRCS
President, Indian Orthopaedic Association
Chairman Research, AO Trauma (Asia Pacific)
Founder President, Indian Biological Orthopaedics Society
Past President, Indian Arthroplasty Association
Past President, Indian Association for Sports Medicine
Past President, Indian Foot and Ankle Society

Professor and Head, Orthopedics
Head, Physical Medicine Department
Postgraduate Institute of Medical Education and Research
Chandigarh, India

Foreword

Since long-time, the art of medicine consisted of proper history taking, thorough physical examination, completed with radiographic investigations.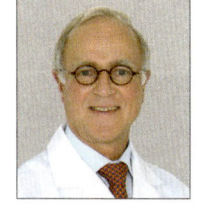

Nowadays we live in a time, where technology brought us important tools help us in the diagnosis and treatment of orthopedic diseases.

It is even suggested, that diagnostic modalities, like MRI, are more secure, than a simple physical examination; it is also well known, that several physical tests, used in daily practice are not so sensitive and specific and thus could perhaps be replaced by the more modern diagnostic tools. But we have also learned, that with the high accuracy of an MRI many orthopedic diseases can be detected, without having any clinical significance. It can lead to over-diagnosis and unnecessary treatment.

Not only for that reason, the core of our profession, continues to consist of the combination of listening to the patient, completed with an accurate physical examination.

Dr Pandey should be complimented with completing the huge tasks of overviewing all possible tests in several areas in orthopedics by selecting the most sensitive, thus most useful tests for daily practice.

The way the content of this book is organized, makes it a very practical tool, not only for the medical students and orthopedic residents, but also for all doctors, who deal with orthopedic patients, as well as physiotherapists.

I can heartily recommend this extensive book on physical examination, it deserves a place on many bookshelves!

W Jaap Willems MD PhD
Orthopedic Surgeon
Chief Shoulder and Elbow Unit, Lairesse Kliniek
Past President (European Society for Surgery of Shoulder and Elbow)
Amsterdam, The Netherlands

Preface

While I was pursuing my MBBS in the 90s, I had difficulties in understanding the musculoskeletal examination due to several reasons. One, fewer books were available and were not structured in the way orthopedic examination was taught and/or be understood. Two, there was barely any description of the basic anatomy, physiology and other facts which are required for the understanding of the joint and its assessment. Three, there were barely few pictures of the tests described. Over the years, the gap between 'requirement versus availability' of the structured, readable and pictorial format of orthopedic examination in print format continued to exist.

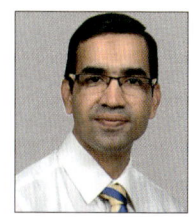

After I started clinical teaching for students as a resident and later as a staff, I always wondered how to simplify the clinical teaching, make it interesting, logical and deliver it in a structured fashion, especially for undergraduates whose interaction in orthopedics remains limited as compared to surgery, medicine, etc. Even for postgraduates, the available material remains less organized and sometimes, too much for basic understanding. Further, available material is quite a bit imaginary and devoid of pictures, which is difficult for a student to understand and apply. Many sections were poorly described such as peripheral nerve injury and spine examination. These two areas need understanding of basics of anatomy and function before the reader embarks the journey of understanding the examination. Certain sections were completely missing such as Amputation stump examination.

In my pursuit to make the clinical teaching simple and structured for students, I decided to pen down the entire basic orthopedic examination in a simple, structured and pictorial format, so that it becomes a 'one-stop basic referral' for musculoskeletal examination. I always believed that pictures and images say a lot than words! At one end, I wanted the book to have a basic understanding for undergraduates and on the other end to have advanced concepts for postgraduates too making it a complete guide for musculoskeletal examination.

After all the chapters were written, each chapter was reviewed by the specialist surgeons in the field to make it perfect for reading and understanding. However, despite multiple revisions of each chapter, paragraphs, word and reviews by another specialist, there is a possibility of some inadvertent error and unwanted omissions. We would welcome all suggestions and constructive criticism in our future reprints and revised editions.

If this simplified, structured, filled in with tips and pearls and pictorial academic material could help a student in understanding the nuances of musculoskeletal examination, I would feel blessed and consider my humble endeavor successful.

Mail your feedback and suggestions at: vivekortho@yahoo.co.in

Vivek Pandey

Acknowledgments

It gives me immense pleasure to acknowledge the efforts of every individual and organization who motivated and helped me in accomplishing my academic work on musculoskeletal examination.

At the onset, I am deeply indebted to my alma mater Kasturba Medical College (KMC), Manipal and its organizational support who has created an excellent academic and clinical environment for teaching. Even though I conceptualized, wrote many chapters and edited the entire work, this academic work was not possible without the help of my colleagues Drs Hitesh, Sujayendra Murali, Naveen Mathai and Sameer Qureshi, who contributed several sections of the book and helped in the perfect shaping of this book. My father, Dr KN Pandey, who has always taught me tenets of life, professionalism and surgical skills too contributed a chapter.

After the text part of the book was over, the most important contributors of this book stepped in that is my two 2nd year residents; Dr Raghavendra Vyas and Dr Sashi Aier. The black and white text would not have been interesting without colorful images wherein both of my handsome residents agreed to model for various clinical tests on multiple occasion amidst their grueling schedule of orthopedics.

A disciple's growth exponentially accelerates if he has the guidance of great mentors! I thank my mentor Prof Sripathi Rao and my lifelong mentor and father Dr KN Pandey, who continue to inspire me about simplified and structured teaching. Further, I have been lucky to have great teachers like Prof(s) Benjamin Joseph, SP Mohanti and Sharath Rao, whose teaching methods had a remarkable effect on my teaching style. Special thanks to Prof Vineet Sharma from KGMC, Lucknow who always encouraged me to continue writing newer materials which can help students. I also thank my senior colleagues Prof Anil Bhat and Shyamsunder Bhat whose day-to-day guidance remains precious. My colleague Prof Kiran Acharya continued to give me invaluable inputs at each stage of book writing, editing and layout over morning coffee.

I am indebted to many of my colleagues who pitched in to review chapters to ensure that each section of the book is up to the mark. I thank Dr Navadgi (Consultant Hip and Knee Surgeon, Swindon, UK) for his valuable opinion in the knee and hip section and Dr KR Prathap Kumar (Consultant Shoulder and Elbow Surgeon, Sunrise Hospital, Kochi), for reviewing the shoulder and elbow section and providing valuable inputs. I thank my colleague Dr Darshan (Asst Prof, MS Ramaiah Medical College, Bengaluru) who is a brilliant wrist and hand surgeon for reviewing wrist and hand section and contributing the wrist instability section. My heartfelt thanks to Dr Nishanth Ampar (Asst Prof, KMC Manipal) and Dr Raghuraj Kundangar (Asst Prof, KMC Manipal), for their worthwhile opinion about the spine section. My senior

Dr Ashwath Acharya (Asso Prof, KMC Manipal) who is very experienced in the field of brachial plexus and peripheral nerve injuries management reviewed the peripheral nerve injury section and gave many useful comments. Vast experience of Dr Kishore Reddy (Musculoskeletal Oncologist, Hyderabad) helped in shaping the bone tumor section.

This work was impossible to complete without the help of my colleagues Drs Naveen Mathai, Sandesh Madi and Jayakrishnan who extensively reviewed the entire manuscript and provided precious comments. During the early days of the writing of each section, few of my interns (Drs Jasleen, Prachi and Tirth) gave me important feedback from the student point of view.

Even though it is the hard work of the author, but this work would not have seen the light of the day without the help of Sri Jitendar P Vij (Group Chairman) and Mr Ankit Vij (Group President) of M/S Jaypee Brothers Medical Publishers (P) Ltd, New Delhi, India and their team. I thank Ms Chetna Malhotra Vohra (Associate Director—Content Strategy), Ms Payal (Senior Manager—Publishing) and Mr Venugopal for giving me patient hearing while I narrated my entire project to them. Once the work on book started; the immense help extended by Ms Ritika Chandna (Development Editor) and Mr Vipin Kaushik (Team Leader—Typesetting Department) at each stage is commendable. Both ensured that all my request were appropriately and timely addressed.

Most importantly, I am indebted towards my patients who have always deposed trust in me. The experience gained from them reflects at each step of this book. I also thank all my students of yesteryears and present whose inquisitiveness for knowledge ensured that I continued to make the teaching simple!

Contents

Basics of History Taking and Examination in Orthopedics

▌ FORMAT FOR ORTHOPEDIC CASE PRESENTATION WITH SIMPLE KNOW-HOWS AND TIPS

Before history taking and examination, it is important that the physician greets the patient and introduces himself/herself to the patient. This helps in building the confidence and cooperation in the physician–patient relationship.

Case presentation starts with basic demographic details.

1. Name
2. Age
3. Sex
4. Occupation
5. Address and
6. Handedness (especially in a case involving the upper limb)

Initial demographic details are informed as "Miss NN, a 26-year-old female from Delhi, left-handed person, software professional by occupation, presents with chief complaints of…"

Chief complaints (in chronological order)

1. A
2. B
3. C
4. D

The chief complaints could be single or multiple. Each complaint should be assessed for onset, duration, progression, aggravating and relieving factors. Further, one can assess any specific points about the same problem; e.g. chills and rigor for fever, radiation in case of pain, etc.

The major complaints in orthopedic patients are:

- Pain
- Swelling
- Difficulty in bearing weight/inability to move a joint
- Deformity
- Shortening or lengthening of a limb
- Instability of the joint
- Locking

- Limp
- *Systemic features*: Fever, weight loss, etc.
- Others

█ HISTORY OF PRESENT ILLNESS

Classically, the history of present illness is always started by stating "Patient was apparently all right … days/weeks/months back when he developed complaint of…"
Next, one must always ask "How did it start"? It means what led to initiation of that complaint or symptom. Was it a traumatic event (minor or major) or was it insidious in onset? The complaints are then elaborated as per the standard assessment protocol.

The fundamental idea of history of present illness (HOPI) assessment is that each chief complaint must be evaluated and described in detail regarding onset, duration, progression, aggravating and relieving factors and other specific points, if any. Once all the chief complaints are well described, the relevant positive and negative history is taken. *The aim of this exercise of detailing HOPI with positive and negative history is to zero in on the possible etiology and pathology of the symptoms in question*.

The possible etiopathology of the symptoms could be
Congenital/Traumatic/Infective/Inflammatory/Neoplastic/Degenerative/Metabolic/Hematological/Neurological/Others

Important Facts about Common Complaints

1. Pain

Apart from elaborating the pain, it is important to understand the nature of pain which could be "*mechanical" pain* or "*rest" pain,* or pain of "*neurological origin."*

- Usually, **mechanical pain** results from loading the joint (standing, walking, turning, running, jumping, etc.). It is usually due to degenerative pathologies like osteoarthritis, spondylosis, tendinopathies, fasciitis, etc.
- Usually, **rest pain** happens even without loading and is often associated with morning stiffness. It is usually due to inflammatory, infective, or tumorous disorders such as rheumatoid arthritis, ankylosing spondylitis, tuberculosis of the joint, malignant tumors, respectively. Any rest pain lasting for more than 3–4 weeks should be thoroughly investigated as "rest pain" could indicate underlying sinister pathology!

However, there are a *few exceptions* to the general rule about rest pain, e.g. shoulder and cervical spine degenerative pathologies. Most shoulder degenerative pathologies (rotator cuff tendinopathy, tear, frozen shoulder, arthritis, calcific tendinitis, etc.) are painful at night and may not hurt much during day time. Also, cervical spine intervertebral disc prolapse with root compression often hurts at night while the patient lies on the side (due to increased root compression). So, even though these conditions are painful at night, they do not indicate any sinister pathology.

- **The pain of neurological origin:** It is usually shooting/dragging type, often associated with tingling and numbness along the course of the nerve. It is often due to nerve compression due to varying etiologies.

2. Swelling

The swelling could be arising from the joint (intra-articular) or elsewhere. The swelling elsewhere could be from any underlying structure and should be evaluated as per the standard assessment. However, while assessing the intra-articular swelling, one must question the timing of onset of swelling especially after trauma.

- *If the intra-articular swelling has arisen immediately after or within a few hours of trauma,* it indicates hemarthrosis. Hemarthrosis is a result of injury to any intra-articular structure that is rich in blood supply (e.g. peripheral meniscal tear, cruciate ligament tear, synovial or capsular tears) or intra-articular fractures.
- *If the intra-articular swelling has arisen 12–24 hours after the injury,* it indicates excess synovial fluid production in the joint following synovial irritation. This could be due to any injury causing synovial irritation like cartilage injury, central or inner meniscal tear, foreign body reaction, chronic synovitis, etc.

3. Inability or difficulty in bearing weight (lower limb)

Normal weight bearing is possible due to the normal linkage between normally innervated "bone–joint–ligament–muscle–tendon–capsule" complexes. Any disturbance in this linkage could lead to inability to bear or difficulty in bearing weight.

- Acute h/o inability to bear weight after acute trauma indicates a significant bone or joint injury (fracture or dislocation), a nerve palsy, complete ligament injury, complete tendon tear, or major capsular disruption.
- If the patient can bear weight after the first acute injury, it "fairly well rules out" any significant bony or soft tissue injury. Nevertheless, in impacted fractures, one can still bear weight! Further; in case of partial injury to ligaments or tendons, the patient can bear weight albeit with difficulty.
- Chronic ligament injuries are more tolerant to weight bearing, i.e. most patients can bear weight easily or can use the limb with minimal difficulty. However, with every fresh episode of injury to the limb superimposed over chronic existing ligament injury, the patient returns to weight bearing or usage of limb faster than the previous occasion.
- A chronic h/o of inability to bear weight on lower limb indicates that there is nonunion of a fracture.

4. Inability or difficulty in moving a joint

The normal sequence to move a joint is completed by a **"normal neuromuscular–tendinous–ligamentous–capsular–bone and joint-soft tissue pathway."** Table 1.1 shows the normal pathway required for joint movement, and how an abnormal condition can affect its working with a few examples.

Table 1.1: Normal pathway required for joint movement, and conditions which can affect its working.	
Normal component	*Pathology which will affect joint movement: A few examples*
Normal central nervous system (CNS) where patient can hear, comprehend, and send the motor command to the spinal cord	Hemiplegia, any other brain disorder affecting its function, Parkinson's, etc.
Normal spinal cord and nerve roots	Spinal cord injury, polio, brachial or lumbar plexus affection, nerve root compression intervertebral disc prolapse
Normal peripheral nerve	Nerve injury
Normal neuromuscular junction	Myasthenia Gravis
Normally functioning muscle	Muscular dystrophy, Myopathies
Normal tendon to transmit the muscle power	Tendinopathy, tendon tear
Normal articulation of joint	Dislocation or subluxation
Normal bone	Acute fracture, non- or malunion
Normal ligaments	Ligament tear
Normal capsule and soft tissue (skin and subcutaneous tissue) to stretch while joint is moving	Adhesive capsulitis (frozen shoulder), postburn scar, scleroderma, etc.

Note: The history should be aimed to find what is leading to difficulty in moving a joint

5. Deformity

It could be **structural or spasmodic**. Structural deformities are not passively correctable, whereas spasmodic ones can be corrected with changed posture or they are spontaneously corrected as pain is relieved.

- *Structural deformities* could be arising from *bone* [congenital malformation (scoliosis), malunion/nonunion of fracture, growth plate disturbance, etc.,] *joint* (dislocated or subluxated), *muscle–tendon contractures* (Volkmann's ischemic contracture), *fascial contractures* (Dupuytren's contracture), *capsular or ligament contractures, skin or scar contractures* (postburn contracture, scleroderma).
- *Spasmodic deformities* are seen in *acute painful musculoskeletal conditions due to muscle spasm,* e.g. paraspinal muscle spasm after acute intervertebral disc prolapse leading to postural scoliosis.

6. Shortening or lengthening of a limb

There could be true or apparent discrepancy in the limb length.

- **True discrepancy** in the limb length is due to "the lengthening or shortening of the bone" due to Traumatic (fracture/dislocation) infective, or metabolic pathology truly altering the length of the bone.
- **Apparent discrepancy** in the limb length is due to a *"deformity"* but there is no true deficit in the limb length when measured. *It looks short or long but not truly long or short!*

7. Instability of the joint

Normally, ligaments provide stability to the joint by linking two *morphologically normal bones* across the joint. So when ligament tears completely, it leads to instability of the joint. Partial ligament tears may not cause instability. Also, an abnormal shape of bony articulation can contribute to instability (e.g. Trochlear dysplasia results in patellar dislocation).

8. Locking

Normally, the joint movement is smooth and it does not get "locked" (fixed in a particular position) because nothing gets in between the two mobile articulating surfaces. So if something loose comes in between the two articulating surfaces, it gets entrapped and stops the smooth gliding of joint surfaces. This leads to joint stuck in a fixed position without patient being able to bend it or straighten it is known as locking. It is usually an intermittent phenomenon as once the loose fragment moves out, the joint gets unlocked.

Some common causes of locking are:

- *Meniscal tear in knee joint*: Bucket handle tears of meniscus
- Loose body in any joint.

> **"Pseudolocking"** is another condition wherein the joint gets stuck in a flexed position. However, this is due to severe pain leading to spasm causing sudden limitation of movement of that joint. A classical example is a patient complaining of such locking with patellofemoral arthritis wherein the knee suddenly gets locked in flexed position.

9. Limp

It is observed in lower limb and it could be due to various causes. The main causes are:

- Limb length discrepancy
- Painful conditions of the lower limb
- Weakness of the Hip abductor mechanism.

10. Systemic features

Fever, weight loss, or loss of appetite, etc.

- Presence of systemic feature indicates that either the local condition observed at the musculoskeletal system is having a systemic influence (e.g. septic arthritis, malignant tumor, etc.) or the local pathology is a culmination of a systemic disease (rheumatoid arthritis).

> *Another important facet of history evaluation is to assess the effect of the disease process on the activities of daily living, walking, squatting, cross-leg sitting, overhead activities, sports, occupation, etc.*

> **A common mistake while taking history of present illness!**
> Often students start with HOPI and then abruptly include treatment history with HOPI. This leads to dilution of assessment of the chief complaints. It could possibly lead to wrong diagnosis especially if the diagnosis established by the previous treatment provider was inaccurate or incomplete. The student may get carried away by "*diagnosis at arrival*" and may stop his own assessment efforts.

The rest of the history goes as per the standard protocol. The questions asked about the rest of the history should have an aim to further investigate the cause of the disease.

- *Past history*
- *Personal history*: Smoking, h/o alcohol intake, sleep, bowel and bladder habit
- *Treatment history*: One can get vital clues about diagnosis with treatment history. However, one must assess it separately and avoid mixing it with HOPI. An exception is a case of trauma wherein treatment history is assessed along with HOPI
- *Family history*
- *Menstrual history*
- *History of allergies.*

At the end of the complete history assessment, the candidate must be able to arrive at a possible conclusion about the etiopathology of the condition. The possible etiologies could be:
- **Congenital:** Present from birth/late presentation of the congenital pathology
- **Traumatic:** H/o trauma
- **Inflammatory:** H/o multiple joint/area involvement, morning stiffness, malaise, and multisystem affection
- **Infective:** H/o fever, purulent discharge from the bone/joint
- **Neoplastic:** H/o slowly or rapidly growing swelling, pain, loss of weight, and loss of appetite
- **Metabolic:** Osteoporosis, Gout and Pseudogout
- **Degenerative:** Mostly age-related osteoarthritis, tendinitis, tendon tear, and spondylosis leading to mechanical pain
- **Hematologic:** Hemophilia and sickle cell anemia
- **Neurological:** H/o tingling, numbness, weakness, burning sensation
- **Others:** Avascular necrosis

EXAMINATION

Prerequisites for examination
A - Acquaintance with the patient
B - Bright/optimal light
C - Consent to examination, comfortable couch, comparison with normal side
D - Devices (measuring tape, knee hammer, goniometer, etc.)
E - Expose the part properly, explain the examination process and methods
F - Female attendant for female patient, Another adult for vulnerable adults, kids and adolescents, (Chaperoning)
G - Gentle palpation, especially during tenderness, movement, and special test maneuver.

The examination starts with general and systemic examination whether it is a short or long case. *The general and systemic examination is mandatory as per the standard protocol. It would be improper to say that I have not done the general and systemic examination.*

- **General examination:** The examination of vital parameters and pallor, icterus, clubbing, cyanosis, lymph nodes and pedal edema in standard fashion.
- **Systemic examination:** *Central nervous system (CNS), cardiovascular system (CVS), respiratory system (RS), abdomen and pelvis.*

Tips to present general and systemic examination findings
- *If the **general and systemic examination findings are normal**,* it can be summarized as "general and systemic examination findings are normal" and the student can proceed to local examination rather than typically repeating pallor, icterus, etc.
- *If the **general and systemic examination findings are abnormal**,* the student can summarize the relevant findings such as "pallor present, patient is hypertensive", etc. rather than narrating the entire systemic examination findings in routine fashion.

- **Local examination**
The standard order of examination in orthopaedic cases is as follows:
  1. **Gait:** In case of lower limb or spine examination
  2. **Attitude:** It is described as the position assumed by each joint and bone at rest which is comfortable to the patient.
  3. **Inspection**

4. **Palpation**
5. **Movements**
6. **Measurement**
7. **Neurovascular examination**
8. **Special tests for individual pathology/region**
9. **Joint above and below**
10. **Lymph node examination.**

Pearls and Pitfalls while Performing Local Examination

1. **While presenting the examination findings:**
   (a) *Adjectives must be avoided unless it has been standardized as grading, e.g. "severe" tenderness. Tenderness is either present or absent but no such grading is discussed in literature. One's "severe tenderness" could be someone else's "moderate"!*
   (b) *The methodology of examination should not be* informed during presentation unless asked for. One must just present the finding.
   (c) *The etiology of the finding should not be discussed* while presenting the finding. It must be left for the discussion.

2. **Inspection**
   While performing inspection, there are many findings that are general in nature (swelling, scar, sinus, ulcer, etc.) and students are already aware how to describe them with their previous exposure in surgery, medicine, and other clinical postings. However, one must look for specifics in orthopaedic case like:
   (a) Deformities
   (b) Limb length discrepancy
   (c) Muscle wasting
   Certain common terms that are used to describe deformity in limbs are described here:
   Varus:
   It implies "part of the body moving closer to the midline." Genu varum means that "genu" or "knee" is the referencing point and the "part," i.e. the leg has moved closer to the midline (Fig. 1.1).
   Valgus:
   It implies "part of body moving away from the midline." Genu valgum means that "genu" or "knee" is the referencing point and the "part," i.e. the leg, has moved away from the midline (Fig. 1.1). Cubitus valgus means that "cubitus," i.e. the elbow is the referencing point and forearm has moved away from the midline.
   Recurvatum:
   It implies hyperextension and is observed in the elbow and knee. It is known as genu recurvatum in the knee. Normally, when the patient stands erect and observed from the side, the axis of the lower limb passes through the center of hip, knee, and ankle. However, in recurvatum, it passes anterior to the knee (Fig. 1.1).
   Flexion deformity:
   It implies that the affected joint cannot be brought into complete extension, passively or actively.

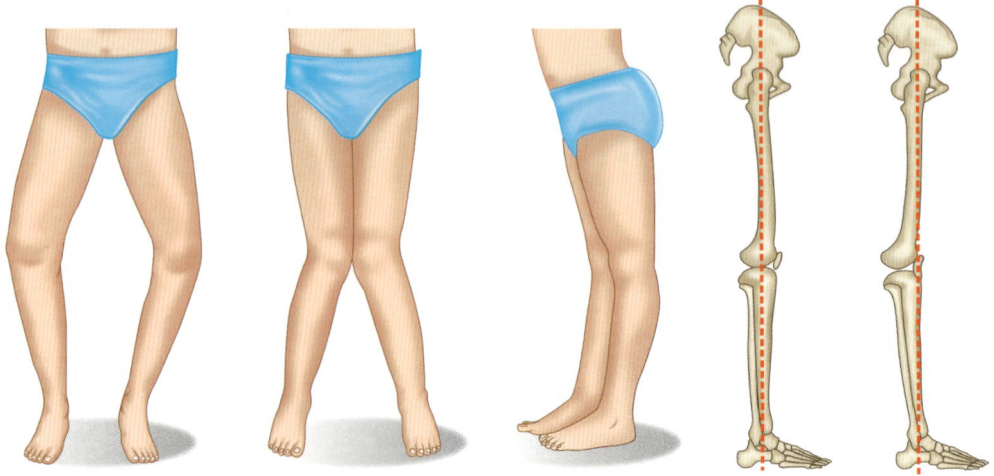

Fig. 1.1: Images demonstrate varus, valgus and recurvatum deformities of the knee joint.

*Ankylosis***:**

Pathological fusion of a joint in a fixed position (flexed or extended) with no movements possible. *(Arthrodesis: Surgical fusion of joint)* .

Principles of deformity assessment.
- *Always stand in the plane perpendicular to the plane of deformity.* E.g. varus and valgus at the knee are a coronal plane deformity. So, stand in the sagittal plane of the patient (in front of the patient) to assess it. Several other examples are:
  1. Scoliosis occurs in the coronal plane: So, stand in sagittal plane, i.e. behind the patient to observe scoliosis
  2. Kyphosis occurs in the sagittal plane: So, stand in the coronal plane, i.e. on the side of patient to observe kyphosis

---

3. Palpation
- *Before palpation, ask the patient to mention the exact site of tenderness* as it helps in localizing the site and type of pathology. Also, this helps the examiner to remain cautious while palpating the tender area.
- The palpation must be done with *due gentleness* especially in tender areas as it can lead to increased pain. Afterward, the patient may not cooperate with the rest of the examination.
- The palpation must follow a sequence of eliciting tenderness over bony prominences, soft tissues and joint line.

4. Movement
- Always check and highlight the deformities before commenting on the range of movement (ROM).
- The ROM is assessed using a goniometer (*The methodology to assess the joint movement using goniometer is discussed at the end of chapter with relevant images*).
- The *total* "ROM" must be mentioned.
- The ROM should be assessed on the following parameters
  (i) Active and passive ROM: Active ROM should be assessed primarily as–
  - It gives an idea whether active movement is possible or not

– Always compare with the normal side.
– If active is not possible, it may indicate nerve palsy, tendon-muscle tear or fracture dislocations, etc.
– Also, it gives a fair assessment of painless or painful range of movement.
– Passive ROM helps in assessing total movement at the joint.

(ii) Painless/painful ROM

(iii) Associated crepitus with ROM: Crepitus indicates rubbing of rough surfaces in arthritis of joint, loose body in the joint; an inflamed bursa or a torn, frayed tendon edge rubbing with another bone.

- ***Extensor lag:*** This is a *specific term used for the knee* wherein the patient can actively flex his knee but while actively extending back, it does not come back to the starting point of flexion. It means that the knee "lags in extension." However, passively the knee can be brought to the starting point of flexion. It occurs due to the weakness in the quadriceps mechanism.

> **How to mention range of movement? An example!**
> *Elbow flexion*: 0°–120°. 0°–100° is painless, whereas the remaining 20° is painful. Further flexion is not possible. Both active and passive movements are the same.

5. Measurement

The objective of limb length measurement is to analyze the discrepancy in limb length, if any, and to assess the segment of discrepancy (arm and forearm/thigh and leg).

Few important points must be ensured while limbs are measured for any discrepancy.

- A preexisting deformity in the limb must be checked and corrected (Eg. squaring the pelvis). A preexisting limb length discrepancy must be asked for, if any.
- The limb measurement is performed between the two predesignated bony landmarks.
- The bony landmarks must be marked with a skin marking pencil.
- The two limbs must be kept in identical positions for measurement.
- The segmental length of the limb must be measured.
- Finally, while mentioning the limb length assessment, the student should inform the discrepancy/normalcy of limb length rather than narrating the individual measurements of bone length and not calculate the final discrepancy.

> **The usual but incorrect way of referring to limb length discrepancy:** "The right femur is 48 cm long, and the right tibia is 32 cm long. The left femur is 48 cm long and the left tibia is 31 cm long." After this statement, many students think that the job is over.
> However, after the measurement of total and segmental lengths of the limb, the *goal* is to measure the "limb length discrepancy" if any. So, the simple way is to calculate the discrepancy, if any, and answer accordingly.
> *So,* **the correct way of describing limb length discrepancy:** "The left lower limb is one cm short compared to the left, and the shortening is in the tibia."
> **If the limbs are equal in length, then informing that "there is no limb length discrepancy" is enough.**

> Remember! During the presentation of the case, the examiner is not interested in the individual measurements of bone length unless asked for.

6. **Neurovascular (NV) examination:** As per the standard neurovascular assessment of the limb.

- **If the NV examination is normal**, it can be informed as *"neurovascular examination is normal."*
- **If the NV examination is abnormal**, then *individual pathological findings should be told.* For example, if the posterior tibial pulse is feeble on the right side but the neurological examination is normal, then it is appropriate to say that "neurological examination is normal. However, posterior tibial artery is feeble on the right side."

7. **Special tests:** The key to the special tests is **explain–demonstrate–interpret–compare**
   "Explain (to patient)–demonstrate (on index side)–interpret (finding)–compare (with normal side)"

8. **Joint above and below:** As per standard examination practice.

One must always assess the joints above and below as the disease or affection of proximal or distal joint may cause radiation of pain to the neighboring joint. (E.g. Hip pathology may lead to radiation of pain in the knee due to the Hilton's law. Another example where bilateral flat foot leads to the knee pain.) However, the pain perceived area may be absolutely normal. Hence, it is vital to examine the neighboring joints.

Further, it can be again summarized as "Joints above and below are normal." However, if there is an abnormal finding in neighboring joint, it should be informed.

9. **Lymph node examination:** It should always be done especially in suspected case of infective, inflammatory and tumorous conditions.

10. **Final diagnosis:** *The final diagnosis should have the following components:*
    - Duration
    - Anatomical Site
    - Side
    - Pathology
    - Etiology
    - Complication, if any.

An example of a complete diagnosis: 11-month-old, right femur shaft nonunion due to road traffic accident with 3-cm shortening of the femur with stiffness of the knee.
Description: 11-month-old (duration) *Right-side* (side) *femur shaft* (anatomical site) *nonunion* (pathology) due *to road traffic accident* (etiology) with *shortening* of femur and stiffness of knee (complication).

- Diagnosis should be based upon **points favoring the diagnosis** from history and examination.
- Diagnosis **must not be given based upon negative points**. *The presence of points against the primary diagnosis must stimulate the student to think about the differential diagnosis.*
- It is not *always* essential to give a differential diagnosis. For example, there will not be any differential diagnosis for fracture femur nonunion. However, there can be differential diagnosis in patients with rheumatoid arthritis of the knee.

11. **Plan the investigations** relevant to "your case" and not a hypothetical case.

Avoid the statement "routine investigations" as no investigation is asked as routine. Every investigation asked for has a specific goal which could help either in corroborating or in confirming the diagnosis or may further help in deciding the surgical fitness of the patient.

12. **Final plan of the treatment**
    It could be conservative or operative. Tell the plan of treatment for your patient that is optimal for the diagnosis.

A NOTE ON TECHNIQUE OF USING A GONIOMETER FOR THE ROM MEASUREMENT

Goniometer: It is an instrument which measures range of motion joint angles of the body.

Technique: The joint's ROM is measured by number of degrees from starting point of a segment to its position at the end of full ROM present at that joint.

A double armed goniometer is used for the ROM measurement wherein stationary arm of the goniometer lies parallel to the stationary segment of the limb and mobile arm of goniometer is placed parallel to the axis of the mobile segment of the limb. ***The center of goniometer lies over the central axis of the joint*** (Fig. 1.2). When all the landmarks are well defined and arms of goniometer are placed parallel to the limb, the accuracy of ROM measurement is high.

Important Tips

- The referencing segment or stationary part of the body should be stable and stationary arm of goniometer should be stable and parallel to the referencing limb. (Figs. 1.3 and 1.4) However; sometimes, there is no referencing segment for the goniometer in cases of the joints which are connected to torso directly; shoulder and hip. In such cases, the referencing segment is the midline of the body, and stationary arm of the goniometer should be placed over or parallel to the imaginary midline axis of the body (Figs. 1.5 and 1.6)
- Look at the goniometer reading and confirm it before it is removed from the body.

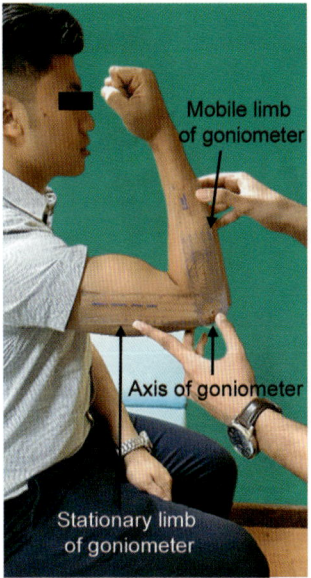

Fig.1.2: ROM measurement of elbow with goniometer.

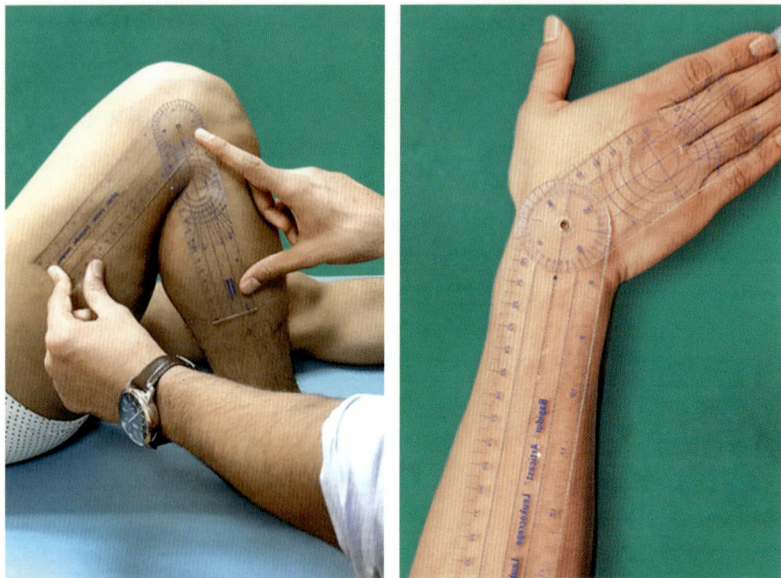

Fig.1.3: ROM measurement of knee flexion (left image) and wrist ulnar deviation (right image) using goniometer. The center of goniometer is over the center of joint.

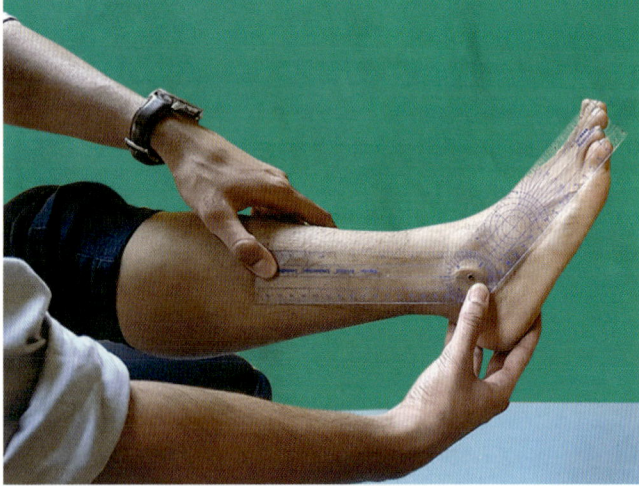

Fig.1.4: ROM measurement of ankle plantar flexion using goniometer with center of goniometer over the center of ankle joint.

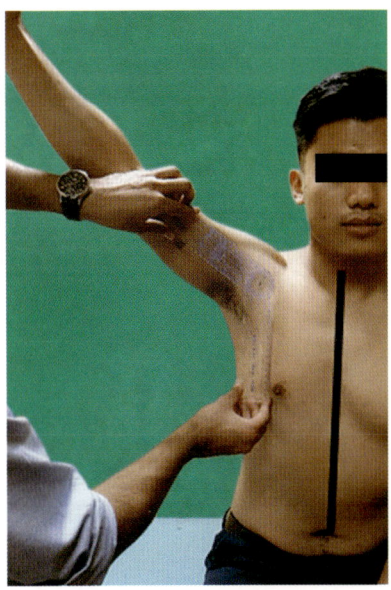

Fig. 1.5: Measurement of shoulder abduction ROM keeping stationary of arm of goniometer parallel to the imaginary midline axis of body (black line) and mobile arm parallel to the abducted arm. The center of goniometer is over the center of the shoulder joint.

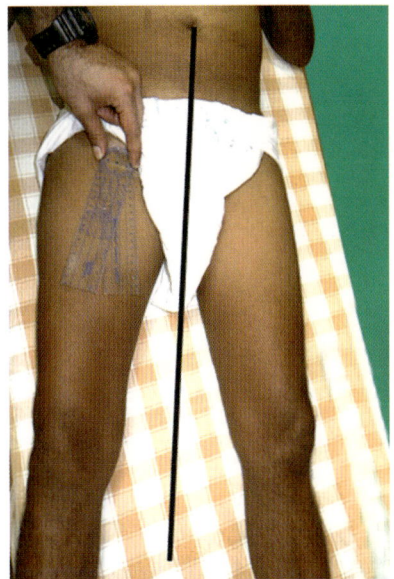

Fig. 1.6: Measurement of hip abduction ROM keeping stationary of arm of goniometer parallel to the imaginary midline axis of body (black line) and mobile arm parallel to the abducted thigh. The center of goniometer is over the hip joint.

Notes

Clinical Evaluation of Acute Injury of Bones and Joints

▊ INTRODUCTION

Patients arriving with a history of trauma to the limb(s), is one of the most frequent scenarios encountered in orthopedics. There are several pertinent points to be probed while taking the history of the injured person.

▊ HISTORY

Age

- Injury in growing children may lead to greenstick fracture or epiphyseal injury.
- Young and adult patients are more prone to high-velocity road traffic accidents.
- Elderly patients are more prone to falls and subsequent fragility fractures (fracture distal radius, neck of femur, intertrochanteric femur fracture or vertebral fracture due to osteoporosis).

Mechanism and Force of Trauma

- The mechanism of trauma entails how the patient sustained the injury, e.g. fall from a height, hit by a vehicle, trivial injury, etc. This can give a clue to the structures injured. For example, fall from a height can cause fracture of calcaneum, tibia, pelvis, and spine.
- Further, the mechanism of injury could be ***direct, indirect, and stress fracture***
  - *The **direct injury** could result in a transverse fracture, comminuted fracture, open fracture, or a crush injury of the limb, whereas indirect injury could result in spiral/oblique fracture.*
    A dashboard injury to the knee can cause posterior dislocation of hip, patella fracture, and injury to the PCL.
  - *An **indirect injury** like forceful muscle contraction over a limb bent in the direction opposite to the action of muscle can also lead to a fracture. For example, forceful quadriceps contraction over a flexed knee can lead to a transverse fracture patella or a peroneus brevis contraction over an inverted foot can lead to fracture of the base of the fifth metatarsal.*
  - ***Stress fracture:*** *A repeated unaccustomed stress over the limb can lead to stress fracture of a bone (march fracture of the second metatarsal, shin splint of tibia).*
- *The **force of trauma***: It must be probed as major trauma or force can certainly cause a fracture. However, if a minor force results in the fracture, this indicates that the bone was diseased before the trauma (osteoporosis, infection, tumor) and such fractures are known as a *pathological fracture.*

Sprain: Stretch and/or tear of a *ligament*.
Strain: An injury to a *muscle and/or tendons*.
Fracture: Discontinuity or break in the anatomical continuity of the *bone*.
Dislocation: When two articular surfaces of *joint* are no more in contact with each other.
Subluxation: When two articular surfaces of *joint* are in partial contact with each other.

Loss of Function of the Limb

After the trauma to the limb, the clinician must probe whether the patient has any difficulty or inability to use the limb or whether he/she finds difficulty or inability to bear weight.

Any such difficulty or inability to use the limb or to bear weight almost always indicates serious soft tissue (ligament/muscle/nerve or combination injury) or bony injury (fracture or dislocation) or both.

The patient with an injured limb will have one or more complaints of:
- Pain
- Swelling
- Deformity
- Inability or difficulty to use the limb.

In case of an open fracture, specific history has to be taken
- *Time since injury:* The longer the duration of open wound which remained unclosed/not debrided (>8 hours), higher is the chance of local infection and morbidity!.
- *High- or low-velocity of trauma accidents:* High-velocity injuries could lead to severe bone and soft tissue damage.
- *Site of accident:* To understand the possible type of contamination. E.g. *Farm accidents* could lead to anerobic infection like *Clostridium welchii*. There can be contamination with lots of mud, grass, organic fertilizers, etc.

▌GENERAL ASSESSMENT

Apart from the history to evaluate the local injuries, one must assess the injuries to the rest of the body and the system (Head and maxillofacial, Chest, Spine and spinal cord, Abdomen and Pelvis) on the lines of the advanced trauma life support (ATLS) protocol.

After the quick general and systemic evaluation, one should focus on local examination. *This chapter will refrain from the detailed general and systemic evaluation of a trauma patient as that is out of the scope of this chapter.*

▌LOCAL EXAMINATION

Attitude

Often a typical attitude of the limb may indicate a specific diagnosis. For example; in a patient of posterior dislocation of the hip, the index hip assumes a position of flexion, adduction, and internal rotation. In a case of fracture neck of femur or intertrochanteric femur, the lower limb appears short and externally rotated.

However, in most of the cases, making a diagnosis merely by the attitude of the limb is not possible. An abnormal attitude merely indicates that the limb is injured.

Inspection

1. **Swelling:** It is a common sign of an injured limb whether it has sustained fracture, dislocation, or a soft tissue injury.
2. **Deformity:** A displaced fracture, dislocation, or a major ligament injury will present as a deformity whereas undisplaced fracture or grade 1 or 2 ligament injury will not have any deformity.
3. **Limb length discrepancy:** Commonly, displaced fracture with overriding of fracture ends or a dislocated joint will present as shortening of limb. In certain situations, the injured limb may appear longer. e.g., Anterior dislocation of the hip.
4. **Condition of overlying skin and the presence of wound, if any:** The skin overlying the site of injury must be thoroughly inspected for any of the following:
   - *Fracture blisters*: It indicates severe injury to the soft tissue envelope and possibly compromised circulation to the soft tissue. This is a contraindication to open reduction and internal fixation (ORIF). One must wait till blisters subside indicating return of optimum skin vascularity.
   - *Ecchymosis*: It indicates the presence of blood in the subcutaneous tissue. For example, an ecchymosis adjacent to the multiligament injured knee is suggestive of major capsular disruption through which joint hematoma leaks out.
   - *Presence of wound*: In case of an open fracture, there is a wound around the site of the fracture. The type of the wound should be ascertained; lacerated wound/incised wound/abrasion/degloving injury. Further assessment of the wound can be done on the basis of Gustilo-Anderson classification of open fractures.

Palpation

Before the palpation is initiated, the clinician should ask the patient about the site of maximum tenderness. *The traumatized limb should be palpated and moved with utmost care* as it causes severe pain.

A limb with fracture has certain specific signs:

1. **Bony tenderness:** The fracture site is tender when palpated through the overlying soft tissue.
2. **Bony crepitus:** A grating sensation is felt when the two ends of the fractured bone are moved. ***However, it is a very painful maneuver; hence, it is never deliberately elicited***. Also, it is absent in undisplaced fracture.
3. **Palpation of a gap** between two ends of the fracture is a certain sign of a fracture.
4. **Abnormal mobility:** When two ends of the fracture are held together, the abnormal mobility at the fracture site can be elicited. However, it is not deliberately elicited as it is quite a painful manoeuver.
5. **Compression test:** This is an indirect tenderness test wherein the pressure is exerted over a single or group of normal bone(s) leading to the tenderness over the fracture site.

   This is classically performed where there are two or more parallel bones and one is fractured (ribs, metatarsal or metacarpals, forearm, leg). The compression of both or more bones together can elicit tenderness over the fracture site. For example, in the case of fracture ribs (one or more), gentle pressure over the sternum with one hand and other over the spine or gently side to side squeezing the rib cage in axilla with both hands cause pain over the fractured rib. Also, gentle squeezing of the hand or foot causes a painful response in case of metatarsal or metacarpal fracture.

6. **Loss of transmitted movements:** The fractured limb fails to transmit the movements performed at the distal segment. For example, if the ankle is rotated in a case of tibia shaft fracture, the proximal tibia will not rotate as there is a break in continuity. Also, if the distal part is elevated, this will not result in the spontaneous lifting of the proximal part due to break in continuity of bone.

Movements

It is always difficult to assess the movement at the joint near the fracture site due to pain and, hence, it can be avoided. Also, no additional information is gathered by eliciting the range of motion.

Measurement

Careful assessment of the longitudinal length of the limb should be done between pre-designated bony landmarks of bones. However, it is usually not performed in acute fractures as maneuvering would be very painful.

The muscle wasting would not be a feature of acute trauma unless there was a preexisting one.

Neurovascular Examination

A thorough neurovascular examination of the extremity is mandatory to rule out any neurovascular deficit.

Joint Above and Below

Careful assessment of the joint above and below is essential to rule out any transmitted injury to the neighboring joints.

Special Tests

The local conditions are often quite painful to perform special tests. However, they can be performed with care, if deemed necessary.

Table showing grade of injury to ligaments and muscle-tendon complex			
Grade	*Degree of damage*	*Clinical finding*	*Prognosis*
Grade I	Minimal disruption	Mild tenderness, no swelling; ROM fine, minimal pain. No functional loss or instability	Excellent healing, No long term impairment
Grade II	Moderate damage	Tenderness with swelling; Bruise ±, Painful ROM. Moderate functional loss and mild instability	Good prognosis, Minimal long term impairment
Grade III	Complete disruption in substance of ligament/ tendon-muscle	Severe tenderness and swelling, Bruise +, Palpable defect may be present, Complete loss of function and instability +	Variable prognosis Might require surgery Longer rehabilitation required

Notes

Clinical Evaluation of Diseased Long Bones

▌ INTRODUCTION

Although the history and examination pattern of the skeletal system follows a standard protocol, the clinical evaluation of the acute traumatized limb is different from nontraumatic conditions. The clinical evaluation of a traumatized limb has been discussed in a separate chapter. This chapter will discuss only chronic nontraumatic conditions (inflammatory, infective, tumors, degenerative, congenital, etc.) or chronic sequel of acute trauma.

▌ HISTORY

Common pathological conditions of long bone could be differentiated with a careful history.

Common complaints
Pain, swelling, inability to bear weight, sinus, fever, loss of weight or appetite

Common complaints—

1. **Pain:** Bone pain without significant trauma is indicative of atraumatic pathology. Infection and tumors are common atraumatic pathologies.
   - *The onset of pain*
     - *Acute* in acute fractures or dislocation, acute infections (osteomyelitis or septic arthritis), acute episodes of metabolic/inflammatory arthritis, or malignant tumors
     - *Insidious* in chronic or slow-growing conditions, such as degenerative arthritis, benign tumors, chronic inflammation or chronic infection.
   - *The character of pain*
     - Throbbing and dull type of pain is suggestive of inflammation or mechanical type, respectively. Shooting or dragging pain often associated with tingling and numbness suggests pain of neural origin.
   - *Activities causing pain*
     - *Pain at rest*: Inflammatory (rheumatoid, gout), infective (osteomyelitis) lesions or malignant tumors (osteosarcoma)
     - *Pain while load bearing/mechanical pain*: Degenerative arthritis.
2. **Swelling**
   - Long-standing, insidious onset swelling of bone without a history of fever is suggestive of benign tumor of bone.

- Acute-onset pain with sudden swelling of the bone is suggestive of malignant tumors of bone or acute osteomyelitis.

3. **Inability to bear weight**
   - The acute h/o inability to bear weight indicates a significant bone or joint injury (fracture or dislocation) or a ligament injury.
   - However, the chronic h/o of inability to bear weight indicates that there is nonunion of a fracture/neuromuscular disorder.
   - Chronic ligament injuries or subluxated joint are more tolerant to weight bearing, i.e. patients with such chronic conditions can bear weight. However, they may have pain, instability, deformity, and restricted ROM.

4. **Sinus**
   The presence of a sinus indicates a focus of dead material inside the soft tissue or bone. It could be a sequestrum, suture material (absorbable or nonabsorbable), a foreign body or presence of underlying cavity.
   - A pus-discharging sinus following a long-standing infection associated with discharge of bony spicules is suggestive of chronic osteomyelitis.
   - H/o open wound must be asked for in a case of persistent discharging sinus which may indicate an old open fracture.

5. **History of fever and other systemic symptoms**
   - Acute high-grade fever with/without toxemia with prior infection of the skin or upper respiratory tract favors acute infection of the bone (acute osteomyelitis) or joint (septic arthritis).
   - Chronic conditions like tuberculosis or even inflammatory conditions may present with low-grade fever.
   - H/o weight loss or loss of appetite may indicate a chronic inflammatory, infective, or malignancy.

6. **Family history** of the similar disorder may be present in multiple osteochondromatosis, osteogenesis imperfecta.

7. **Past, personal, and treatment history:** Relevant questions must be asked for.

8. **Menstrual history:** Important in postmenopausal osteoporotic fractures.

GENERAL AND SYSTEMIC EXAMINATION

It forms an integral part of the examination in nontraumatic conditions such as tumors, inflammatory, metabolic, neuropathic, or infective conditions because such conditions are either culmination of a systemic disease on a joint (rheumatoid disease) or bone or the condition itself can cast a systemic influence (metastasis after osteosarcoma). Hence, a detailed systemic and general examination is important.

LOCAL EXAMINATION

1. Attitude

2. Inspection

Alignment of the limb and deformity, if any
- Findings from the front, side, and back of the affected limb should be noted. It must be compared with normal limb.

- Sagittal, coronal, and rotation malalignments of the limb must be recorded.
- The site, side, and anatomical area of the deformity must be recorded.

Skin
- The skin around the affected bone and nearby joint must be visualized carefully for any scar, sinus, or ulcer. Also, the skin changes distal to the injured site may be present in complex regional pain syndrome. The trophic changes of the distal part are suggestive of associated vascular affection.
- Scar healing must be described as primary healing or secondary healing (read scar examination).
- Sinus must be inspected for active discharge or healed sinus (read sinus examination). Bony spicules from the sinus are suggestive of chronic osteomyelitis.

Swelling
- Note whether it is generalized (neurofibromatosis and multiple exostoses) or localised; Bony or soft tissue swelling.
- Occasionally swelling may be present in the nearby joint due to sympathetic effusion.

Muscle wasting
- Wasting should be best inspected by comparing both limbs. Wasting is present in chronic pathology.

Length of the limb
- Check the comparative length of the limb—whether short, long, or equal.

3. Palpation

Temperature
- The raised temperature around the affected site must raise suspicion of infection/inflammation/tumor of the local bone.

Tenderness
- The site of tenderness gives an idea of the underlying abnormalities of the long bone.
- The tenderness may be present in an acute fracture, infection of bone, inflammation, and malignant tumor or arthritis.
- Tenderness is absent in malunion, nonunion, and neuropathic conditions (Charcot's arthropathy).

Step
- Palpable step over the shaft of a long bone is suggestive of its discontinuity. It is an important sign for the diagnosis of fracture or gap nonunion of the long bone.

Bony thickening
- Localized abnormal thickening of the bone is suggestive of old healed fracture or chronic osteomyelitis.

Loss of transmitted movement
- If one moves one end of the long bone, the other end too moves. It is termed as 'transmitted movement. If one end moves without the other end of the long bone, it indicates discontinuity of the long bone.
- Loss of transmitted movement is noted in nonunion of a fracture.

Crepitus
- Classically, nonunion is said to have no crepitus due to rounded and soft fracture ends.
- *It must not be checked in acute condition.*
- However, a joint crepitus indicates rough joint surface due to arthritis or presence of a loose body in the joint.
  The crepitus of arthritis is usually fixed, i.e. it is elicited at the same sector of range of motion every time when the joint is moved, whereas crepitus elicited in the presence of a loose body is variable. It is elicited whenever the loose body is caught between the articulating surfaces and may not be felt if the loose body escapes from getting caught between the two joint surfaces.

Sinus
- Active or quiescent sinus should be differentiated. A little pressure over surrounding tissue may lead to discharge of purulent material from the mouth of the sinus.
- A sinus due to chronic osteomyelitis is always fixed to the underlying bone.
- The quality and quantity of the discharge must be noted.
- Bony spicules from the sinus are suggestive of chronic osteomyelitis *(read chapter on scar, sinus and ulcer examination).*

Scar and ulcer
- Standard examination *(read Chapter on scar, sinus and ulcer examination).*

4. Movement
- Normal movements of nearby joints (proximal and distal) must be examined and noted. Restriction of the nearby joints (stiffness) may be present in long-standing non-union, malunion, or any adjacent bony pathology.
  Any painless, abnormally excessive movements at a joint that is swollen and deformed, is suggestive of neuropathic joint or Charcot's arthropathy.
- Abnormal movements at long bone are pathological. Abnormal movements should be examined in all three planes. The abnormal mobility of the long bone is suggestive of nonunion. It is absent in union of the bone (including normal union and malunion).

5. Measurement
- The length of the bone should be compared with the opposite side.
- The length of the bone/limb can be normal, increased, or decreased compared to the opposite side. Limb shortening may be present in nonunion, malunion, and chronic osteomyelitis or a pathological fracture.
- The length of both bones should be measured separately in an upper limb for arm and forearm and lower limb for thigh and leg to know the segmental length and discrepancy in the actual segment.
- Measurement of muscle girth may reveal wasting on diseased side.

6. Neurovascular, Joint above and below, Lymph Node, and Distal Part of Limb Examination
It is necessary to examine the distal neurovascular structures, joints above and below, lymph node, and swelling of distal extremity.

- Neurovascular examination.
- Lymph node enlargement may be present in a chronic infection or a malignant tumor.
- The swelling of the distal limb may be present due to the pressure effect over the venous system due to tumor compressing the venous system. It is also seen in the infection, inflammation, or post-traumatic conditions. Multiple surgeries can scar lymphatic and venous system of the limb leading to the distal swelling. Ruptured Baker's cyst can produce deep vein thrombosis (DVT) like clinical picture in the limb. Nevertheless, localized musculoskeletal system affection causes unilateral swelling of the limb. Bilateral swelling of the lower limb is usually due to the systemic causes (cardiac, renal, hepatic, cor pulmonale, low albumin levels, etc.).

▌ DIFFERENTIAL DIAGNOSIS

Common conditions affecting long bone with salient features:

1. **Malunion**
   - H/o fall/accident or trauma followed by fracture
   - No weight bearing or limb usage for at least 3–6 weeks after injury
   - Nonprogressive deformity, mostly painless
   - Unidirectional/multidirectional deformity
   - Loss of function of limb +/-
   - Absence of tenderness, gap, step, crepitation, abnormal mobility
   - Bony thickening present at the fracture site.

2. **Nonunion**
   - H/o fall/accident or trauma followed by fracture
   - Presently; loss of function, not able to bear weight or use the limb properly
   - Absence of pain and tenderness
   - Presence of gap, step; absence of crepitus at nonunion site
   - Classic "painless abnormal mobility" at the nonunion site.

3. **Chronic osteomyelitis**
   - H/o prior infection
   - H/o pus discharging sinus, bony spicules
   - Pain (tenderness) may be present or absent
   - Bony thickening and irregularity present around the sinus
   - Sinus is fixed to the underlying bone
   - Absence of gap, step, crepitation, abnormal mobility unless associated pathological fracture.

4. **Pathological fracture (following infection, osteogenesis imperfecta, tumor, etc.)**
   - H/o fracture with minimal/trivial trauma
   - No weight bearing/loss of function after the trivial trauma
   - Pain is present in acute condition followed by absence of pain in chronic condition
   - *Acute stage*: Presence of gap, step, crepitation, abnormal mobility
   - *Chronic*: Step and abnormal mobility present
   - Bony thickening may be present in a chronic condition.

Notes

Clinical Evaluation of the Shoulder Joint

■ BRIEF ANATOMY AND FUNCTION OF THE SHOULDER JOINT

1. **Basic osteology**
   - The shoulder joint (glenohumeral joint) is formed by the articulation of the humeral head and the glenoid cavity. However, functionally it is a combination of four joints, namely:
     o Glenohumeral joint (GHJ)
     o Acromioclavicular joint (ACJ)
     o Sternoclavicular joint (SCJ)
     o Scapulothoracic joint (STJ).

   > Any disease or affection at any of the other three joints other than GHJ affects the function of the entire shoulder girdle, as when GHJ moves, there is also movement at the other three joints and vice versa. In addition, STJ is only a physiological and *not* an anatomical joint, as it does not have a synovial cavity.

2. **Stabilizing structures of GHJ**
   (a) *Ligaments*: Anterior, middle and inferior glenohumeral ligaments
   (b) *Labrum*: Fibrocartilaginous structure circumscribing the glenoid cavity
   (c) *Capsule*
   (d) *Rotator cuff* and other surrounding muscles
   (e) *Bony conformity of articulating surfaces and negative pressure of joint.*

3. **Type of joint:**
   GHJ (synovial, ball and socket), ACJ (synovial, plane), SCJ (synovial, plane).

4. **Movements:**
   Flexion, extension, abduction, adduction, external and internal rotation.

5. **Other facts:**
   Both ACJ and SCJ have an articular disc. The ACJ is stabilized by AC joint capsule and coracoclavicular ligaments (conoid and trapezoid).

6. **Important muscles around shoulder (Table 4.1).**

Table 4.1: Important muscles around the shoulder joint; their insertion, nerve supply, and action.

Muscle	Insertion	Nerve supply	Principal action at the shoulder joint
Deltoid	Over upper one-third of the shaft humerus	Axillary nerve	Abductor Flexor Extensor
Subscapularis	Lesser tuberosity	Upper and lower subscapularis nerve	Internal rotator
Supraspinatus	Greater tuberosity	Suprascapular nerve	Abductor
Infraspinatus	Greater tuberosity	Suprascapular nerve	External rotator
Teres minor	Greater tuberosity	Axillary nerve	External rotator
Latissimus dorsi	Floor of intertubercular groove of humerus	Thoracodorsal nerve	Extensor, adductor and internal rotator
Trapezius	Posterior border of lateral one-third of the clavicle, acromion process and spine of the scapula	Spinal accessory nerve	Rotation, retraction, elevation and depression of scapula
Serratus anterior	Costal aspect of medial margin of the scapula	Long thoracic nerve	Protracts and stabilizes scapula, assists in upward rotation
Pectoralis major	Lateral lip of the bicipital groove	Lateral and medial pectoral nerve	Clavicular head—flexion of humerus Sternocoastal head—adduction of humerus

Overall function of the rotator cuff (subscapularis, supraspinatus, infraspinatus and teres minor) is "centralization of the humeral head into the glenoid cavity." This enables the deltoid to efficiently elevate and abduct the arm, while the head remains centralized in the glenoid during entire range of motion.

Common conditions affecting the shoulder

- **Degenerative: MOST COMMON CATEGORY**
  - Rotator cuff tendinopathy
  - Frozen shoulder
  - Calcific tendinitis
  - Rotator cuff tear
  - Acromioclavicular arthritis
  - Rotator cuff arthropathy
  - Glenohumeral arthritis
- **Traumatic:** Dislocation, Fractures, associated brachial plexus injury
- **Congenital:** Sprengel shoulder
- **Infections:** Tuberculosis and septic arthritis
- **Inflammatory:** Rheumatoid arthritis
- **Metabolic:** Gouty/pseudogout arthritis
- **Neurological:** Charcot's shoulder, Winging of scapula
- **Neoplastic:** Benign/malignant tumors

> **Common shoulder pathologies in various age groups**
> - **Infants and young ones**
>   - Sprengel deformity, Klippel–Feil syndrome, Cleidocranial dysostosis
>   - Septic arthritis, osteomyelitis
> - **15–35 years**
>   - Shoulder instability (glenohumeral and acromioclavicular)
>   - SLAP tears
> - **35–55 years**
>   - Rotator cuff tendinopathy, partial cuff tears
>   - Frozen shoulder
>   - Calcific tendinitis
>   - Acromioclavicular arthritis
> - **More than 55 years**
>   - Rotator cuff tear
>   - Glenohumeral arthritis
>   - Rotator cuff arthropathy

▌ HISTORY AND ITS EVALUATION

Chief Complaints

Patients with shoulder pathology often come up with certain specific complaints:
- Pain
- Difficulty in movement/overhead activities/reaching back
- Subluxation or dislocation
- Cannot throw the ball/an object
- *Others*: Catching and locking.

1. **Pain:** It is the most common complaint.
   - **(A)** *Onset:* Mostly insidious in onset. However, a few conditions can cause acute pain:
     - *Calcific tendinitis*: Acute, severe pain
     - *Traumatic*: H/o frank trauma
     - Acute infection.
   - **(B)** *Timing of pain:* Though pain is often encountered during movements, most shoulder conditions cause pain in the night, which further increases with attempted sleeping on the affected shoulder. Many patients complain that they have not slept on the affected side for weeks or months. *It is a very specific sign of a shoulder pathology especially degenerative ones.*
   - **(C)** *Radiation:* The shoulder pain radiates to the tip of deltoid insertion, and sometimes, up to the elbow or the mid forearm. Rarely, it radiates towards neck or scapula. *If there is radiation of pain towards the fingers, then the origin of the pain is usually from the cervical spine or it is a neurological disorder.*
   - **(D)** *Aggravating factor:* Usually in the night/while lying on the index side/during attempted movements.
2. **Difficulty in movements:** The patient may find difficulty in moving their shoulder because of pain, stiffness, cuff tear, loss of power (nerve affection), the joint not being in place (dislocated or subluxated), fracture, etc. *(Read Chapter 1 for the inability or difficulty in moving a joint).*

(A) **Pain:** Arising out of any shoulder pathology (arthritis, tendinopathy, bursitis, labral tear, fracture, etc.).

(B) **Stiffness:** The tissues around the shoulder are tight, e.g. frozen shoulder (primary or secondary).

(C) **Rotator cuff tear:** Chronic tendinopathy renders the tendon weaker, followed by smaller tears, which later become bigger and cause a loss of power to move the joint, especially forward flexion, abduction and rotations. These patients often give history of chronic shoulder pain (months to years) with/without history of minor/major trauma. In addition, a major trauma can cause an acute rotator cuff tear, leading to an inability or difficulty in moving the shoulder.

(D) **Loss of power (nerve injury/paralysis)**
- Traumatic brachial plexus injury: H/o road traffic accident (RTA) or fall over the tip of shoulder
- Suprascapular nerve compressive neuropathy due to a ganglion in the spinoglenoid notch leading to Supra- and Infraspinatus palsy
- *Spinal accessory nerve injury*: Lymph node biopsy from posterior triangle leading to Trapezius palsy
- *Axillary nerve injury*: Especially after RTA/acute shoulder dislocation leading to Deltoid and Teres Minor palsy.

(E) **Joint not in place or broken levers (bone):** A dislocation/subluxation/fracture of the shoulder.

3. **Primary or recurrent dislocation/subluxation of the shoulder**

   Mostly, in such cases, the patient himself/herself comes up with a specific history of dislocation or subluxation. The primary event that caused the dislocation (traumatic vs nontraumatic) should be noted, as the pathology in these two situations is different. Also, confirm whether the dislocation happen after major trauma or did it happen without any specific trauma? Traumatic dislocations "may require surgical repair" whereas atraumatic dislocations often require extensive physiotherapy.

4. **Unable to throw an object**

   Sometimes, a patient reports a difficulty or inability to throw an object overhead (like a cricket ball from the boundary or a stone) or a difficulty in performing a smash while playing badminton. However, underarm throwing may not be difficult. This complaint is mostly seen in young patients (<40 years), especially those who play overhead sports. The possible cause for such a problem is likely:
   - Superior labral anterior-posterior (SLAP) tear
   - Weakness in external or internal rotators
   - Sometimes, tight posterior capsule.

5. **Catching or locking**

   It might be observed in instability, labral tears or loose bodies.

6. **History of neck pain**

   The history should always include query regarding complaints of neck pain, as neck pain with radiation towards the shoulder and scapula is often confused with shoulder pain. However when patient is asked to show the exact site of pain; in case of neck pain, the patient keeps his hand on the neck or the scapula or suprascapular region; whereas in case of shoulder pain, the patient keeps his hand over the shoulder. This helps in differentiating between neck and shoulder pain.

Also, the neck pain due to disc prolapse or spondylitis can radiate till the tip of the thumb and the index finger, whereas shoulder pain usually does not radiate below the elbow.

7. **Limitation of activity**

   It should be asked for reaching back, combing hair, dressing/undressing, reaching overhead objects, etc.

8. **Occupational history**

   It is important in shoulder pathology as workers with overhead activities are more prone to rotator cuff pathology. Overhead athletes often suffer from superior labral tears (SLAP). Weight lifters often suffer from ACJ arthritis. Those who train hard on the bench press may suffer from anteroinferior labral tears.

Past History

Apart from all other illnesses, the history of "diabetes and thyroid dysfunction" is most important in painful degenerative conditions of the shoulder. There is a strong association between shoulder pain (especially frozen shoulder) and these two "dysfunctions." Also, epileptics can suffer from primary/recurrent shoulder dislocations, especially posterior dislocation. Further, one must not forget that cardiac origin pain can radiate to left shoulder giving rise to confusion in diagnosis. Furthermore, subdiaphragmatic pathologies like chronic liver, gallbladder and splenic affections can lead to referred pain over the shoulder.

Personal, Treatment, Family, Menstrual and Allergy History

It should be evaluated as per the standard protocol.

▌ CLINICAL EVALUATION

General and Systemic Examination

As per the standard protocol.

Local Examination

After obtaining informed consent, privacy and chaperone for the patients and a female attender for female patient, the local examination must be performed after exposing the upper half of the body (adequately covered private parts in female).

Attitude

The shoulder is examined in a sitting or standing position. The attitude of the index shoulder and upper limb should be described in the standard fashion (e.g. The patient is sitting on a stool with right shoulder drooped, arm adducted and internally rotated, elbow flexed, forearm mid-prone and wrist in neutral).

Inspection

General findings:

Swelling, scar, and sinus should be described as per the standard descriptions.

Specific findings:

(A) From front (Fig. 4.1)

1. Shoulder contour: The contour of shoulder is maintained by deltoid and underlying head of humerus. Deltoid wasting/dislocated head will cause loss of contour (Fig. 4.2).
2. Deltoid wasting (Fig. 4.3).
3. Shoulder drooping.
4. Swelling/prominence of Sternoclavicular joint, ACJ or other areas.

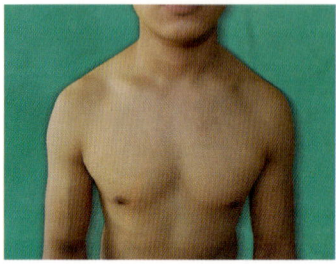
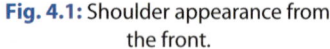
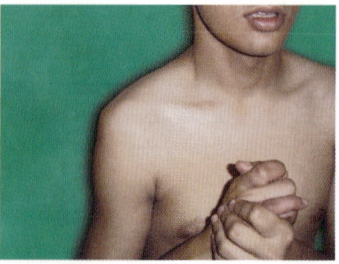
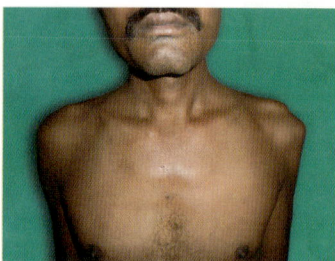

Fig. 4.1: Shoulder appearance from the front.   **Fig. 4.2:** Loss of right shoulder contour due to anterior dislocation shoulder.   **Fig. 4.3:** Loss of left shoulder contour due to deltoid wasting.

(B) From side (Fig. 4.4)

1. *Dorsal spine curvature*: Kyphosis
2. *Shoulder from side over deltoid area, ACJ.*

(C) From back (Fig. 4.5)

1. ***Spine and its curvature:*** *Scoliosis (if any), Hairline (low/normal), Neck (any tilt)*
2. ***Muscle wasting:*** Supraspinatus, Infraspinatus, Deltoid or other periscapular muscles (trapezius, serratus anterior, and latissimus dorsi) (Fig. 4.6)
3. ***Scapula (comparative)***
   - *Level of scapula*: Higher or lower (Fig. 4.7)
   - Distance of medial border of scapula from spine
   - *Winging*:
     - *Inferior and lateral*: Trapezius palsy
     - *Superior and medial*: Serratus anterior palsy
   - *Scapular dyskinesia*: Implies "dysfunctional movement of scapula"

   Method to elicit scapular dyskinesia: While patient is standing or sitting, the examiner stands behind the patient. Now, patient is asked to completely forward flex his shoulder upto 180° a couple of times. Observe the movement of both scapulae from behind.

Dyskinetic scapula

Normally, when patient is asked to perform forward flexion from 0-180° repeatedly , both scapulae move symmetrically. However, any shoulder girdle muscle weakness, shoulder pathologies (cuff tear, labral tear, impingement, etc.) nerve injury or proprioceptive imbalance would lead to asymmetric movement of scapula, which is known as scapular dyskinesia (primary/secondary)

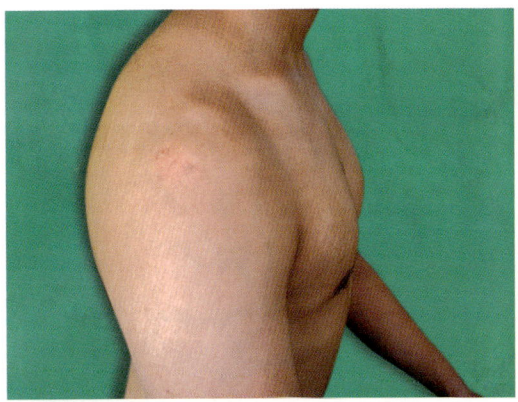

Fig. 4.4: Shoulder and spine appearance from the side.

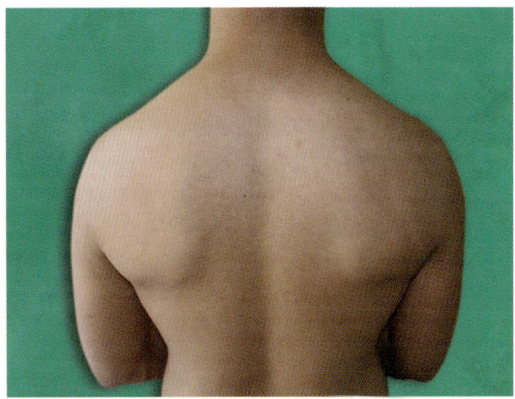

Fig. 4.5: Neck, Shoulder, Spine and Scapulae appearance from the back.

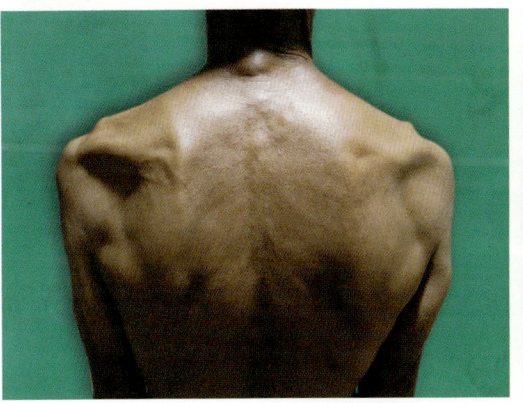

Fig. 4.6: Muscle wasting of supra- and infraspinatus of both sides (left more than right).

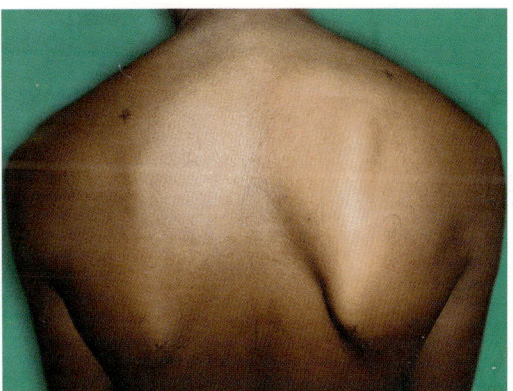

Fig. 4.7: Altered scapula symmetry.

Palpation

1. **Local rise in temperature:** Palpate from the dorsum of the hand over both the shoulders to compare for any rise in local temperature.
2. **Tenderness:** Always palpate in a sequence to feel for tenderness over major soft tissue, bony landmarks and joint lines (Figs. 4.8A to C).
   - *Sternoclavicular joint* (1)
   - *Clavicle* (2)
   - *Acromioclavicular joint* (3)
   - *Coracoid process (4)*: Below the lateral third of the clavicle
   - *Anterior joint line* (5) (Figs. 4.9A to C)
   - *Lesser tuberosity* (6)
   - *Bicipital groove (7)*: Just lateral to the lesser tuberosity

- *Greater tuberosity* (8)
- *Acromion* (9)
- *Spine of scapula* (10)
- *Medial border of scapula* (11)
- *Inferior angle* (12)
- *Lateral border* (13)
- *Posterior joint line* (14) (Figs. 4.10A to C)
- *Axilla*: Any abnormal mass, lymph node, etc.

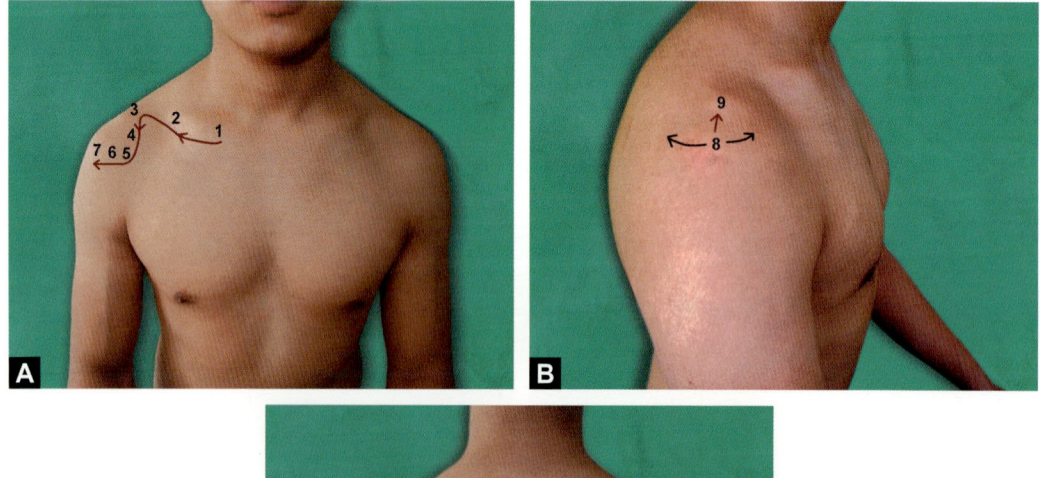

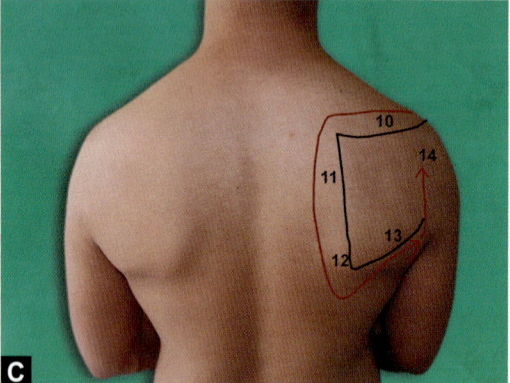

Figs. 4.8A to C: Shoulder palpation (in sequence).

Method to palpate anterior shoulder joint line:

Patient is sitting or standing. Examiner can palpate the anterior joint line of the right shoulder by keeping his left thumb *just lateral to the tip of the coracoid process*, while the right hand holds the elbow and the proximal part of forearm to rotate the humerus, and feels the rotating head over the glenoid. This confirms the position of the thumb over the joint line (Figs. 4.9A to C).

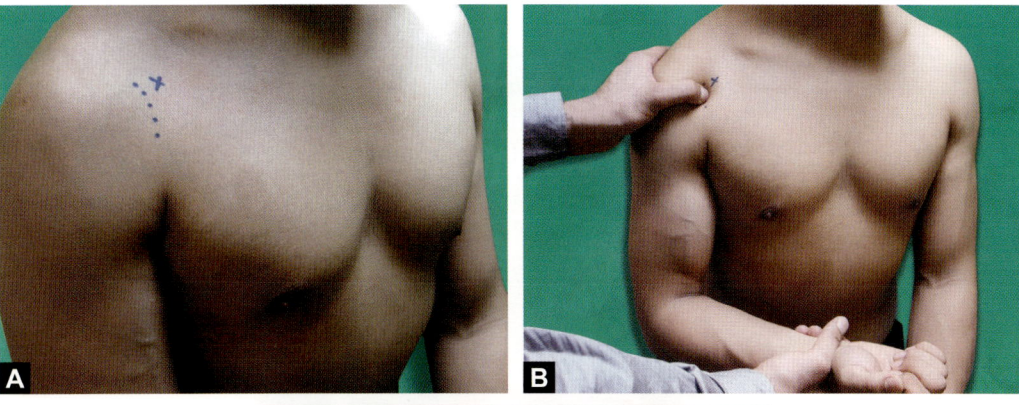

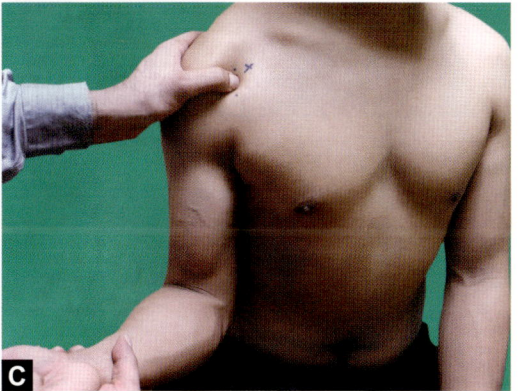

Figs. 4.9A to C: Palpation technique of the anterior joint line (X denotes coracoid process and dashed line as anterior joint line).

Method to palpate posterior shoulder joint line:

The posterior joint line is located *3 cm medial and inferior to the posterior angle of the acromion* (Figs. 4.10A to C). Hold the elbow-proximal forearm junction like above and rotate the arm while index finger/thumb feels the joint line.

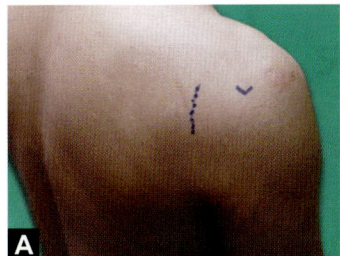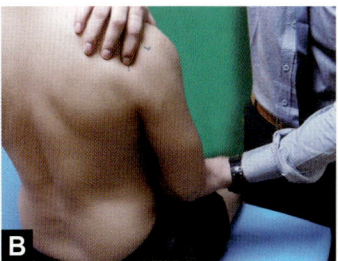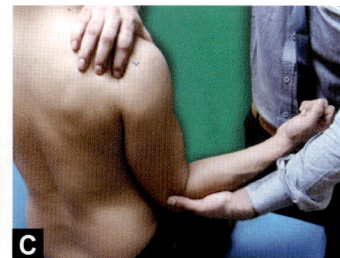

Figs. 4.10A to C: (A to C) Palpation technique of the posterior joint line (V denotes posterior acromion angle and dashed line as posterior joint line).

3. **Hyperlaxity of the joints:** Look for hyperlaxity of the joints and grade it according to the *Beighton hypermobility score*.

The Beighton score uses a nine-point system (Table 4.2) wherein the clinician assesses *thumb and little finger dorsiflexion, elbow and knee hyperextension and ability to touch the ground with the palm with forward flexion at the spine* (Figs. 4.11A to C).

The scoring is done bilaterally, except for the ability to flex forward. The score is either 1 or 0 for an activity if it could be performed or not. The maximum score in a hyperlax person would be 9. Usually, a Beighton score of 4/9 or greater is considered to be *significant. (Note: Presence of hypermobility is not akin to instability).*

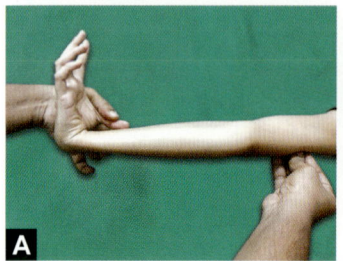 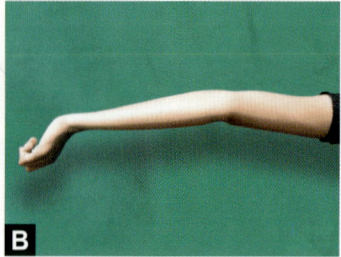 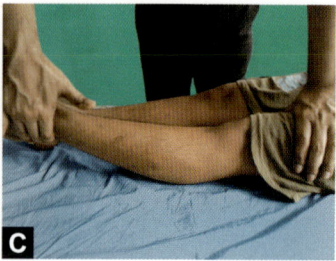

Figs. 4.11A to C: Hyperlaxity assessment.

Table 4.2: Components of the Beighton score.	
Joint/Area	**Finding**
Thumb; right, and left side	Passive apposition to the flexor aspect of forearm
Little finger; right and left side	Passive dorsiflexion at metacarpophalangeal joints (MCP) beyond 90°
Elbow; right and left side	Hyperextension beyond 10°
Knee; right and left side	Hyperextension beyond 10°
Forward flexion of spine with knee extended	Touch the ground with palm flat

Movements

- Active range of movement (ROM) should be assessed, followed by passive ROM (Figs. 4.12A to E).

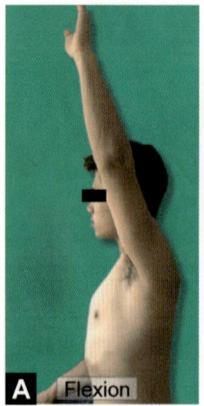 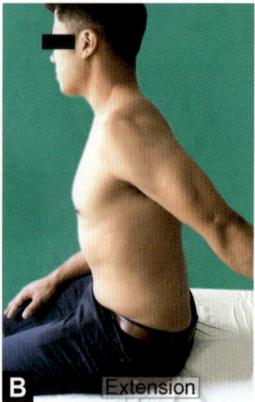 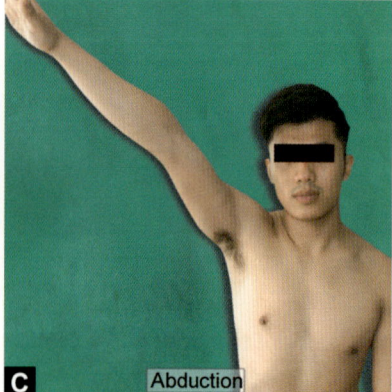

A Flexion   B Extension   C Abduction

Figs. 4.12A to C

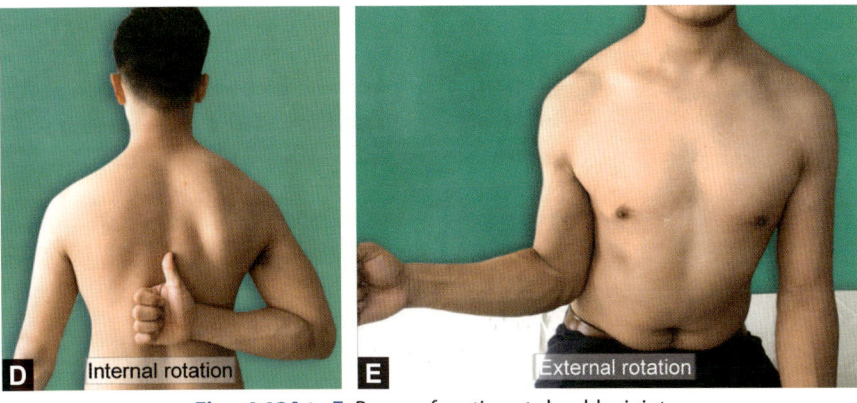

Figs. 4.12A to E: Range of motion at shoulder joint.

- Always compare with the normal side.

Before the ROM of the shoulder is performed, one must understand two concepts:

Normal ROM at shoulder joint	
1. *Flexion:* 0-180°	5. *External rotation (with arm adducted to chest wall):* 0-70°
2. *Extension:* 0-60°	
3. *Abduction:* 0-180°	6. *Internal rotation:* Thumb reaching up to D6/D7 vertebra spinous process
4. *Adduction:* 0-60°	

Two general rules while performing shoulder ROM are:

1. When the shoulder moves in flexion–extension or abduction–adduction, there is always movement at the GHJ along with movement at the STJ. Hence, one must minimize the movement at the STJ to assess the true ROM at the GHJ by firmly keeping the hand over the scapula to avoid movement at the STJ (Figs. 4.13A and B).

   However, after 90° of flexion or abduction, the STJ movement cannot be prevented any further, and then the STJ movement interplays with glenohumeral movement in the ratio of 1:2 (30° of ST ROM to 60° of GH ROM).

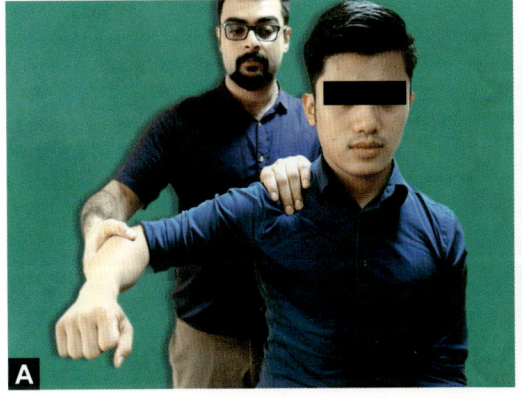
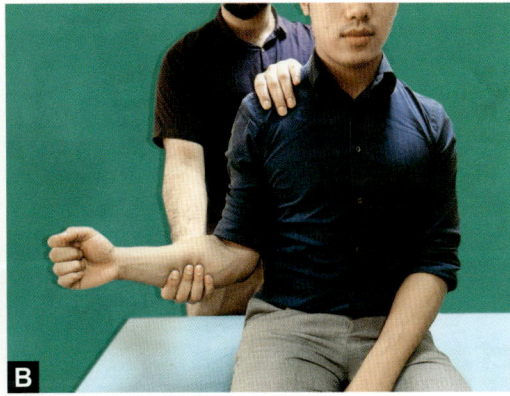

Figs. 4.13A and B: Shoulder movement after stabilizing scapula.

2. Shoulder movements such as abduction-adduction and flexion-extension are elicited in the plane of or perpendicular to the scapula respectively. The scapular plane lies 30° anterior to the coronal plane of the body as the scapula is tilted 30° forward. *Hence, flexion–extension is performed in a plane perpendicular to the scapular plane while abduction–adduction is in the plane of the scapula.*

Crepitus and click are elicited during passive range of movement (ROM) of the shoulder, assessed while keeping the hand over the moving shoulder through the available ROM.

Crepitus may suggest	*Click may suggest*
• Subacromial bursitis, loose body	• Labral tear
• Rotator cuff tear	• Biceps subluxation from groove
• Glenohumeral arthritis	

Assessment of movement can often give a clue to the diagnosis.
- *Gross restriction of both active and passive:* Frozen shoulder, Glenohumeral arthritis
- *Restriction of only active ROM:* Rotator cuff tear, nerve injury
- *Both active and passive are terminally restricted and painful:* Rotator cuff tendinopathy, Impingement syndrome, subacromial bursitis
- *Painful movements (active/passive) in mid-abduction arc of 60–120°:* Painful arc syndrome.

Measurements

The measurements are performed over both upper limbs for comparison (Fig. 4.14).
- *"The arm length"* is measured from the anterolateral angle of the acromion to the lateral epicondyle.
- *"Forearm length"* from the lateral epicondyle to the tip of the radial styloid process.
- *"Measure the arm and forearm circumference"*: In an adult, it should be checked 10 cm above the tip of the olecranon (for arm muscle bulk) and 10 cm below the tip of the olecranon (for forearm muscle bulk) on both sides for comparison.

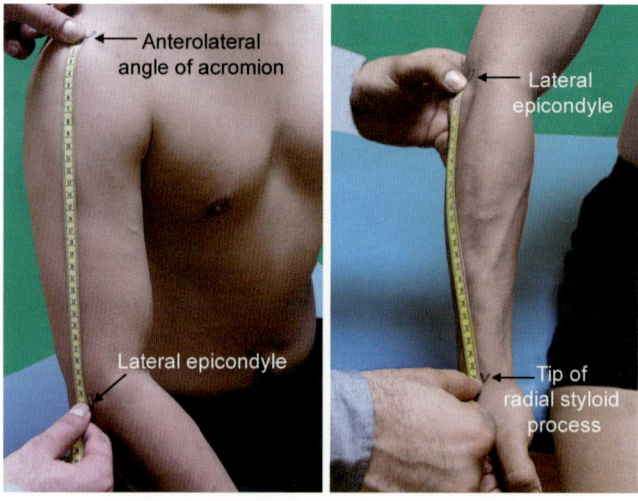

Fig. 4.14: Upper limb length measurement.

Neurovascular Examination of the Upper Limbs

As per the standard protocol.

Special Tests

(A) For shoulder instability: Anterior, Posterior and Inferior

(i) *Anterior instability*

1. *Apprehension test*

Method: While patient is standing, the examiner stands behind the patient's index shoulder. The shoulder is gradually brought in 90° abduction (AB) and 90° external rotation (ER). For right shoulder, the examiner's right hand supports the elbow (which can further rotate the arm externally). The fingers of the left hand are kept in front of the anterior joint line of the shoulder, while the thumb is kept over the posterior part of the head of the humerus. Then, the head is gently pushed forward by the left thumb (Fig. 4.15). This pushes the head of the humerus out in AB–ER position leading to the apprehension over the face of the patient. However, the fingers in front of shoulder prevent the further outward movement of the head of the humerus.

Interpretation:[*] Positive apprehension test indicates anteroinferior instability due to a torn and lax anteroinferior capsulolabral complex (Bankart lesion), with or without anteroinferior bony defect in glenoid.

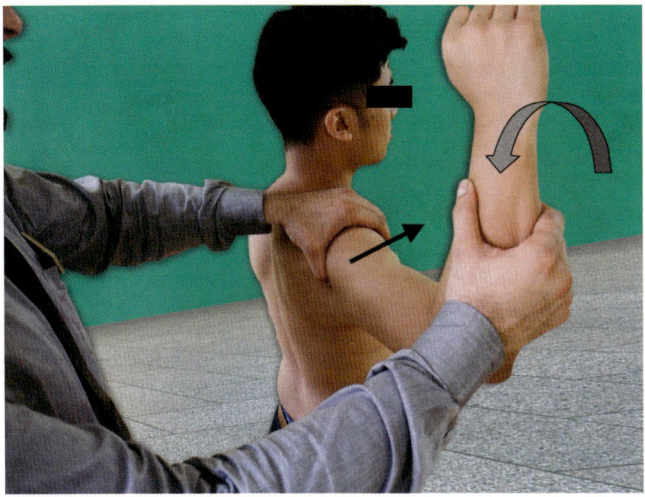

Fig. 4.15: Apprehension test.

* Caution: Sometimes, a shoulder can dislocate while performing an apprehension test, which could be very painful for the patient. Hence, relocation–release test is now preferred.

2. *Relocation–release test*

Method: This test is done with the patient lies supine on the couch. For right shoulder, the right arm is taken in 90° AB and 90° ER, whereas the midarm lies against the edge of the couch (Fig. 4.16). The examiner holds the right elbow by his left hand and keeps his right hand over the patient's right shoulder. The examiner's right hand is used to push (relocate, black arrow) the head posteriorly in reduced position in glenoid while the arm is kept in AB–ER position. Gradually, the extension at the shoulder is increased by pushing elbow downwards by left hand of examiner, while mid-arm stays against the edge of the couch, whereas right hand in front of the shoulder keeps the shoulder relocated. Then, the examiner gently releases his hand in front of the shoulder to let the head of the humerus move anteriorly (*never remove the hand completely from the anterior aspect of the shoulder, but just relax the anterior pressure*). This leads to the apprehension (of impending dislocation), noted over the face of the patient.Now, again press the right hand against the head of humerus and releasing the pressure over the elbow. This again reduces the head in joint (relocates) and apprehension over the face of patient disappears. This maneuver is repeated several times to confirm the finding.

Interpretation: The release of examiner's hand from the front of shoulder causes the release of the head anteriorly, and makes the patient apprehensive of dislocation. During this maneuver, presence of either pain or apprehension or both are significant. It implies anteroinferior instability due to **torn and lax** anteroinferior capsulolabral complex (Bankart lesion) with or without bony defect in anterior glenoid.

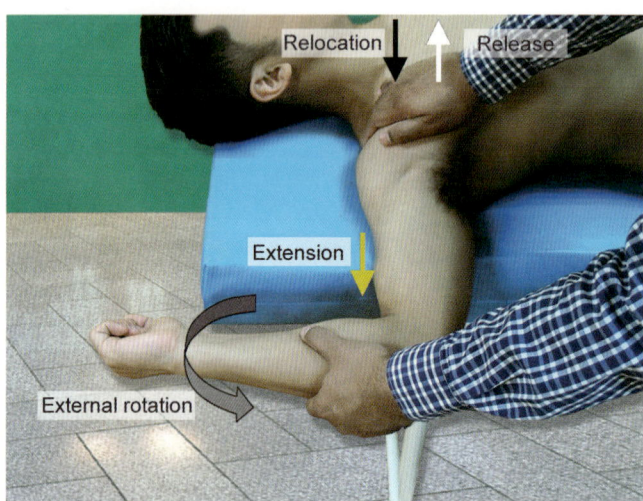

Fig. 4.16: Relocation–release test.

(ii) *For posterior instability*

1. *Jerk test (Figs. 4.17A and B)*

Method: The patient remains in a sitting/standing position. While stabilizing the scapula with one hand, the index arm is brought in 90° abduction, 90° internal rotation and *axially loaded towards the glenoid fossa* (black arrow) (Figs. 4.17A and B). Further, the arm is gradually brought in horizontal adduction. This subluxates or dislocates the head posteriorly with a jerk. Again, taking arm back to the plane of the body/scapula reduces the head with another jerk.

Interpretation: In posteriorly unstable shoulders, the axially loaded posteriorly directed force subluxes or dislocates the head posteriorly which reduces with a jerk when the arm is brought back in the plane of the body or scapula. This implies posterior instability due to posteroinferior labral tear with or without bony defect in glenoid.

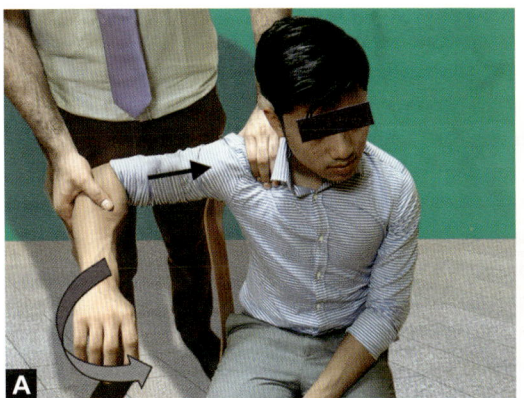 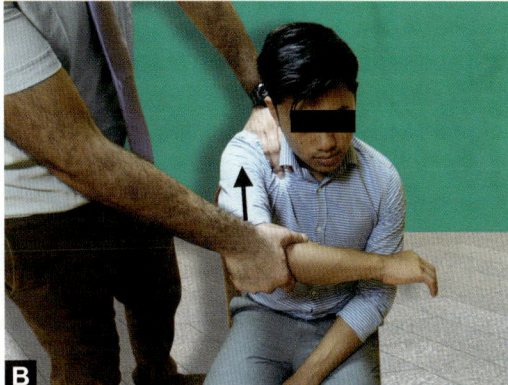

Figs. 4.17A and B: Jerk test.

(iii) *For inferior instability*

1. *Sulcus sign*

Method: Patient remains in a sitting/standing position. It can also be performed in a supine position too. The index *arm hangs by the side of the chest in the neutral rotation* while the elbow is kept flexed at 90° (Fig. 4.18). Now, a downward traction is applied to the arm by holding the elbow (black arrow).

Interpretation: If there appears a sulcus just below the acromion more than a finger breadth (white arrow), it indicates a positive sulcus sign. It implies lax or torn superior glenohumeral and coracohumeral ligaments leading to inferior instability of the GHJ.

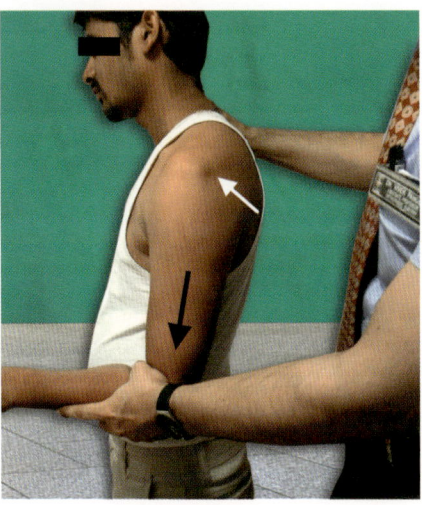

Fig. 4.18: Sulcus sign. White arrow shows sulcus appearing below the acromion.

(B) For impingement and subacromial bursitis

1. ***Neer's impingement sign:*** To test impingement in the subacromial space.

   Method: In a normal shoulder, the shoulder can be gradually forward flexed till 180° without pain (Fig. 4.19).

   Interpretation: In patients with impingement, he/she would complain of pain usually after 140°–150° of flexion indicating impingement.

   (Note: Read about impingement at the end of special test description).

2. ***Neer's impingement test:*** To confirm impingement in the subacromial space, and rule out pain from other source.

   Method: First, 2–5 mL of xylocaine is injected into the subacromial space. Then, Neer's sign is performed after few minutes.

   Interpretation: If Neer's sign is negative, it implies that the pain was due to impingement of structures present in the subacromial space only. If Neer's sign is still positive, it implies that the source of the pain is not in the subacromial space.

   (Remember: The sign is performed before the test)

3. ***Hawkin's sign:*** To test "subacromial bursitis."

   Method: The shoulder is brought in 90° forward flexion followed by elbow flexion to 90°. Then, the shoulder is gently internally rotated (Fig. 4.20).

   Interpretation: Pain in internal rotation is suggestive of subacromial bursitis.

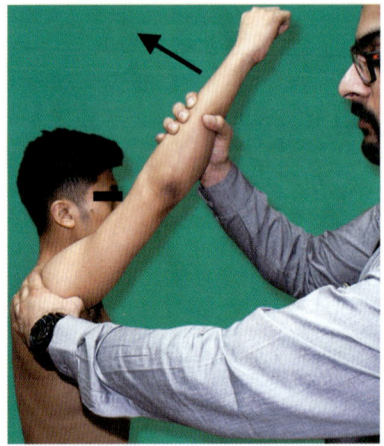

Fig. 4.19: Neer's sign.

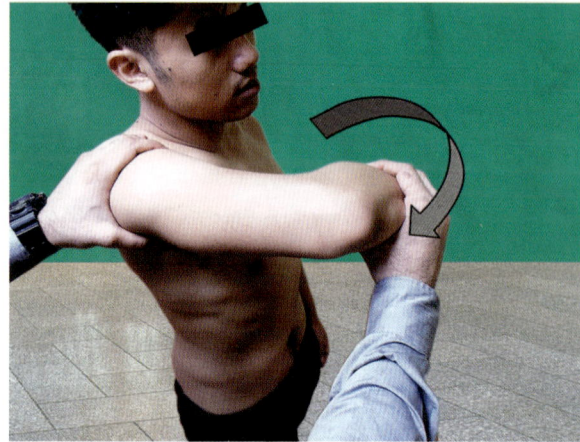

Fig. 4.20: Hawkin's sign.

(C) For rotator cuff tear

Normally, all the cuff tests are performed in standing or sitting. However, other than Gerber's lift off, all cuff tests can be performed supine too.

1. ***Supraspinatus (SS) tear:*** *Full can test*

   Method: The patient is seated or standing. The shoulder is elevated 60°–70° in scapular plane and externally rotated such that the *thumb points upwards (holding a full can of cola).* Then, the examiner applies a downward pressure just above the wrist while the patient resists it by lifting his arm upwards (Fig. 4.21). *(Note: Ensure that patient does not flexes his elbow or shrugs his shoulder to perform this test)*

   Interpretation: Any weakness with/without pain in this maneuver is suggestive of supraspinatus tear.

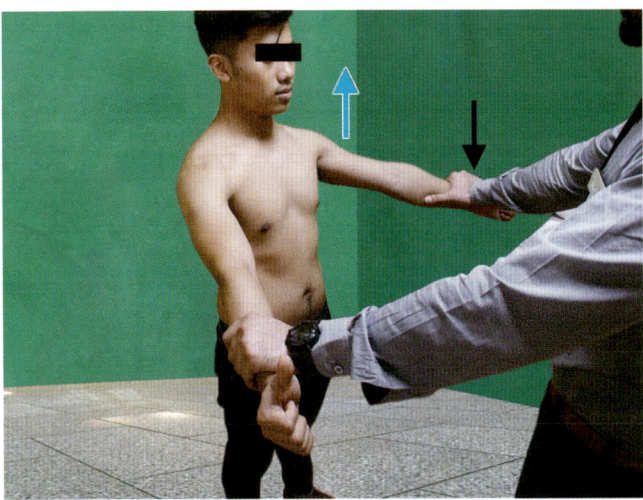

Fig. 4.21: Full can test.

2. **Supraspinatus tear:** *Empty can test (Jobe's supraspinatus test)*

    Method: The patient is seated or standing. The shoulder is elevated 60°–70° in scapular plane and internally rotated such that the *thumb points downwards (as if emptying a full can of cola)*. Then, the examiner applies a downward pressure just above the wrist while the patient resists it by lifting his arm upwards.

    Interpretation: Any pain and weakness in this maneuver is suggestive of supraspinatus tear. It is also positive in partial supraspinatus tear, rotator cuff tendinopathy, subacromial bursitis and impingement.

> - ***If the full can test is painful and weak***, there is no need to repeat the empty can test as latter is a provocative test.
> - If the full can test is quite strong in strength and not very painful, then the empty can test must be performed. ***Now, if the empty can test is painful and weak***, it may indicate a partial cuff tear or rotator cuff tendinopathy.

(Note: Empty can test is more provocative for pain than full can test.)

> **Drop arm test for supraspinatus tear**
> While patient in sitting/standing, examiner stands behind the patient and passively abducts arm to 90° supporting arm at the level of elbow. Then, release the elbow support and ask patient to gently lower the arm by the side of chest. Test is positive if there is pain while lowering the arm, sudden dropping of the arm or weakness in maintaining arm position during lowering (with or without pain), suggesting injury to the supraspinatus.

3. **Infraspinatus tear:** **External rotation lag test**

    This test is performed in 0° adduction and 90° abduction.

    Method in 0° adduction: The patient is seated or standing. The shoulder is kept adducted to the chest and externally rotated, and then it is released with a jerk (Figs. 4.22A and B).

    Interpretation: If the shoulder returns in internal rotation abruptly, it indicates weakness of external rotators, i.e. infraspinatus tear.

Method in 90° abduction: The shoulder is brought in 90° abduction and full ER and the patient is asked to hold in that position.

Interpretation: If the patient is unable to maintain that position and the arm falls in internal rotation, it indicates a weakness/tear in the infraspinatus.

> Another way to assess infraspinatus is to ask patient to externally rotate shoulder against resistance while arm stays in 0° adduction.

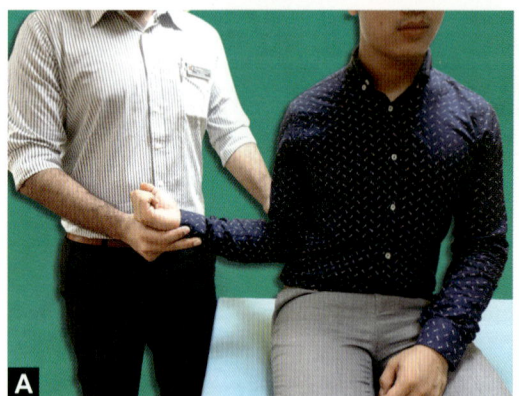
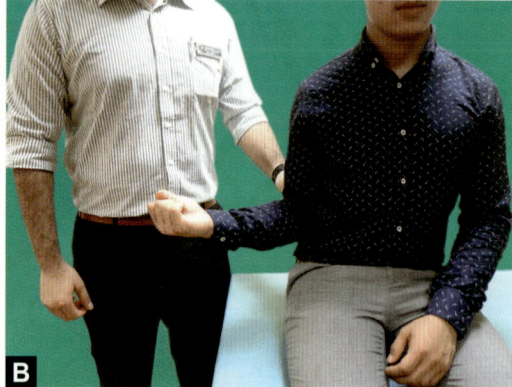

Figs. 4.22A and B: External rotation lag sign.

4. ***Subscapularis tear:*** *Belly press sign (Napoleon sign)*

   Method: The patient is seated or standing. The patient is asked to press his belly with both hands, and is asked to bring his elbows forward (blue arrow) while examiner pushes the elbow backward (white arrow) (Figs. 4.23A and B).

   Interpretation: If subscapularis is normal, the patient would be able to bring his elbows forward against resistance. Also, the angle between the wrist and the forearm would be almost 0°. However, any weakness or tear of subscapularis leads to the elbow falling backward or the patient would be unable to resist forward movement of the elbow. This produces an angle (α) between the wrist and forearm, indicating subscapularis tear.

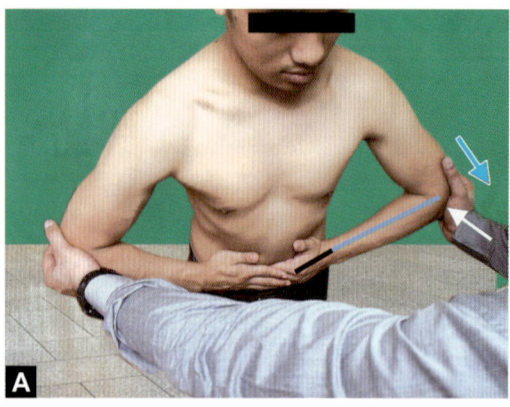
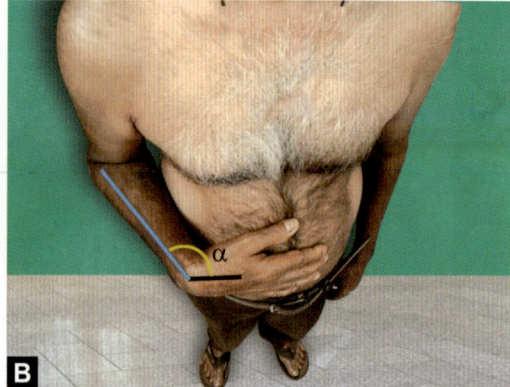

Figs. 4.23A and B: Belly press test (A) Normal; (B) Abnormal.

5. **Subscapularis tear:** *Gerber's lift off test*

   Method: The patient is seated or standing. The patient is asked to keep his hand at the lumbosacral junction and lift it away from it (green arrow). In a normally functioning Subscapularis, he would move his hand away from lumbosacral junction (Figs. 4.24A and B).

   Interpretation: In case of subscapularis tear, patient would be unable to take his/her hand away from the back or would not be able to resist examiner pushing his hand towards back.

   (Note: This test is difficult to perform if the patient is unable to do internal rotation.)

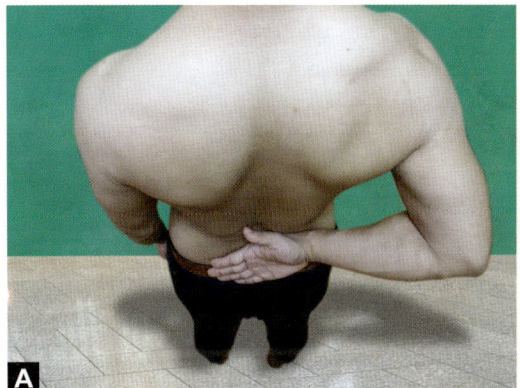 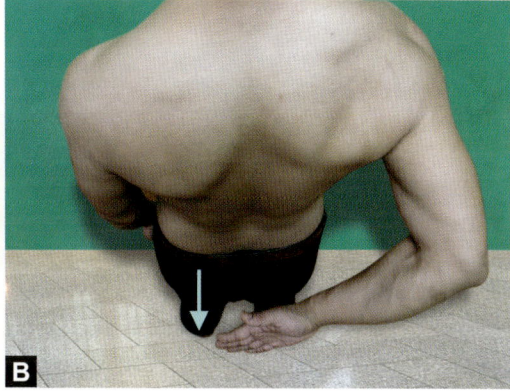

Figs. 4.24A and B: Gerber's test.

Often, in a massive cuff tear of supraspinatus with infraspinatus/subscapularis, or both, the patient may present with *Pseudoparalysis wherein* they may not be able to actively flex or abduct their shoulder beyond 40°–50°.

6. **Teres minor tear:** *Hornblower's sign (Patte's test)*

   Method: The patient is seated or standing. The examiner places the patient's arm at 90° in the scapular plane and elbow in 90° flexion. Now, the patient is asked to externally rotate against the resistance (Figs. 4.25A and B).

   Interpretation: The test is positive if the patient is unable to perform resisted ER and the arm falls in internal rotation and assumes a *"position of horn blower"* (Figs. 4.25A and B).

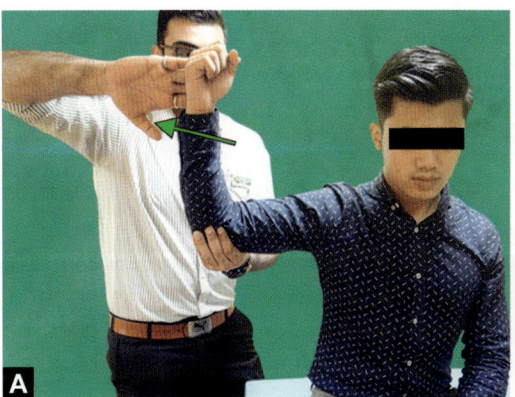 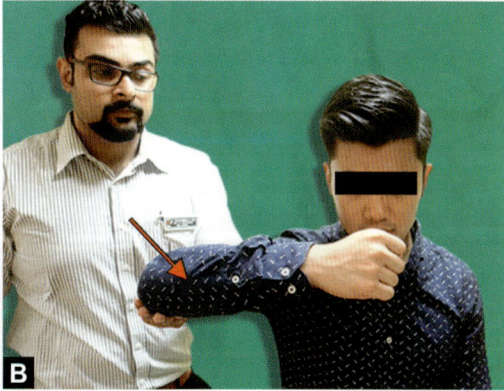

Figs. 4.25A and B: Hornblower sign.

(D) For superior labral anterior–posterior tear

1. *O'Brien test*

Method: While the patient is standing or supine, the shoulder is brought to 90° forward flexion, horizontally adducted by 10° and then internally rotated completely, so that the thumb points downwards. Then the patient is asked to flex his arm upwards (blue arrow), while the examiner gives downward resistance at the distal forearm (black arrow) (Fig. 4.26).

Interpretation: With SLAP tear, the patient is unable to resist downward resistance exerted by the examiner with/without pain.

(Note: Usually SLAP tear is seen in young patients with complaints of pain and inability or difficulty to throw objects.)

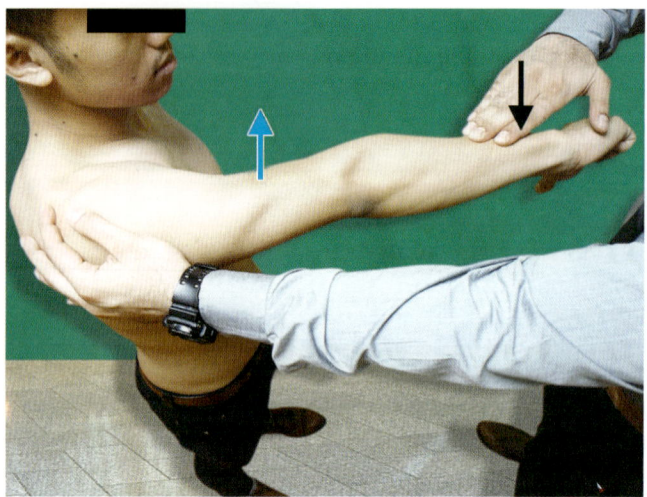

Fig. 4.26: O'Brien test.

2. *Crank test (Liu's test)*

Method: While the patient is standing or supine, the shoulder is brought in 160° abduction and elbow flexed to 90°, the arm is axially loaded, and the shoulder is internally and externally rotated several times.

Interpretation: With SLAP tear, the patient complains of pain while examiner may feel clicks.

(E) For biceps tendon pathology: Bicipital tendinitis

1. *Speed's test*

Method: While the patient is standing or supine, the shoulder is brought in 90° flexion with neutral in abduction or adduction and the forearm in full supination. Then, the patient is asked to further flex the shoulder while the examiner gives resistance against flexion (Fig. 4.27).

Interpretation: Any tenderness in the bicipital groove or anterior aspect of arm along the course of biceps tendon is considered to be sensitive for bicipital tendinitis.

(Self reading: Yergason Test)

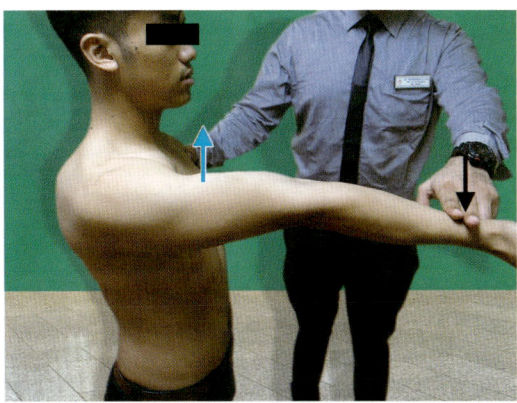

Fig. 4.27: Speed's test.

(F) For acromioclavicular joint arthritis

1. *Acromioclavicular joint tenderness:* It is quite sensitive and specific for ACJ arthritis. Palpate the AC joint for any tenderness.

2. *Cross chest adduction test (Scarf test)*

    Method: While the patient is standing or supine, the patient's elbow is hyperflexed and the shoulder is brought in 90° flexion. Now, the shoulder is horizontally adducted across the chest by pushing the elbow (black arrow), and the hand is made to touch the opposite shoulder (Fig. 4.28).

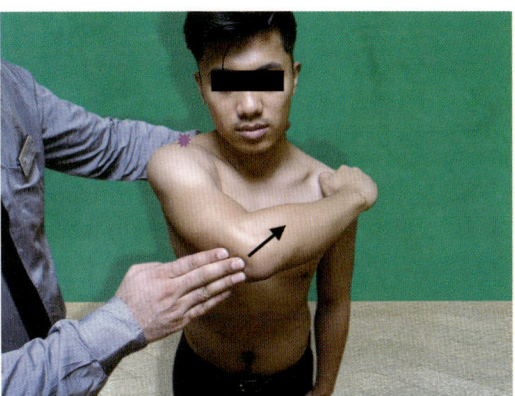

Fig. 4.28: Cross chest adduction test.

Interpretation: In case of ACJ arthritis, the patient complains of pain over the ACJ area with this maneuver (pink star).

(*Note: If this maneuver leads to pain anywhere else, especially posteriorly, and not over the ACJ, it is not suggestive of ACJ arthritis. In fact, it may suggest posterior capsule tightness.*)

Examination of the Joint Above and Below

- Standard cervical spine and elbow joint examination.

Examination of the Lymph Nodes

- Examination of lymph nodes of the neck and the axilla.

A note on impingement in the shoulder.

The term impingement is often used in shoulder pathology, which occur in the subacromial space. So, what does it mean?

Normally, the subacromial space is formed by

1. **Floor:** Top of the greater tuberosity
2. **Roof:** Undersurface of the acromion
3. **Front:** Coracoacromial ligament (CAL)
4. **Contents:** Supraspinatus, infraspinatus and subacromial bursa

In normal conditions, while the shoulder moves in flexion and abduction, the subacromial space narrows. However, the contents move smoothly between the floor and roof due to normal anatomy and the biomechanics of the shoulder joint, and get easily cleared without getting "impinged" between floor, roof or CAL.

However, in certain pathological conditions, the contents find it difficult to negotiate this tight subacromial space during shoulder elevation and get "impinged," causing pain.

1. **Thickening of contents:** In cuff tendinopathy, subacromial bursitis
2. **Downward projection of acromion in** Type 3 acromion, anterior or lateral spur of acromion: Volume of the subacromial space decreases.
3. **Malunion or nonunion of greater tuberosity:** Volume of the subacromial space decreases.
4. **Weak cuff muscles:** It leads to superior migration of humerus, thereby reduction in subacromial space, leading to impingement of cuff.
5. **Hypertrophied CAL:** Volume of the subacromial space decreases.
6. **Asynchronous movement of scapula (scapular dyskinesia):** This alters the acromial tilt and changes the subacromial space volume dynamically.

Hence, impingement is not a specific diagnosis but indicates a syndrome. *One need*s to find out the exact etiology for the impingement of the structures and treat accordingly.

Shoulder examination proforma

1. **Attitude**
2. **Inspection**
   - **General findings:** *All areas for Skin overlying, Swelling, scar, sinus*
   - **Specifics findings of inspection**
     (a) From front
       - Shoulder contour, Muscle wasting (Deltoid), Shoulder drooping, Swelling/prominence of SCJ/ACJ/other areas
     (b) From side
       - Dorsal spine Kyphosis (normal/altered), shoulder from lateral aspect
     (c) From back
       - Spine and its curvature, any deformity, neck, hairline level
       - Muscle wasting: Supra- and infraspinatus, Deltoid, other periscapular muscles
       - Scapula: Level, distance of medial border from spine, winging, scapular dyskinesia
3. **Palpation**
   - Local rise in temperature
   - Tenderness: Soft tissue and bony landmarks, joint line
   - Hyperlaxity of joints
   - Confirmation of palpatory characteristics of swelling, scar, sinus
4. **Movements: Active and passive**
   - Flexion, extension, abduction, adduction, external and internal rotation
   - Crepitus, clicks; if any
5. **Measurements:** Limb length, arm-forearm circumference
6. **Neurovascular examination**
7. **Special tests**
   (a) *Stability tests*: Apprehension test, relocation-release test, Jerk test, Sulcus sign
   (b) *Impingement tests*: Neer's sign, Hawkins test
   (c) *Rotator cuff integrity signs*: Supraspinatus (Full can and Empty can test), Infraspinatus (External rotation lag test), Teres Minor (Hornblower sign), Subscapularis (Gerber's lift-off, Belly press test)
   (d) *SLAP tear test*: O'Brien test, Crank test
   (e) *Biceps tendon pathology*: Speed's test, Yergason test
   (f) *ACJ pathology*: ACJ tenderness, Cross chest adduction test
8. **Joint above (cervical spine) and below (elbow)**
9. **Lymph node examination.**

Common conditions affecting the shoulder with their salient features

1. **Recurrent anterior dislocation (traumatic)**
   - *Affects young patients*: May be associated ligament laxity
   - *Presents with*: Mostly traumatic episodes (TUBS), occasionally atraumatic (AMBRII)
   - *Pathology*: Antero-inferior labral tear (Bankart lesion) along with posterolateral head of Humerus impaction injury (Hill Sachs lesion)
   - *Clinically*: Apprehension and relocation-release test positive, signs of ligament laxity ±
   - *Diagnosis*: Magnetic resonance imaging (MRI), CT scan
   - *Treatment*: Rehabilitation, may need surgical stabilization: Arthroscopic/open Bankart repair or Latarjet procedure
   - *(Note: Posterior dislocation is often seen in epileptics, after electric shock!)*

   > **TUBS:** **T**raumatic, **U**nidirectional, **B**ankart lesion, often needs **S**urgical stabilization
   > **AMBRII:** **A**traumatic, **M**ultidirectional, **B**ilateral, **R**ehabilitation is primary treatment, if surgery required—**I**nferior capsular shift and rotator **I**nterval closure is performed.

2. **Frozen shoulder/adhesive capsulitis/periarthritis shoulder**
   - *Affects* the middle-aged: 40–55 years
   - *Presents with*: Pain and *severe loss of ROM* (active and passive); inability in overhead activities, reaching behind head and back
   - *Pathology*: Inflammation followed by contracture of coracohumeral ligament (CHL), capsule and synovium
   - *Three clinicopathological stages* affecting CHL, capsule and synovium
     - **Freezing (0–6 months)**: Severe pain, gradual loss of ROM
     - **Frozen (6–12 months)**: Pain decreases, profound loss of ROM
     - **Tha*wing (12–18 months)***: Further decrease in pain, ROM starts improving
   - *Clinically*: *Global (in all directions) loss of ROM, painful ROM*
   - *Diagnosis*: MRI/USG
   - *Treatment*: Nonsteroidal anti-inflammatory drugs (NSAIDs), physiotherapy, intra-articular steroid injection, manipulation under general anesthesia or arthroscopic capsular release.

3. **Rotator cuff tendinopathy**
   - *Affects* the middle-aged: 40–55 years
   - *Presents with*: *Mostly pain and mild loss of ROM* at extremes of ROM (active and passive)
   - *Pathology*: Tendinopathy of rotator cuff, especially supraspinatus
   - *Clinically*: Neer's and Hawkin's signs positive, terminally decreased ROM, Empty can test +
   - **Cuff integrity test**: Equivocal but mostly negative for any substantial weakness
   - *Diagnosis*: MRI/USG
   - *Treatment*: NSAIDs, physiotherapy, subacromial steroid injection, rarely arthroscopic subacromial decompression with debridement of frayed tendon and subacromial bursa excision.

4. **Rotator cuff tear**
   - *Affects*: Old age, 50 years onwards unless traumatic tear which can happen at any age
   - *Presents with*: Pain with difficulty in elevating arm. Sometimes, pseudopalsy!
   - *Pathology*: Tear of one or more rotator cuff tendons from its attachment over the tuberosity. The tear could be traumatic or degenerative; the latter is more common than the former.

- *Clinically*:
  - Loss of active movements but usually passive ROM is preserved (unless secondary stiffness)
  - Full can, ER lag test and belly press sign are positive depending upon which tendon is torn
- *Diagnosis*: MRI/USG
- *Treatment*:
  - **Small size tear:** Conservative treatment; NSAIDs, physiotherapy
  - **Medium-large size tears** or ones which do not respond to rehabilitation need surgical repair

5. **Acromioclavicular joint arthritis**
   - *Affects*: Adults, manual workers: mostly after 45 years
   - *Presents with*: Pain with active abduction usually beyond 90° abduction
   - *Pathology*: Acromioclavicular joint arthritis
   - *Clinically:* Tenderness + over ACJ, cross chest adduction +
   - *Diagnosis*: Plain X-ray, MRI
   - *Treatment*: Conservative; NSAIDs, physiotherapy, intra-ACJ steroid injection, activity modification; Open/arthroscopic excision of ACJ if conservative treatment fails

6. **Glenohumeral joint arthritis**
   - *Affects*: Older patients, mostly > 65 years
   - *Presents with*: Pain and difficulty in movement (similar to frozen shoulder but duration is longer; never recovers unlike frozen shoulder, and age is usually more than that of frozen shoulder).
   - *Pathology*: Glenohumeral joint arthritis with loss of cartilage
   - *Clinically*:
     - Tenderness + over the joint line
     - Crepitus while ROM (it is not a feature of primary frozen shoulder)
     - Both active and passive ROM are decreased
   - *Diagnosis*: Plain X-ray, computed tomography (CT) scan, and MRI
   - *Treatment*: Conservative; NSAIDs, physiotherapy, intra-articular steroid injection, activity modification, arthroscopic debridement of GH joint for early stages of GH arthritis; *total shoulder replacement for advanced cases*

7. **Painful arc syndrome (PAS)**
   - It is *not* an isolated diagnosis per se but is a syndrome, as many pathological conditions can cause painful arc syndrome.
   - It is characterized by an arc of painful abduction (classically 60°–120°) during complete abduction of 0°–180° wherein the initial and later part of abduction is painless. It happens because, during the arc of 60°–120°, the subacromial space is quite tight. In case of normal structures in the subacromial space (bursa, cuff, greater tuberosity), the structures are able to navigate easily in the space between tuberosity and the undersurface of the acromion. However, any pathology affecting these structures can cause PAS.
   - *The following conditions can cause PAS*:
     - Subacromial bursitis (thick bursa)
     - Rotator cuff tendinopathy (thick, frayed tendon)
     - Rotator cuff tears (floating, free margins of cuff)

- Greater tuberosity avulsion malunion or nonunion (narrowed space)
- Acromial spur (narrowed subacromial space)

The clinical features, diagnosis, and treatment of PAS are dependent upon the underlying condition.

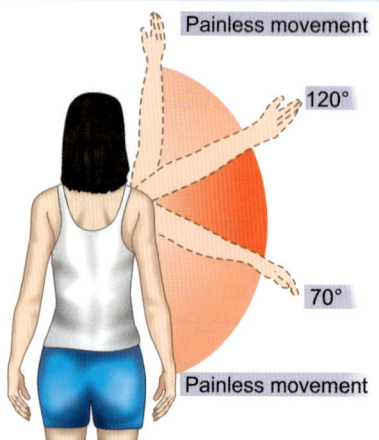

8. **Rotator cuff arthropathy**
   - *Affects*: 65–70+ years
   - *Presents with*: Pain and *inability to elevate the arm (Pseudopalsy)*
   - *Pathology*: A complete tear of supraspinatus and infraspinatus and arthritis of GHJ.
   - *Clinically*: Gross wasting of cuff muscles, all cuff tests are positive, crepitus.
   - *Diagnosis*: MRI, CT scan; X-ray shows the superior migration of the humeral head and arthritis of the GH joint.
   - *Treatment*: NSAIDs, physiotherapy, subacromial steroid injection; definitive treatment is *reverse shoulder arthroplasty*

9. *Superior labral Anterior posterior (SLAP) tear*
   - *Affects*: Young adults, overhead athletes. Often after fall on outstretched hand, traction force on shoulder
   - *Presents with*: Inability to overhead throw an object, pain +/-
   - *Pathology*: Tear in the superior labrum near biceps attachment. May extend further anterior and posterior or lower down
   - *Clinically*: O'Brien's test +, clicks +/-
   - *Diagnosis*: Clinical, MRI
   - *Treatment*: NSAIDs, physiotherapy, arthroscopic SLAP repair

10. *Calcific tendonitis*
    - *Affects*: 4-6th decade
    - *Presents with*: Acute, severe pain. Patients present within a day or two of complaint.
    - *Pathology*: Calcific deposits in degenerated cuff
    - *Clinically*: Very painful and grossly restricted ROM: Almost "Pseudoparalysis"
    - *Diagnosis*: X-ray
    - *Treatment*: NSAIDs, USG guided Barbotage, Subacromial steroid injection, rarely arthroscopy

Notes

Clinical Evaluation of the Elbow Joint

Chapter **5**

BRIEF ANATOMY AND FUNCTION OF THE ELBOW JOINT

1. **Basic osteology:**
   - The elbow joint is composed of the **humeroulnar articulation**, which is formed by the distal end of the humerus (trochlea) and the proximal end of ulna (trochlear notch); and the **humeroradial articulation**, which is formed by the capitulum and the radial head.
   - **Lateral condyle of the elbow** is formed by the *lateral epicondyle, the capitulum, and the lateral half of the trochlea.*
   - The articulating surface of the distal humerus is tilted 30 degrees anteriorly with respect to the shaft.
2. **Static stabilizing structures (ligaments) (Fig. 5.1):**
   - Medial and lateral sides are supported by the ulnar and radial collateral ligaments.
   - *Medial collateral ligament components*: Anterior, posterior and transverse bands.
   - *Ligament components-lateral side*: Radial collateral ligament, lateral ulnar collateral ligament, annular ligament.

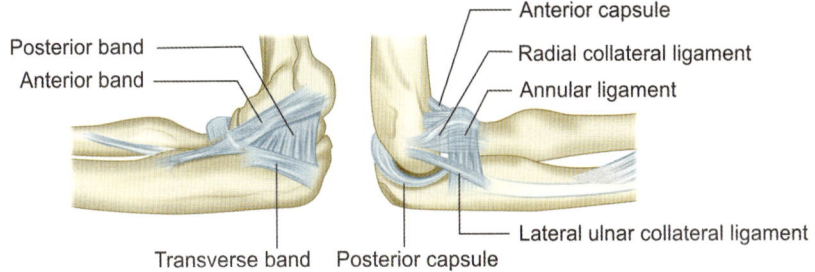

Fig. 5.1: Ligaments of the elbow joint.

3. **Type of joint:**
   - The elbow is a synovial hinge joint, whereas the superior radioulnar joint is a pivot joint.
4. **Movements:**
   - *Elbow joint*: Flexion–extension
   - *Superior radioulnar joint*: Pronation–supination

5. **Other facts:**
   - *Normal alignment* for the elbow (carrying angle) in extension is 7°–15° of the valgus.
   - *Classic three bony points* **are:** the lateral epicondyle, tip of the olecranon and the medial epicondyle. These three points form a triangle in a flexed elbow, whereas, it lies in a straight line in an extended elbow.
   - *Anconeus triangle:* Formed by joining the lateral epicondyle, the radial head and the tip of the olecranon. The center of the anconeus triangle represents the radiohumeral joint
6. **Important muscles around the elbow joint; their insertion, nerve supply, and action**
   - Common extensors originate from the lateral epicondyle, whereas common flexors originate from the medial epicondyle (Table 5.1)

Table 5.1: Important muscles around elbow joint; their insertion, nerve supply, and action.

Muscle	Insertion	Nerve supply	Principal action
Brachialis	Tuberosity of the ulna	Musculocutaneous nerve	Primary flexor of elbow
Biceps	Bicipital tuberosity of radius	Musculocutaneous nerve	Flexor of the elbow, Supinator of the forearm
Brachioradialis	Just above the radial styloid process	Radial nerve	Weak flexor of the elbow, supinator of the forearm
Triceps	Tip of the olecranon	Radial nerve	Extensor of the elbow
Anconeus	Posterior surface of ulna	Radial nerve	Weak extensor of elbow prevents capsular pinching in olecranon fossa
Pronator teres	Over upper one-third of shaft of radius	Median nerve	Pronator of the forearm
Supinator	Upper third of the radius	Posterior interosseous nerve	Supinator of the forearm

Common conditions affecting the elbow

1. *Traumatic:* Old fractures leading to deformities like cubitus varus/valgus, 2° arthritis, Post-traumatic stiffness, Myositis ossificans, Ligament injury leading to elbow instability, Tardy ulnar nerve palsy
2. *Degenerative:* Tennis elbow, Golfer's elbow, Olecranon bursitis, Cubital tunnel syndrome, Supinator tunnel syndrome
3. *Infections:* Septic arthritis, Tuberculosis
4. *Inflammatory:* Rheumatoid arthritis
5. *Metabolic:* Gout, Pseudo gout

HISTORY AND ITS EVALUATION

Chief Complaints

The patients with elbow pathology often come up with certain specific complaints:

- *Pain*
- *Stiffness/difficulty in movement*
- *Swelling*
- *Deformity*
- *Instability*
- *Tingling and numbness*

1. **Pain:** It could be acute or chronic.
   - Acute pain reflects trauma, acute infection or exacerbation of a chronic condition.
   - Constant 'night pain', disrupting sleep for a few weeks should raise the raise suspicion of infection, inflammation, or malignancy.
   - Generalized pain from elbow may indicate an intra-articular pathology, such as infection/inflammation/arthritis.
   - Localized pain like–
     - *Lateral side pain* could be due to tennis elbow, Lateral collateral ligament injury, radial tunnel syndrome
     - *Medial side pain* could be due to golfers' elbow, ulnar nerve affection or ulnar collateral ligament injury
     - *Posterior over olecranon*: Olecranon bursitis
     - *Anterior*: Bicipitoradial bursitis.

2. **Stiffness/difficulty in movement:** It could be due to pain, deformity, swelling, post-traumatic stiffness or mechanical block.
     - *Mechanical block*: Myositis ossificans, loose body

3. **Swelling:** It could arise within the joint or from an extra-articular source (bone, tendon, nerve, vessels, etc.).
   However, within the joint, the causes of swelling to swelling are joint effusion or synovial hypertrophy, or both. Most intra-articular swellings are observed over para-olecranon area or Anconeus triangle.

4. **Deformity:** Mostly post-traumatic (cubitus varus/valgus).
     - *Cubitus varus*: Malunited supracondylar fracture of the humerus
     - *Cubitus valgus*: Nonunion of lateral condyle fracture of the humerus
     - *Flexion deformity*: Post-traumatic stiffness, Prolonged immobilization, inflammatory (e.g. Rheumatoid arthritis) or infective (e.g. Tubercular arthritis)

5. **Instability:** It is seen in overhead throwers and pitchers. Post-traumatic causes (posterior dislocation of elbow) or overuse is another possibility.

6. **Tingling, numbness:** The tingling and numbness in the forearm and hand could be due to nerve affection around the elbow, which may be seen in cubital tunnel syndrome (ulnar nerve) or radial tunnel syndrome (posterior interosseous nerve).

Elaboration of Trauma Episode

- Most often, trauma precedes several elbow pathologies such as deformities (cubitus varus, valgus, and flexion) and stiffness. Young children present with cubitus varus deformity, with treated/untreated fractures of the supracondylar humerus.

- The **mechanism of injury** is important for the diagnosis of distal humerus fracture (fall on outstretched hand).
- ***Details of treatment*:** Incomplete, inadequate or no treatment could lead to malunion or nonunion of the fracture of the distal humerus. An unreduced radial head fracture can restrict pronation and supination of the forearm.
- ***History of massage to the elbow*:** Often present in case of myositis ossificans.
- *Progressive deformity of the elbow*: Malunion is usually nonprogressive unless associated with involvement of growth plate in growing children/avascular necrosis of the distal humerus. Progressive cubitus valgus is usually seen in nonunion of the lateral condyle.

Past, Personal, Treatment, Family, Menstrual and Allergy History

It should be evaluated as per the standard protocol. Assessment of occupation may give an idea about overuse of elbow leading to pain (tennis elbow, etc.).

▌ CLINICAL EVALUATION

General and Systemic Examination

As per the standard protocol.

It is important in systemic diseases affecting the elbow joint, such as inflammatory arthritis, tuberculosis, etc.

Local Examination

Attitude

The elbow is examined with the patient sitting/standing and the attitude can be described in the standard fashion.

Inspection

General findings
- A swelling, scar, sinus or an ulcer should be described as per the standard description.

Specific findings:

(A) **From front (Fig. 5.2A)**

1. ***Carrying angle*:** It is the angle formed between the longitudinal axis of the arm and forearm with the *elbow in neutral extension* and the *forearm in full supination (Fig. 5.2B)*. The normal carrying angle in the female is 8°–14°, and 4°–8° in the male.

> "Carrying angle is *always* checked in a completely extended elbow and supinated forearm. Hence, it should not be commented upon in cases with flexion deformity of the elbow or when forearm cannot be completely supinated.

> **Cubitus varus:** Extended forearm is deviated towards midline of the body. Often seen after malunited supracondylar fracture in children.
> **Cubitus valgus:** Extended forearm is deviated away from the midline of the body. Often seen in nonunion of lateral condyle of the humerus.

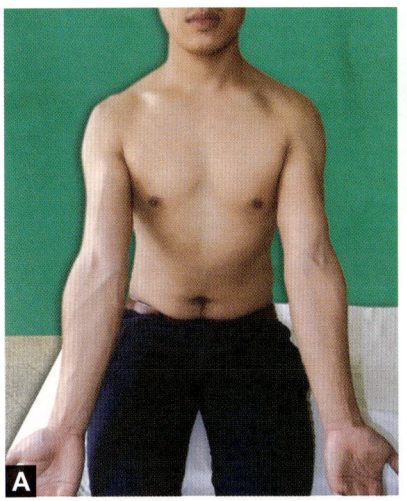 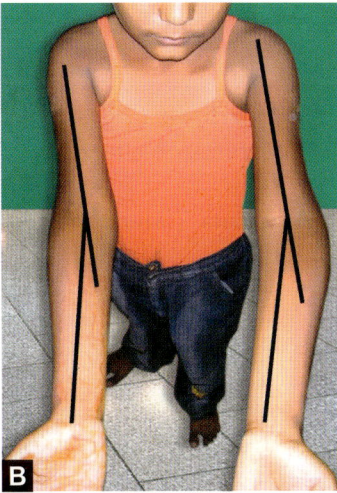

Figs. 5.2A and B: (A) Elbow from front. (B) Normal carrying angle in extension of right elbow. Left elbow shows Cubitus Varus with decreased/reversed carrying angle.

2. *Muscle wasting*: Note wasting of muscles of the arm and forearm, if any. It indicates chronic pathology.
3. *Limb length discrepancy*: It should be noted in an extended elbow.

(B) Observed from side:
From the side view, the axis of arm and forearm should be parallel in full extension. If it is not possible, it indicates a flexion deformity or recurvatum of the elbow (Fig. 5.2C).
1. **Sagittal plane deformity:**
   • Flexion/recurvatum
2. **Anconeus triangle swelling:**
   • It is a triangle formed over the lateral aspect in a 90° flexed elbow by joining three bony landmarks: *lateral epicondyle* (blue circle), *radial head* (orange circle) and the *tip of olecranon process* (yellow circle) (Fig. 5.2D). The center of the anconeus triangle (green star) forms the center of the radiocapitellar joint.

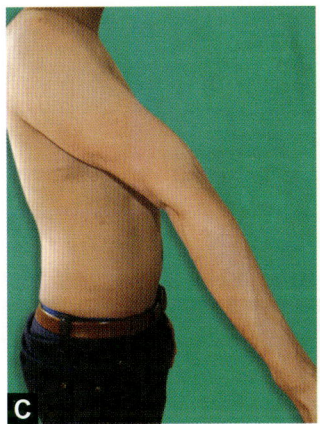 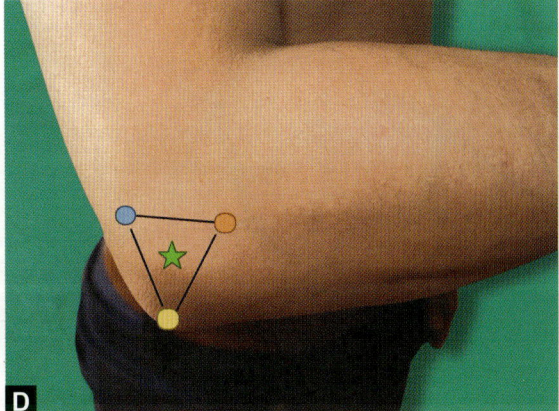

Figs. 5.2C and D: (C) Elbow from side (recurvatum). (D) Anconeus triangle

- Any visible swelling in anconeus triangle is suggestive of swelling arising from the elbow joint.

(C) Observed from back: (Fig. 5.3A)
1. **Position of Olecranon:** It alters in posterior dislocation of the elbow/fracture of the Olecranon.
2. **Three bony points (lateral and medial epicondyle and tip of the olecranon) relationship**

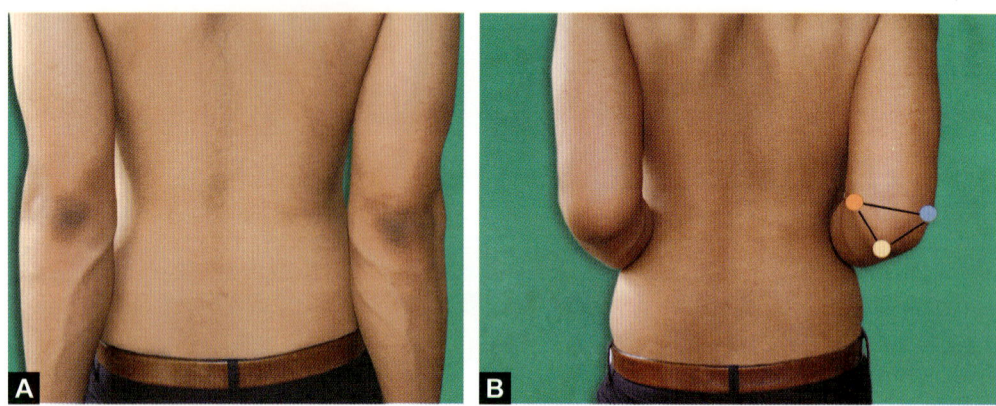

Figs. 5.3A and B: (A) Elbow from back. (B) Three bony point relationship.

- *In extended elbow*: Three points fall in a *straight line*
- *In 90° flexion*: Three points form a *triangle (scalene) (Fig. 5.3B)*
3. **Para-olecranon fossa for swelling**
   - Normally, there is a hollow on either side of the olecranon which is obliterated in the presence of intra-articular swelling (effusion/synovial hypertrophy/both).

Palpation

Palpation of the joint line, soft tissues and bony landmarks and ascertaining relationship between important bony landmark is the key aim of palpation.
1. **Check for rise in local temperature**
2. **Palpation of normal bony landmarks**

Supracondylar ridges, two epicondyles, olecranon process, the relationship between olecranon tip and epicondyles, radial head, proximal ulna and the lower end of the humerus.

These landmarks should be palpated for their position, relationship and presence of bony irregularity and thickness (*see* Figs. 5.7A and B).

(i) Palpation of the supracondylar ridges and two epicondyles—medial and lateral

Method: It is easy to feel the supracondylar ridges in a 90° flexed elbow. One must feel for the sharp supracondylar ridges over the lateral aspect of the distal end of the humerus using the index, middle and ring fingers by moving in an anterior–posterior direction. Once the ridge is felt, gradually descend over the ridge with the index finger alone. The first, most prominent point felt is the epicondyle, medial or lateral. The medial ridge is difficult to palpate as it is located in a plane deeper when compared to the lateral.

(ii) Palpation of the tip of olecranon process

Method: It is palpated by placing the index finger over the proximal part of posterior ulnar border which is subcutaneous. Then, the index finger is gradually moved proximally. The most prominent point felt is the tip of the olecranon process.

(iii) Ascertaining three bony point (two epicondyles and tip of olecranon) relationship

Method: Three bony points *"fall in straight line in an extended elbow"*, whereas the same form a *"scalene triangle in 90° flexion"* (Fig. 5.3B).

Nevertheless, it is immaterial what kind of triangle they form, **but the triangles of the two elbows should be compared with each other** (the measurement of each side of the triangle should be compared to that of the normal side) to ascertain the abnormality, if any.

> - *Conditions altering the three bony point relationship* (any condition where any of these three points are displaced):
>   1. Posterior dislocation of the elbow
>   2. Lateral/medial epicondyle fracture
>   3. Intercondylar fracture of the elbow
>   4. Olecranon fracture
> - *Condition where the three bony point relationship is maintained*
>   1. Malunited supracondylar fracture humerus

(iv) Palpation of the radial head

Method: Keep the elbow in 90° flexion to facilitate palpation of the radial head.

It is palpated about 1 cm below the lateral epicondyle (blue circle) along the shaft of the radius. Further confirmation of radial head is done by pronating–supinating the forearm, during which the radial head can be felt rotating under the palpating thumb (Figs. 5.4A and B).

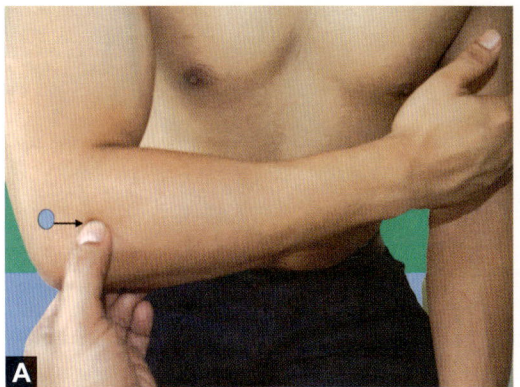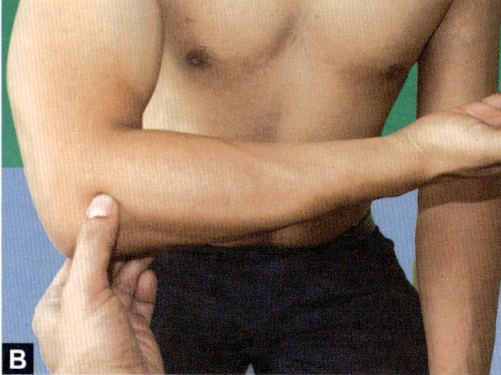

Figs. 5.4A and B: (A and B) Radial head palpation with forearm in alternating pronation-supination.

Altered radial head position is seen in dislocated/subluxated radial head. Palpate for tenderness and irregularity of the radial head (seen in fractures).

(v) Palpation of the anconeus triangle: A swelling present in this triangle is suggestive of an intra-articular pathology (synovial hypertrophy/effusion/both). Also, palpate for tenderness.

3. *Palpation of elbow joint line, anterior and posterior*

Method for palpation of anterior joint line of the elbow (Fig. 5.5): Palpate the lateral epicondyle (orange circle) and medial epicondyle (blue circle). Then, select a point 1 cm below the lateral epicondyle and 2 cm below the medial epicondyle. Join these two points from medial to lateral (blue hashed line). This is the surface landmark for the anterior joint line of the elbow. Palpate along this line for tenderness. The anterior joint line is difficult to palpate due to multiple soft tissues in the cubital fossa.

Method for palpation of posterior joint line of the elbow: It is along the para-olecranon margins for the ulnotrochlear joint (black curvilinear line in Figure 5.6) and just above the radial head in the anconeus triangle for the radiocapitellar joint. Palpate along this line for tenderness over the posterior joint line which indicates intra-articular pathology (arthritis).

> Feel for tenderness and synovial hypertrophy of the elbow joint, especially along the posterior joint line along the para-olecranon fossa.

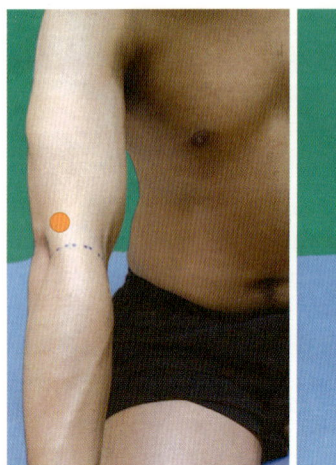 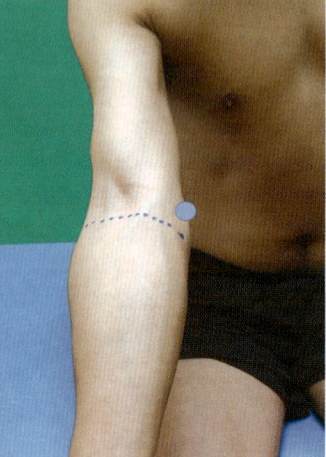 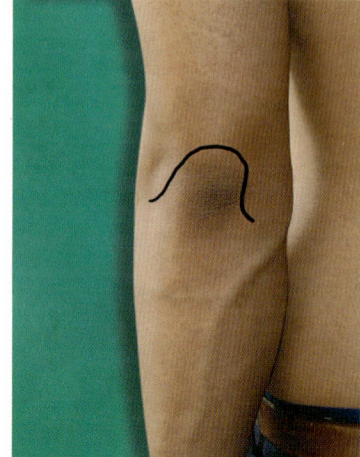

Fig. 5.5: Anterior joint line.   **Fig. 5.6:** Posterior joint line.

4. *Abnormal bony mass:*
Palpation of an abnormal hard bony mass on the anterior aspect or on the sides of the elbow indicates myositis ossificans or a tumorous pathology.

5. *Cubital fossa:*
"Hook test"-Ask patient to actively supinate a 90° flexed elbow. This makes distal biceps tendon (DBT) taut in the cubital fossa like a cord, and examiner can hook his index finger under the taut DBT from the lateral side. In case of DBT rupture, hooking of DBT with finger is not possible as there is no cord like structure to palpate or hook.

6. *Palpate the Ulnar nerve* behind the medial epicondyle

7. *Palpation of the flexor, extensor tendon attachment* over the epicondyles and triceps tendon over the olecranon.

8. *Palpate for features of ligament laxity* (Read Beighton score from Shoulder examination)

9. *Palpation of swelling, scar, sinus and ulcer, if any,* and its relevant description.

Tenderness over specific bony points may be suggestive of a specific pathology.
Lateral epicondyle: Tennis elbow
Medial epicondyle: Golfer's elbow
Radial head: Fracture
Olecranon process: Olecranon bursitis
Generalized over both joint lines: Arthritis/infection

Movements at the Elbow and Radioulnar Joint

- Flexion and extension can be checked in the standard fashion (Figs. 5.7A and B). The normal ROM is mentioned in Box 5.1. However, conventionally while commenting about the ROM; only flexion is mentioned unless there is hyperextension.
  (Note: Same is true for all hinge joints like knee, PIP, DIP joint of finger and toes etc with ROM of flexion and extension. Only flexion is mentioned unless there is hyperextension)
- Pronation and supination of the forearm (radioulnar joint) should be checked by keeping both the arm and the elbow by the side of the chest and the elbow flexed to 900. With pen gripped in the patient's hand vertically and forearm in mid-prone, ask the patient to pronate and supinate. Note the arc of pronation–supination by the movement of the pen (Figs. 5.8A and B). *Restriction of pronation–supination indicates the involvement of the radioulnar joint.*

Box 5.1: Movements at elbow and radioulnar joint: Normal range
Flexion: 0°–145°. (It may be few degrees less or more depending upon the bulk of elbow and forearm. *Functional elbow flexion requirement is 30–130°)*
Hyperextension, if any: Normally 0° but occasionally it could be up to 10°–20° (especially in children)
Pronation at RU joint: 0°–70°
Supination at RU joint: 0°–90° *(functional pronation-supination requirement is 50-50° each)*

Crepitus is elicited during passive range of movement (ROM) of the elbow and forearm while keeping the hand over the moving elbow, through the available range of movement.

Some important conclusions while performing range of motion (ROM) of the elbow.
- *Exaggerated extension with restricted flexion*: Quite typical in extension type malunion of the supracondylar fracture.
- *Restriction of flexion and extension in elbow*: Possible intra-articular pathology (infection, inflammation, intra-articular fracture malunion) or extra-articular mechanical block (myositis ossificans). The latter can cause only flexion deficit as well.
Note: Cubitus varus is often associated with increased internal rotation at the shoulder with decreased external rotation, which is suggestive of malunited supracondylar fracture of the humerus.
Note: *While informing active elbow ROM; Say flexion 0–140°. Do not say extension 140-0°. The latter term is avoided. Only hyperextension is mention, if any. Follow same rule for knee, PIP and DIP joint.*

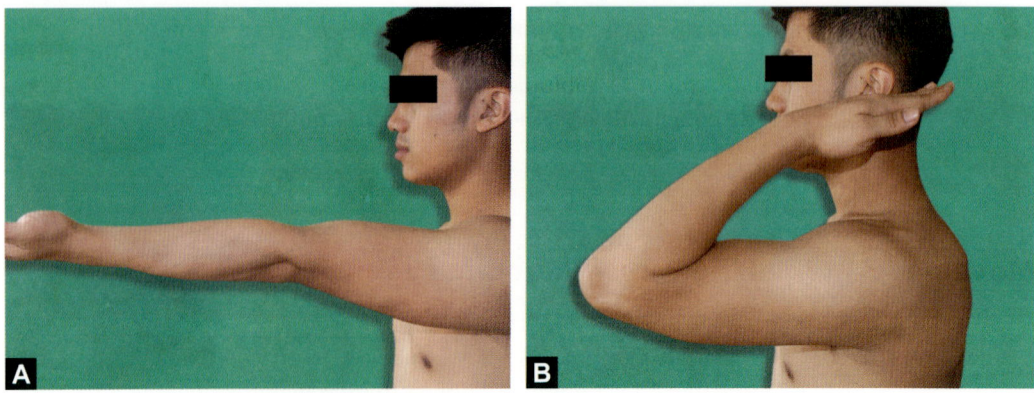

Figs. 5.7A and B: Normal elbow extension and flexion.

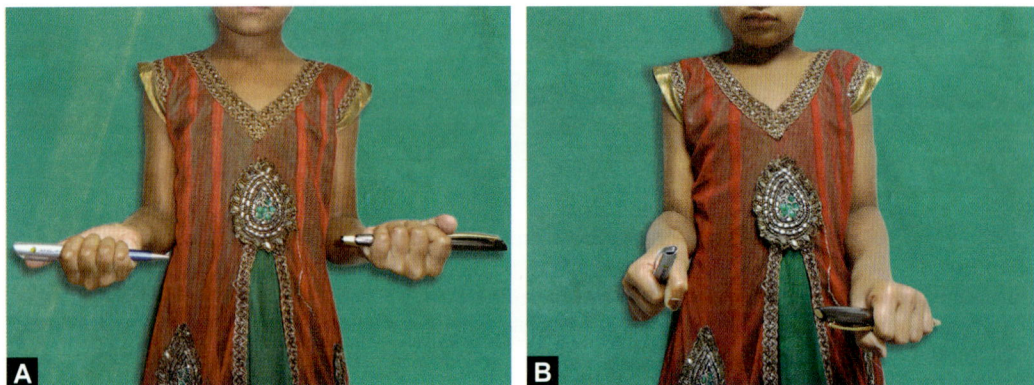

Figs. 5.8A and B: Supination and pronation at the radioulnar joint.

Measurement

1. **Limb length discrepancy**

   Arm length: From the anterolateral angle of the acromion to the lateral epicondyle (Fig. 5.9).

   Forearm length: From the lateral epicondyle to the tip of the radial styloid process (Fig. 5.9).

2. **Carrying angle**

   It is the inner angle between the long axis of the arm and forearm. The normal carrying angle is 4°–8° in males and 8°–14° in females.

   Prerequisite: The elbow should be fully extendible and the forearm should be fully supinated. *Carrying angle cannot be accurately assessed if there is a flexion deformity at the elbow joint or if forearm cannot be supinated (see Fig. 5.11).*

   Method to measure: Keeping the elbow fully extended and forearm supinated, draw the midline long axis of the arm and forearm with skin-marking pencil. Extend the forearm axis line upwards and arm axis line downwards so that the two lines bisect each other over the anterior aspect of the cubital fossa. Now place the center of goniometer at the anterior aspect of the cubital fossa over the bisected point, and align the two limbs of goniometer along arm and forearm midline axis. The inner angle between the intersection of two lines is the carrying angle (Fig. 5.10).

3. Wasting of arm and forearm muscles: It should be looked for, at 10 cm above the tip of the olecranon and 10 cm below the tip of the olecranon for arm and forearm muscle wasting respectively on both sides.

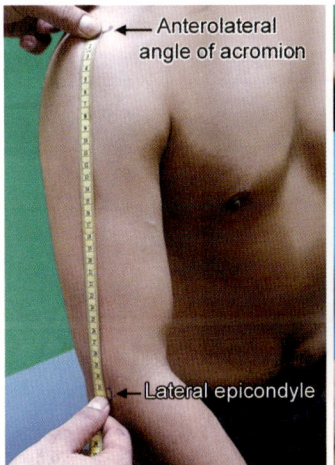
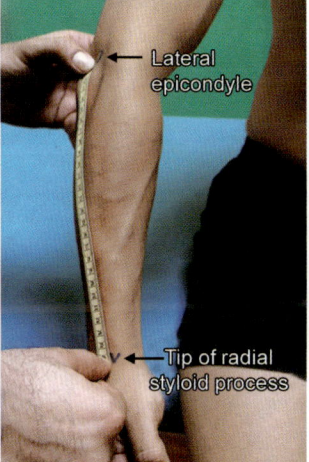
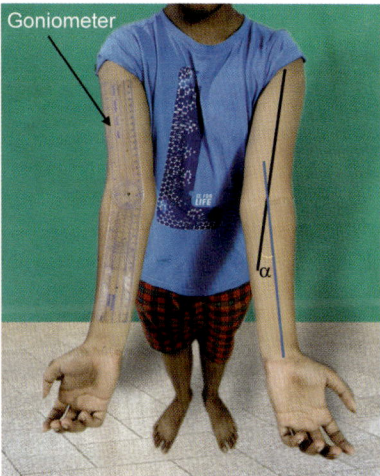

Fig. 5.9: Upper limb length measurement.

Fig. 5.10: Carrying angle measurement.

Neurovascular Examination of the Upper Limb

As per the standard assessment protocol.

Special Tests

(A) For Tennis elbow

1. *Cozen's test*

Method: With the patient seated and the right elbow flexed to 90°, the examiner palpates the patient's lateral epicondyle with the thumb of his left hand. All the while, the elbow stabilised by the examiner by holding it. Then the forearm is pronated, the wrist is dorsiflexed and radially deviated. Then, the examiner palmar flexes the patient's wrist passively, with his right hand and the patient is asked to resist this maneuver by attempting dorsiflexion (Fig. 5.11). This produces pain over the lateral epicondyle.

2. *Mill's test*

   Method: In a seated patient with a 90° flexed elbow, the lateral epicondyle is palpated with the thumb and elbow is stabilised by the examiner. Then, the wrist of the patient is forcibly palmar flexed while pronating the forearm and extending the elbow. This produces pain over the lateral epicondyle area.

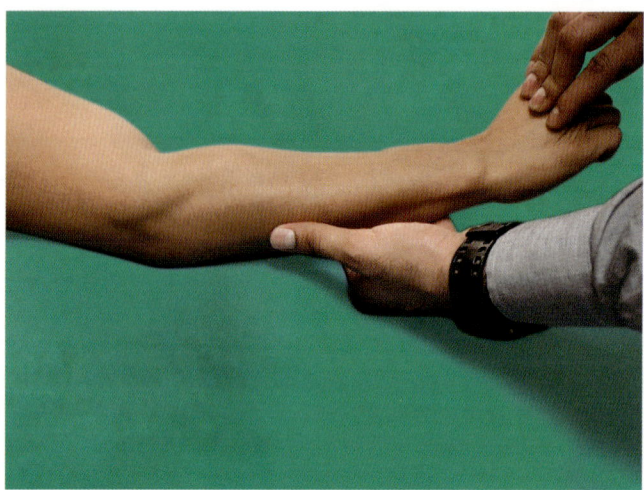

Fig. 5.11: Cozen's test.

(B) For Golfer's elbow

1. ***Reverse Cozen's test***

   Method: With the patient seated, the medial epicondyle is palpated with the thumb of one hand while keeping the elbow in 90° flexion; elbow is stabilised by holding it. Then the forearm is supinated, and wrist is kept in palmar flexion and slight ulnar deviation. Then examiner pushes the wrist downwards (dorsiflexion) and patient is asked to resist the attempt of dorsiflexion by pushing it towards palmarflexion. This produces pain over the medial epicondyle.

(C) For elbow instability

1. ***Valgus and varus stress test for ulnar (medial) and radial (lateral) collateral ligament integrity***

   Method: The test is done in standing, sitting or supine position. With forearm fully supinated, the elbow is kept in 20° flexion to unlock the olecranon tip from the olecranon fossa. For the right elbow, the examiner holds the patient's elbow with his left hand index finger and thumb over the medial and lateral joint line respectively to assess the medial or lateral opening of the joint when valgus or varus stress is applied. Now, valgus/varus stress is applied by the right hand holding the forearm (Fig. 5.12).

   Interpretation: Pain and excess medial/lateral opening in comparison to the normal side indicates medial (ulnar) collateral or lateral (radial) collateral ligament injury.

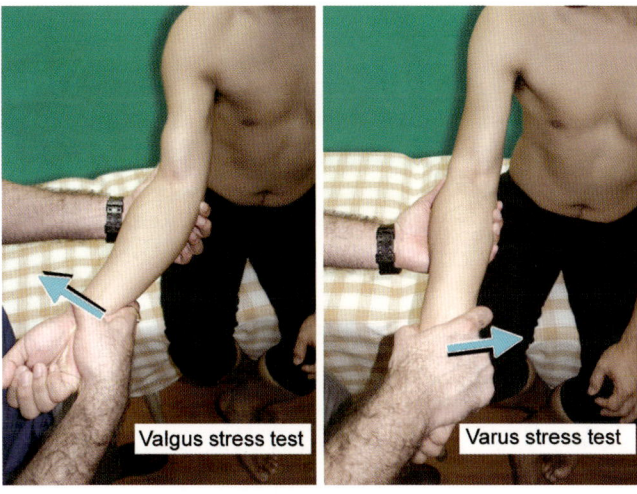

Fig. 5.12: Valgus and varus stress tests.

2. **Posterolateral rotatory pivot shift test (O'Driscoll):** It is due to an injury to the "lateral ulnar collateral ligament."

   Method: The patient lies supine with the shoulder flexed to 90°–100°, the elbow flexed to 90°–100° and the forearm fully supinated. While standing at the head end of the patient or facing the patient, the examiner holds the distal arm with one hand and the distal forearm with another. Now the examiner applies valgus stress and the elbow is gradually extended. The elbow suddenly subluxes in 20°–40° of flexion (Fig. 5.13).

   Interpretation: Posterolateral instability of the elbow.

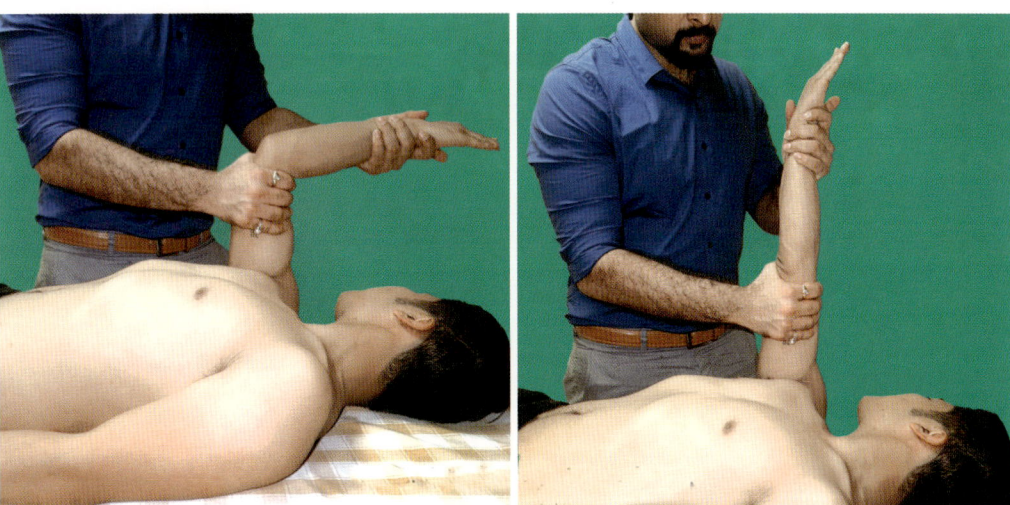

Fig. 5.13: Posterolateral rotatory pivot shift test.

3. ***Moving valgus stress test:*** For posteromedial instability due to medial collateral ligament (MCL) injury.

   Method: The patient is seated with the shoulder abducted to 90° and externally rotated. Now, the examiner places the elbow in full flexion and the forearm in full supination. Subsequently, hold the patient's hand and apply valgus stress while extending the elbow in the full arc of movement.

   Interpretation: Patient will complain of pain on medial side of the elbow and subjective instability during 70°–120° of ROM, if there is a tear of the MCL.

Examination of the Joint Above and Below

- Standard assessment of Shoulder joint, cervical spine and wrist-hand joint.

Regional Lymph Nodes of Cubital Fossa (Supratrochlear) and Axilla

Elbow examination proforma

1. **Attitude**
2. **Inspection**
   - **General findings:** *All areas for Skin overlying, Swelling, scar, sinus*
   - **Specifics findings of inspection**
     - **(a) From front**
       - Carrying angle, cubitus varus/valgus, any other deformity, muscle wasting, limb length discrepancy, cubital fossa
     - **(b) From side**
       - Sagittal plane deformity: flexion/recurvatum deformity, Anconeus triangle
     - **(c) From back**
       - Position of olecranon, para-olecranon swelling, three bony point relationship in extension-flexion
3. **Palpation**
   - Local rise in temperature
   - Tenderness: Soft tissue and bony landmarks, Joint line, Anconeus triangle
   - Three bony point relationship, Ulnar nerve, cubital fossa, Hook test
   - Hyperlaxity of joints
   - *Confirmation of palpatory characteristics of swelling, scar and sinus*
4. **Movements: Active and passive**
   - Elbow joint: Flexion, extension
   - Radioulnar joint: Pronation, supination
   - Crepitus, clicks; if any
5. **Measurements: Limb length, arm-forearm circumference, carrying angle, three bony point relationship measurements**
6. **Neurovascular examination**
7. **Special tests**
   - (a) *Tennis elbow tests*: **Cozen's and Mill's test**
   - (b) *Golfer's elbow test*: **Reverse Cozen's test**
   - (c) *Elbow instability test*: **Varus and valgus stress test, Posterolateral rotary pivot shift test, Moving valgus stress test.**
8. **Joint above (Shoulder, cervical spine) and below (wrist-hand)**
9. **Lymph node examination.**

Common conditions affecting the elbow with their salient features

1. **Cubitus varus due to malunited supracondylar fracture of the humerus:**
   - *Affects*: Children after a fall
   - *Presents with*: Painless deformity at the elbow following H/O fall on outstretched hand, not treated/inadequately treated fracture
   - *Pathology*: Malunited supracondylar fracture of the humerus
   - *Clinically*
     – Cubitus varus deformity (progressive/non-progressive)
     – Decreased or reversed carrying angle
     – Three-bony-point relation is maintained
     – Irregular supracondylar ridges and supracondylar area
     – Internal rotation of the shoulder is more whereas external rotation is decreased as compared to normal side
     – Sometimes, flexion of the elbow is restricted; whereas extension of the elbow, exaggerated
   - *Diagnosis*: X-ray
   - *Treatment*: Conservative, corrective osteotomy (Modified French)
2. **Cubitus valgus due to fracture nonunion of lateral condyle of humerus:**
   - *Affects*: Mostly affects children, can present in adults too
   - *Presents with*: Deformity of the elbow following a fall on the outstretched hand. Often from an untreated/inadequately treated fracture
   - *Pathology*: Nonunion of the lateral condyle of the humerus
   - *Clinically*:
     – Cubitus Valgus deformity; sometimes, painful, progressive
     – Irregular supracondylar ridges on the lateral aspect
     – Palpable step on the lateral distal humerus, three bony points relation is not maintained
     – Elbow flexion and extension may be affected
     – Ulnar nerve palsy may be present at a later stage *(tardy ulnar nerve palsy)*
   - *Diagnosis*: X-ray (fishtail deformity)
   - *Treatment*: Anterior transposition of the ulnar nerve, corrective osteotomy for deformity, internal fixation of the lateral condyle nonunion
3. **Tubercular arthritis:**
   - *Affects*: Any age
   - *Presents with*: Painful elbow with swelling, H/o contact with patient affected by tuberculosis
   - *Pathology*: TB of the elbow; synovitis/arthritis/deformity
   - *Clinically*: Flexion deformity of the elbow, joint line tenderness, synovial thickening, restriction of flexion and extension, marked wasting of the muscles of the arm and forearm
   - *Diagnosis*: X-ray, synovial or bone biopsy
   - *Treatment*: Anti-tuberculosis chemotherapy (ATT), synovectomy, arthrodesis
4. **Rheumatoid arthritis (RA) of the elbow:**
   - *Affects*: Young females
   - *Presents with*: Painful elbow with h/o morning stiffness, other joint involvement
   - *Pathology*: RA; stage—synovitis/arthritis/deformity
   - *Clinically*: Flexion deformity of the elbow, synovial hypertrophy, tender joint line, ROM restricted, marked wasting of the arm and forearm muscles

- **Diagnosis**: X-ray, other tests for RA [RA factor and anti-cyclic citrullinated peptide (anti-CCP)]
- **Treatment**: Disease-modifying antirheumatic drugs (DMARDs), synovectomy, arthrodesis, joint replacement

5. **Myositis ossificans:**
   - **Affects**: Any age
   - **Presents with**: Painless loss of movements of the elbow, H/o trauma/head injury, aggressive physiotherapy (passive mobilization), massage
   - **Pathology:** Bony mass in the muscle (most commonly, Brachialis)
   - **Clinically**: Bony mass palpable on the anterior aspect of the elbow, usually presents as a painless mechanical block during flexion
   - **Diagnosis**: X-ray
   - **Treatment**: Wait and watch, bony mass excision. Watch for recurrence!

6. **Tennis elbow (lateral epicondylitis):**
   - **Affects**: Middle-aged patients
   - **Presents with**: Painful elbow during activities
   - **Pathology**: Tendinosis of extensor carpi radialis brevis (ECRB)
   - **Clinically**: Tender lateral epicondyle, Mill's test and Cozen's test +
   - **Diagnosis**: Mostly clinical, ultrasound (USG), and magnetic resonance imaging (MRI)
   - **Treatment**: Conservative, open/arthroscopic debridement

   > **Radial/supinator tunnel syndrome:** It is a condition which closely mimics tennis elbow in its presentation, wherein the patient complains of mechanical pain over the lateral aspect of the elbow. Also, the patient complains of radiating pain toward the hand with occasional tingling. However, the tenderness is not over the lateral epicondyle but a few centimeters below, over the proximal part of the radius, where the posterior interosseous nerve (PIN) enters the supinator tunnel. The pressure over this area produces tingling along the course of superficial radial nerve. It is due to the PIN entrapment in the supinator muscle.

7. **Golfer's elbow (medial epicondylitis):**
   - **Affects**: Middle-aged patients, less common than tennis elbow but more difficult to treat
   - **Presents with**: Painful elbow during activities, especially those which require flexion of the wrist
   - **Pathology**: Tendinosis of the flexor pronator mass
   - **Clinically**: Tender medial epicondyle
     - Pain with resisted forearm pronation and wrist flexion
     - May be associated with features of valgus instability of the elbow and ulnar neuritis
   - **Diagnosis**: Mostly clinical, USG, and MRI
   - **Treatment**: Conservative, open/arthroscopic debridement

8. **Student's elbow/minor's elbow (olecranon bursitis):**
   - **Affects**: Young students whose elbow rubs against the table/chair while writing
   - **Presents with**: Painful swelling over the back of elbow
   - **Pathology**: Friction bursitis of olecranon bursa
   - **Clinically**: Painful swelling over the olecranon. Rule out hyperuricemia
   - **Diagnosis**: USG and MRI
   - **Treatment**: Activity modification, aspiration, excision of bursa

9. **Elbow/cubital tunnel syndrome:**
   - *Affects*: The middle-aged, and the elderly, those who sleep with a flexed elbow or perform activities, where excessive flexion of the elbow is required or with excessive cell phone usage
   - *Presents with*: Pain around the elbow and tingling along ulnar nerve
   - *Pathology*: *Ulnar nerve entrapment* within the two heads of flexor carpi ulnaris or arcade of Struthers/Osborne ligament and MCL/osteophytes of an arthritic elbow
   - *Clinically*: Pain over the elbow with ulnar nerve compression signs
   - *Diagnosis*: X-ray, nerve conduction velocity (NCV) study
   - *Treatment*: Conservative, activity modification, anterior transposition of the ulnar nerve, release of the ligaments or osteophytes.

10. **Elbow instability:**
    - *Seen after*: Trauma, inflammatory arthritis, repeated overhead movements or overuse (pitching, volleyball, and tennis)
    - *Presents with*: Pain, clicking or catching with elbow extension (while pushing off from chair), loss of velocity or throwing ability
    - *Pathology*: Varus instability due to injury to the lateral collateral ligament (LCL) mostly due to trauma, while medial collateral injury is seen in overuse in overhead activities.
    - *Clinically*: Pain over LUCL/MCL, varus/valgus stress test +
    - *Diagnosis*: Magnetic resonance imaging
    - *Treatment*: Activity modification, splints, ligament reconstruction

11. **Terrible triad of the elbow:**
    - A traumatic condition
    - Combination of elbow dislocation, coronoid fracture and radial head/neck fracture

12. **Little league elbow:**
    - Term used for adolescent elbow overuse injury due to repetitive valgus overloading
    - Comprises of medial epicondyle stress fracture, ulnar collateral ligament injury and flexor–pronator mass strain

13. **Pulled elbow:**
    - Seen in children less than 5 years
    - Occurs when children are pulled or lifted by their forearm; radial head subluxes inferiorly under annular ligament
    - Child cries incessantly and keeps arm and forearm still
    - *Managed by*: Pronation–supination along with flexion at the elbow reduces the subluxation with a "clunk"

14. **Congenital radioulnar synostosis:**
    - Restricted pronation–supination since childhood.

15. **Old Monteggia fracture dislocation:**
    - Seen after trauma
    - Present with deformity and limitation with pronation and supination
    - *Clinically*: Deformity of the forearm, radial head dislocation, limitation of the pronation-supination movements
    - *Diagnosis*: X-rays
    - *Treatment*: Ulnar osteotomy, internal fixation and radial head relocation

Notes

Clinical Evaluation of the Wrist and Hand

Chapter 6

▌BRIEF ANATOMY AND FUNCTION OF THE WRIST JOINT

1. **Basic osteology of wrist**
   - A total of 27 bones form the wrist and hand (and three nerves, radial, median, and ulnar, enter the hand).
   - Wrist joint is ***not a single joint*** but formed by combinations of many bones and joints.
     - Radiocarpal (True wrist joint: formed by distal Radius, proximal row of carpus and articular disc overlying the Ulna)
     - Distal radioulnar joint (DRUJ)
     - Intercarpal.
   - Various bones that take part in formation of anatomical area of wrist are:
     - Distal end of radius and ulna
     - Eight carpal bones
       - *Proximal row (radial to ulnar)*: Scaphoid, lunate, triquetral, and pisiform
       - *Distal row (radial to ulnar)*: Trapezium, trapezoid, capitate, and hamate.
2. **Static stabilizing structures of wrist**
   - Radiocarpal, ulnocarpal, and various intercarpal ligaments bind all these bones together to provide stability to the wrist.
   - Ulnar side of the wrist has triangular fibrocartilage complex (TFCC).
     - Triangular fibrocartilage complex function
       - Load transmission across the wrist
       - Rotation of wrist by stabilizing DRUJ.

Triangular fibrocartilage complex (TFCC) components.
• Triangular fibrocartilage disc
• Radioulnar (dorsal and volar) ligaments
• Ulnocarpal (ulnolunate and ulnotriquetral) ligaments
• Extensor carpi ulnaris (ECU) sheath
• Ulnar collateral ligament
• Meniscal homologue

3. **Retinaculum around wrist**

   Two retinaculum are: (1) Flexor retinaculum (FR) and (2) Extensor retinaculum (ER).
   - **Flexor retinaculum** is on volar side of the wrist with its attachment on four carpals (Fig. 6.1). Nine tendons and one nerve passes underneath FR.

- ○ *The median nerve* passes *under the FR* whereas the *ulnar nerve* passes *outside the FR* through "Guyon's canal" (located between hook of hamate and pisiform).
- **Extensor retinaculum** is on the dorsum of the wrist which runs from distal radius to pisiform and triquetrum (and not ulna). It has six compartments through which various tendons, nerves, and arteries traverse (Table 6.1 and Fig. 6.2).

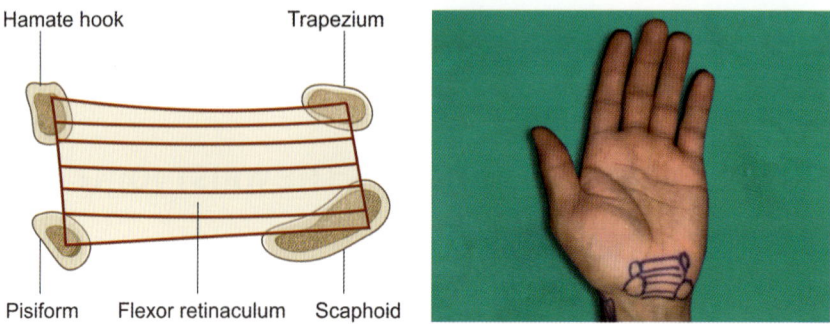

Fig. 6.1: Anatomy of flexor retinaculum (FR) attachment.

> **Structures under flexor retinaculum (nine tendons and one nerve).**
> 1. Median nerve
> 2. All four flexor superficialis tendons
> 3. All four flexor digitorum profundus tendons
> 4. Flexor pollicis longus

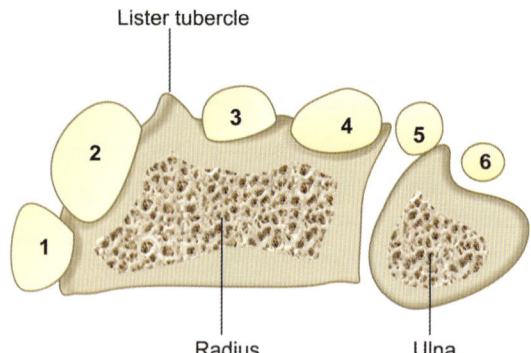

Fig. 6.2: Six compartments: From radial to ulnar side.

Table 6.1: Six compartments through which various tendons, nerves, and arteries run.

From radial to ulnar side					
1st	**2nd**	**3rd**	**4th**	**5th**	**6th**
APL and EPB	ECRL and ECRB	EPL	ED, EI, PIN, and PIA	EDM	ECU

(APL: Abductor pollicis longus; EPB: Extensor pollicis brevis; ECRL and ECRB: Extensor carpi radialis longus and brevis; EPL: Extensor pollicis longus; ED: Extensor digitorum; EI: Extensor indicis; EDM: Extensor digiti minimi; ECU: Extensor carpi ulnaris; PIN: Posterior interosseous nerve; PIA: Posterior interosseous artery)

4. **Anatomical snuffbox:** Radial side of the wrist has anatomical snuffbox which is bounded radially by Abductor pollicis longus (APL) and Extensor pollicis brevis (EPB) and ulnar side by Extensor pollicis longus (EPL). The floor is formed by scaphoid and tip of the distal radius. It contains Cephalic vein, Radial artery, and superficial branch of the Radial nerve.
5. **Type of joint (wrist):** Ellipsoid type synovial joint allowing movement in two axis.
6. **Movements:** Principal movements which occur at the wrist are:
   - Palmar flexion
   - Dorsiflexion
   - Radial deviation
   - Ulnar deviation
7. **Important muscles around wrist joint (Table 6.2).**

Table 6.2: Important muscles around wrist joint, their insertion, nerve supply, and action.

Muscle	Insertion	Nerve supply	Action
FCR	Palmar aspect of second MC base	Median	Palmar flexion
ECRL	Dorsal aspect of second MC base	Radial	Dorsiflexion and radial deviation
ECRB	Dorsal aspect of third MC base	Radial	Dorsiflexion and radial deviation
FCU	Pisiform, hook of hamate and fifth MC	Ulnar	Palmar flexion and ulnar deviation
ECU	Dorsoulnar aspect of fifth MC	PIN	Dorsiflexion and ulnar deviation

(FCR: Flexor carpi radialis; ECRL: Extensor carpi radialis longus; ECRB: Extensor carpi radialis brevis; FCU: Flexor carpi ulnaris; ECU: Extensor carpi ulnaris; MC: Metacarpal; PIN: Posterior interosseous nerve).

▌ BRIEF ANATOMY AND FUNCTION OF THE HAND

1. **Basic osteology**
Five metacarpals in hand; each finger has proximal, middle, and distal phalanx, whereas thumb has proximal and distal phalanx only.
2. **Muscles, ligaments, and tendons**
   - There are extrinsic and intrinsic muscles of the hand: Extrinsic muscles originate from the forearm but insert over bones of the wrist and hand, whereas intrinsic muscle has both its origin and insertion over bones of the wrist and hand.
   - Palmar aponeurosis covers the volar aspect of the hand.
   - Various pulleys support the flexor tendons while it crosses the phalanx.
   - Extensor tendon forms an extensor expansion on the dorsum of fingers, which allows lumbricals and interossei to cause metacarpophalangeal (MCP) flexion and interphalangeal (IP) extension.
   - Many ligaments provide support to the various joints of the hand (extensor ligaments, retinacular ligament, extensor expansion, MCP collateral ligaments, volar plate, deep transverse ligament, etc.)
3. **Type of joint:** All are synovial joints
   - *Intercarpal*: Gliding joint
   - *Carpometacarpal*: Gliding joint
   - *Metacarpophalangeal joints*: Condyloid joint
   - *Interphalangeal joint*: Hinge joint

4. Movements:

- *Metacarpophalangeal joint of fingers*: Flexion, extension, abduction, and adduction
- *Interphalangeal joint of fingers*: Flexion, extension
- *Thumb MCP joint*: Predominantly Flexion, extension; minor adduction, abduction
- *Thumb IP joint*: Flexion, extension

5. Three basic functions of the hand:

1. Pinch
2. Grasp
3. Hook

6. Important muscles of the hand (Table 6.3).

	Table 6.3: Important muscles of the hand, nerve supply, and their action.		
Area	**Important muscles**	**Action**	**Nerve supply**
Thenar eminence	APB, Opponens pollicis, FPB	Abduction, opposition of thumb, and flexion of thumb at MCP joint, respectively	Recurrent branch of median nerve
	Adductor pollicis	Adduction of thumb	Deep branch of ulnar nerve
Hypothenar eminence	Opponens digiti minimi, Flexor digiti minimi, Abductor digiti minimi	Opposition, flexion at MCP joint and abduction of little finger respectively	
Central	Dorsal interossei	*Finger abductors away from middle finger*, Flexion at MCP and extension at IP joint along with Lumbricals	
	Palmar interossei	*Finger adductors toward middle finger*, Flexion at MCP and extension at IP joint along with Lumbricals	
	Ulnar "two" lumbrical	*"With the help of interossei"*—Flexion at MCP, extension at IP joint	
	Radial "two" lumbrical	*"With the help of interossei"*—Flexion at MCP, extension at IP joint	Recurrent branch of median nerve
Other important extrinsic muscles of volar aspect			
	FPL	Flexion of thumb at IP joint	Median nerve
	FDS	Flexion of all fingers at PIP joint	
	FDP lateral two tendons	Flexion of index and middle finger at DIP joint	
	FDP medial two tendons	Flexion of ring and little fingers at DIP joint	Ulnar nerve
Other important extrinsic muscles of dorsal aspect			
	EPL	Extension at thumb IP joint	Posterior interosseous nerve
	ED	Extension at finger (2nd–5th) MCP joint	
	EI	Extension at index finger MCP joint	

(APB: Abductor pollicis brevis; FPB: Flexor pollicis brevis; FPL: Flexor pollicis longus; FDS and FDP: Flexor digitorum superficialis and profundus; MCP: Metacarpophalangeal; IP: Interphalangeal; PIP: Proximal interphalangeal; DIP: Distal interphalangeal)

An interesting fact: Lumbrical muscle originates from "tendons of flexor digitorum profundus (FDP)" and inserts on extensor expansion.

▌HISTORY AND ITS EVALUATION

Chief Complaints

- **Pain**
- **Swelling**
- **Difficulty in movement**
- **Deformity**
- **Clicks around the wrist**

1. **Pain:** It is the most common complaint.
   - Acute or insidious in onset
     - *Acute pain*: Trauma, acute infection, acute inflammation
     - *Insidious*: Arthritis, chronic infection, chronic tendinopathy, chronic ligament injuries and tumors
   - Infection, inflammation and tumors may cause night pain
   - Night pain is also seen in carpal tunnel syndrome radiating to the thumb and radial $3^{1/2}$ fingers.

Often, the clue to the possible diagnosis is according to the location of the pain which is summarized in Table 6.4.

Structures/ area affected	Tendon	Bone	Joint	Ligament	Nerve	Others
Radial side	De Quervain's tenosynovitis (Tendons: APL, EPB)	Scaphoid fracture Radius fracture	CMC arthritis	Scapho-lunate ligament tear	Neuroma of superficial branch of radial nerve	
Dorsal aspect	Extensor tenosynovitis	Lunate fracture/ Dislocation, Keinbock's disease	DRUJ instability, arthritis			Ganglion cyst
Ulnar side	FCU and ECU tendinitis	Ulnar styloid #		TFCC injury, Lunato-triquetral ligament tear	Ulnar nerve compression in Guyon's canal, Ulnar nerve neuritis	
Volar aspect	Flexor tendon tenosynovitis	Hamate fracture			Carpal tunnel syndrome	Ganglion cyst

Table 6.4: Common causes of wrist pain according to the location around the wrist.

(CMC: Carpometacarpal; DRUJ: Distal radioulnar joint; FCU: Flexor carpi ulnaris; ECU: Extensor carpi ulnaris)

2. **Swelling:**
   - *Localized:* Ganglion, usually seen on dorsum of the wrist
   - *Diffuse:*
     - ○ Traumatic injury
     - ○ *Infection:* Tuberculosis
     - ○ *Inflammatory:* Rheumatoid
     - ○ Tumors
     - ○ *Others:* Reflex sympathetic dystrophy, Ganglion
3. **Difficulty in movements:** Any difficulty in movement at the wrist and hand joints could be due to the following common reasons
   - *Pain:* Arising out of any pathology
   - *Stiffness:* Post-traumatic, reflex sympathetic dystrophy (RSD), and arthritis (rheumatoid)
   - *Loss of power:* Nerve palsy, tendon rupture/tear
4. **Deformity:** It could be due to
   - *Congenital:* Madelung deformity
   - *Traumatic:* Malunited colles' fracture leads to manus valgus deformity, Mallet finger
   - *Infections:* Tuberculosis
   - *Rheumatoid:* Manus valgus and various finger deformities
5. **Clicks around the wrist**
   - Carpal instability
   - TFCC injury
   - Tendon snapping.

> *After assessment of chief complaints, always assess 'how current problem of wrist and hand has affected the ADL of the patient'.*

CLINICAL EVALUATION

General and Systemic Examination

As per the standard protocol.

Local Examination

Attitude

Usually, wrist examination is performed in sitting. The attitude of the wrist and hand can be described in a standard fashion.

Inspection

Inspect the wrist and hand from volar and dorsal aspect.

General findings
   - *Skin changes:* Seen in complex regional pain syndrome (CRPS) (Figs. 6.3A and B)
   - Swelling, scars, sinus, and ulcers as per the standard description.

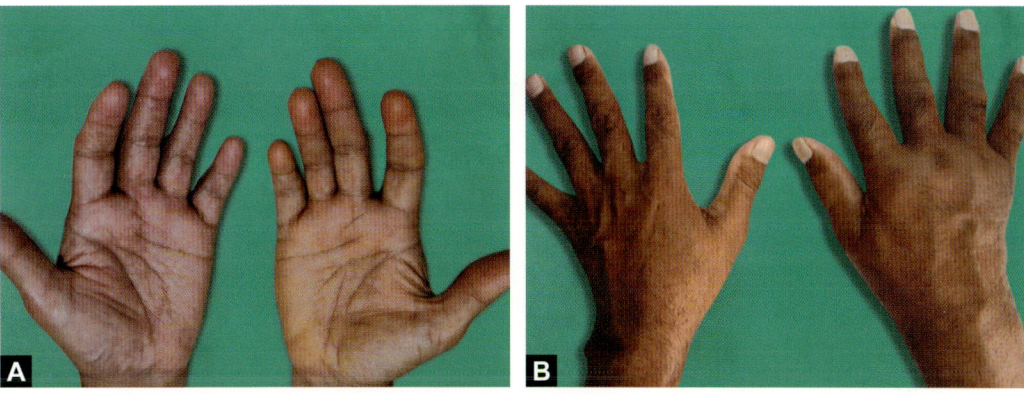

Figs. 6.3A and B: (A and B) Skin changes in CRPS (shiny, reddish/bluish/mottled, hair loss) over left hand (A) and right hand (B).

Specifics to look at wrist, palm (volar and dorsal), and fingers

(A) Wrist
1. *Deformity:* Manus valgus, dinner fork deformity, subluxation of the wrist, or radial deviation in rheumatoid arthritis (RA) (Figs. 6.4A and B)
2. *Swelling:* Ganglion is often seen over dorsum or volar aspect of the wrist (Figs. 6.4C)
3. *DRUJ:* Swelling/subluxation

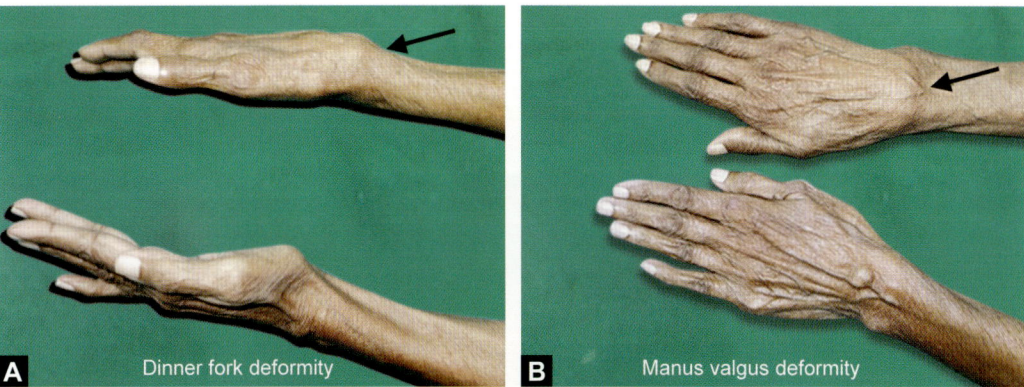

Dinner fork deformity

Manus valgus deformity

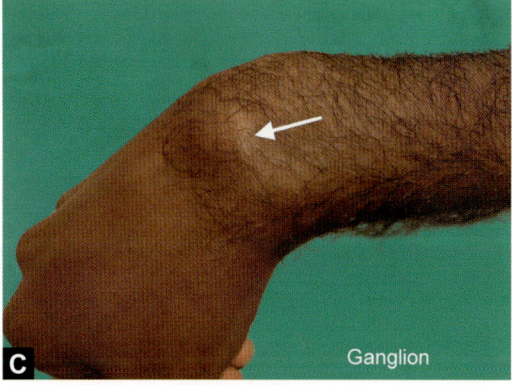

Ganglion

Figs. 6.4A to C: (A to C) Various deformities and ganglion in the wrist.

(B) Palmar and dorsal aspect of hand
1. *Contractures of palmar fascia:* Dupuytren's contracture (Figs. 6.5A and B)
2. *Muscle wasting:* Interossei, thenar, hypothenar eminence, and forearm (Figs. 6.6A to D)

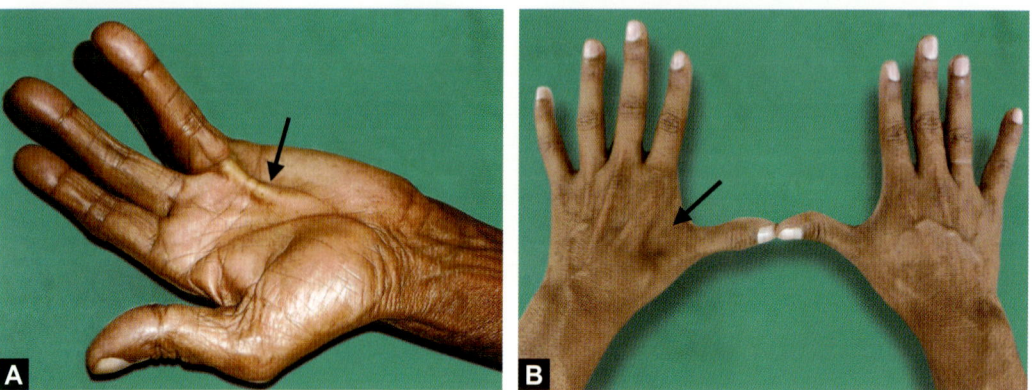

Figs. 6.5A and B: (A) Dupuytren's contracture. (B) Wasting of interosseous muscle of left hand (arrow).

(C) Fingers
1. *Deformity:* Various deformities of RA (Figs. 6.6 A1, A2, B1, B2), psoriatic arthritis, claw hand (hyperextension at MCP, hyperflexion at PIP and DIP), and mallet finger
2. *Swelling:* Bouchard and Heberden nodes at PIP and DIP joint, respectively, in case of osteoarthritis of hand (Fig. 6.6C)
3. *Nail changes:* Psoriasis (pitting, ridging, crumbling, and separation of nail) (Fig. 6.6D).

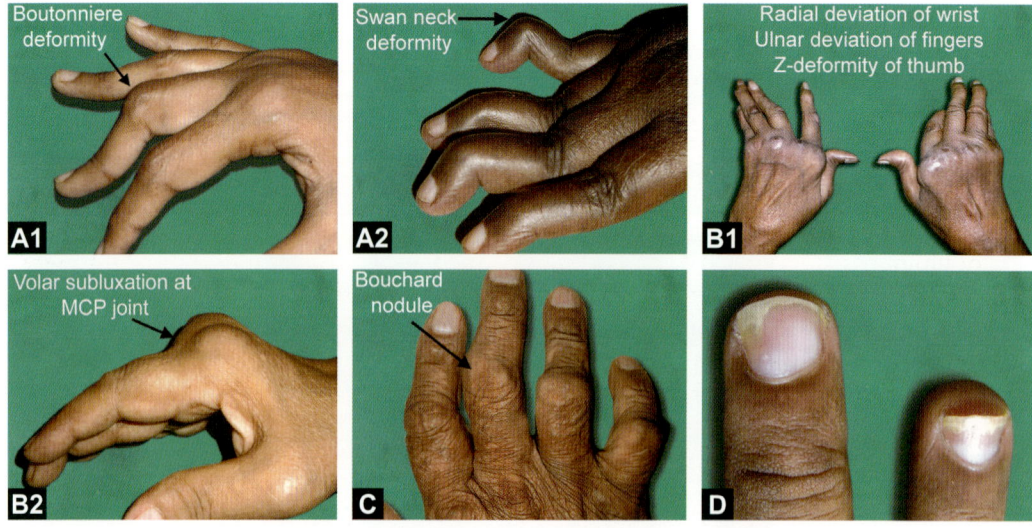

Figs. 6.6A to D: (A1, A2, B1, B2) Various deformities of wrist and hand in Rheumatoid arthritis. (C) Bouchard nodules. (D) Pitting, ridging and nail separation.

4. **Cascade sign:** When all the fingers are flexed at MCP and IP joints, they all converge toward the scaphoid tubercle (Fig. 6.7). However, if one or more fingers do not converge, it indicates malalignment of the fingers due to malunion or nonunion of phalanx or metacarpals.

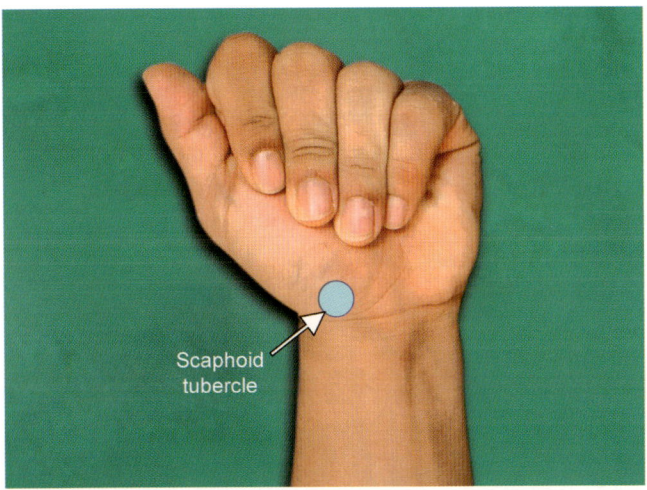

Fig. 6.7: Cascade of fingers pointing towards scaphoid tubercle.

Various classical wrist and hand deformities in Rheumatoid arthritis (RA) and Psoriasis.
Rheumatoid arthritis: MCP and PIP swelling, Boutonniere and Swan-neck deformity, ulnar drifting of fingers, Z deformity of thumb, volar subluxation at MCP, dorsal DRUJ subluxation, and radial deviation at wrist.
(Boutonniere deformity: Hyperflexion at PIP and hyperextension at DIP)
(Swan-neck deformity: Hyperextension at PIP and hyperflexion at DIP)
Psoriasis: Sausage-shaped digit (swelling at PIP), DIP deformity, nail changes
(MCP: Metacarpophalangeal; PIP: Proximal interphalangeal; DRUJ: Distal radioulnar joint; DIP: Distal interphalangeal)

Palpation

(A) **The local rise in temperature:** Rise in local temperature is seen in inflammatory, infective, or tumor conditions. However, hand may feel cold in ischemic conditions like Raynaud's disease, and thoracic outlet syndrome with a vascular component. Warm or cold feeling with altered sweating pattern in hand is common in CRPS.

(B) **Tenderness around wrist:** Always palpate in a sequence "around wrist" to look for tender spots in the following area. It is better to start on dorsoradial side from anatomical snuffbox (Fig. 6.8) and proceed in a circular fashion ulnar-wards and come back to the original point. Important landmarks to palpate are mentioned below (Figs. 6.9A and B). The method to palpate these landmarks are mentioned in Box 6.1.

1. *Anatomical snuffbox:* Tender in scaphoid fracture
2. *Tip of radial styloid process:* Tender in radial styloid fracture
3. *1" proximal to the radial styloid process for tenderness over the tendons of APL and EPB:* In De Quervain's tenosynovitis.

4. *The distal end of radius*
5. *Distal radioulnar joint*
6. *Lunate*
7. *Capitate*
8. *The distal end of ulna*
9. *Tip of ulnar styloid process*
10. *Triangular fibrocartilage complex area:* Foveal tenderness
11. *Extensor carpi ulnaris (ECU) and flexor carpi ulnaris (FCU) tendon sheath:* Resisted palmar flexion with ulnar deviation makes the FCU taut on volar side, whereas ulnar deviation with extension makes ECU taut just ulnar-wards to the tip of ulnar styloid process.
12. *Volar aspect of the wrist*
    - Median and ulnar nerve
    - Pisiform (PS)
    - Hook of hamate (HM)
    - Scaphoid tubercle (ST).

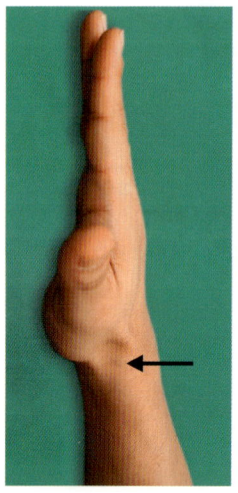
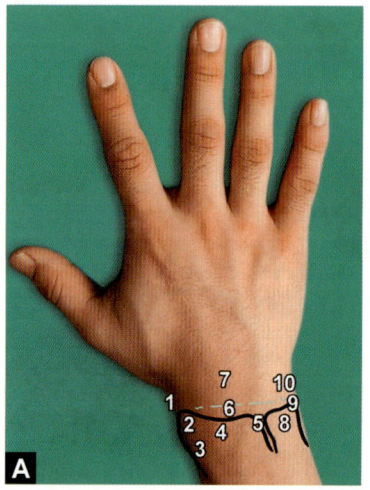
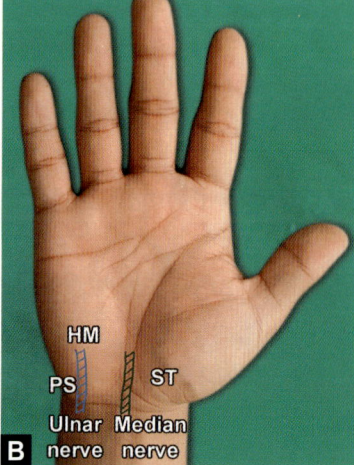

Fig. 6.8: Anatomical snuffbox (arrow).

Figs. 6.9A and B: Palpation of various landmarks on volar and dorsal surface of wrist (Green dash line represents wrist joint line).

Box 6.1: Method to palpate important carpal bones.
- *Scaphoid*: In the anatomical snuffbox. The distal tubercle of scaphoid is palpated over the thenar eminence.
- *Lunate*: Palmar flexing the wrist makes the lunate prominent over dorsum of the wrist just distal to the dorsal lip of distal radius almost in the line of third metacarpal.
- *Capitate*: Just distal to Lunate in the line of third metacarpal.
- *Pisiform*: Make the Flexor carpi ulnaris (FCU) tendon prominent, go along it, and it ends over the prominent pisiform bone.
- *Trapezium*: Just proximal to the first metacarpal base.
- *Trapezoid*: Between Trapezium and Capitate (from dorsal side) in the line of second metacarpal.
- *Hamate*: Hook of Hamate is palpated over the hypothenar eminence.

(C) Wrist joint line tenderness: It is easy to palpate the dorsal joint line of the wrist.
Method: Palpate the Lister's tubercle over the dorsum of the distal radius and move distally. The wrist joint line is felt 1 cm distal to the Lister's tubercle along the interstyloid line (green dashed line in Figure 6.9A).
Another method: The patient's right hand is grasped with the examiner's right hand holding the first and second metacarpal. Then, the examiner uses his thumb of the left hand and palpates the second and third metacarpal shaft and further palpates proximally moving over the metacarpals while the right hand alternately dorsiflexes and palmar-flexes the wrist. The dorsal wrist joint line is felt close to the interstyloid line with the left thumb.

(D) Feel for any synovial hypertrophy or swelling of the wrist joint at the joint line

(E) Radial and ulnar styloid process relationship: The radial styloid process tip is 8–14 mm distal to the ulnar styloid process. Any disturbance in this relationship is an indicator of deformed distal radius/malunited distal radius or ulna fracture.
Method: The radial styloid process lies in the anatomical snuffbox over the lowermost end of the distal radius, and the ulnar styloid process is the distal-most end of the ulna over the ulnar border where it is seen as a prominence, dorsally. On palpation of both styloid processes, radial must lie distal to the ulnar. *This must be compared with the normal side* (Fig. 6.10).

(F) Tenderness of all other areas of hand

- Thenar and hypothenar eminence, all metacarpals
- *Palmar fascia*: Thickened in Dupuytren's contracture
- *Dorsal and volar tendon palpation*: Feel for any tenderness (tenosynovitis). The nodules of trigger finger are typically felt over the volar aspect of MCP joint
- Metacarpophalangeal and IP joints, phalanx
- *Pulp of all fingers*: Pulp space infections
- *Nail beds*: Tender in glomus tumor and paronychia.

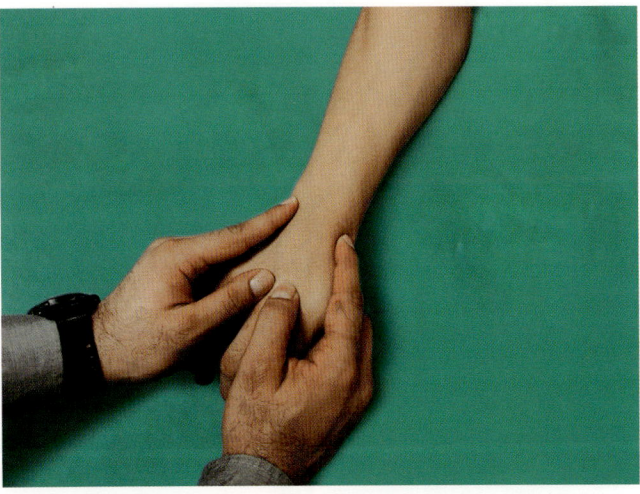

Fig. 6.10: Relationship between two styloid process.

Movements

Check range of movements (ROM) of the wrist (Figs. 6.11A to D), thumb (Figs. 6.12 A to D) and other joints of the fingers (Boxes 6.2 and 6.3). *For passive ROM of the wrist; hold distal part of forearm with one hand and 2nd–5th metacarpal with one hand to elicit various ROM.*

- Active followed by passive **ROM of wrist**
- Painless or painful
- **Movement of the thumb** (Figs. 6.12A to D)
  - Flexion, extension, adduction, abduction, opposition, and circumduction
- **Movement at MCP, IP**
  - Metacarpophalangeal joint allows flexion–extension–adduction–abduction
  - Interphalangeal joint allows flexion–extension.
- Also compare the ***pinch, grasp, and hook strength of the hand*** with the normal side to assess the functional strength of the hand.
- Wrist joint crepitus is felt with hand kept over the wrist while moving the joint through various ROMs. Similarly, DRUJ crepitus is felt while forearm rotations or while eliciting the piano key sign.

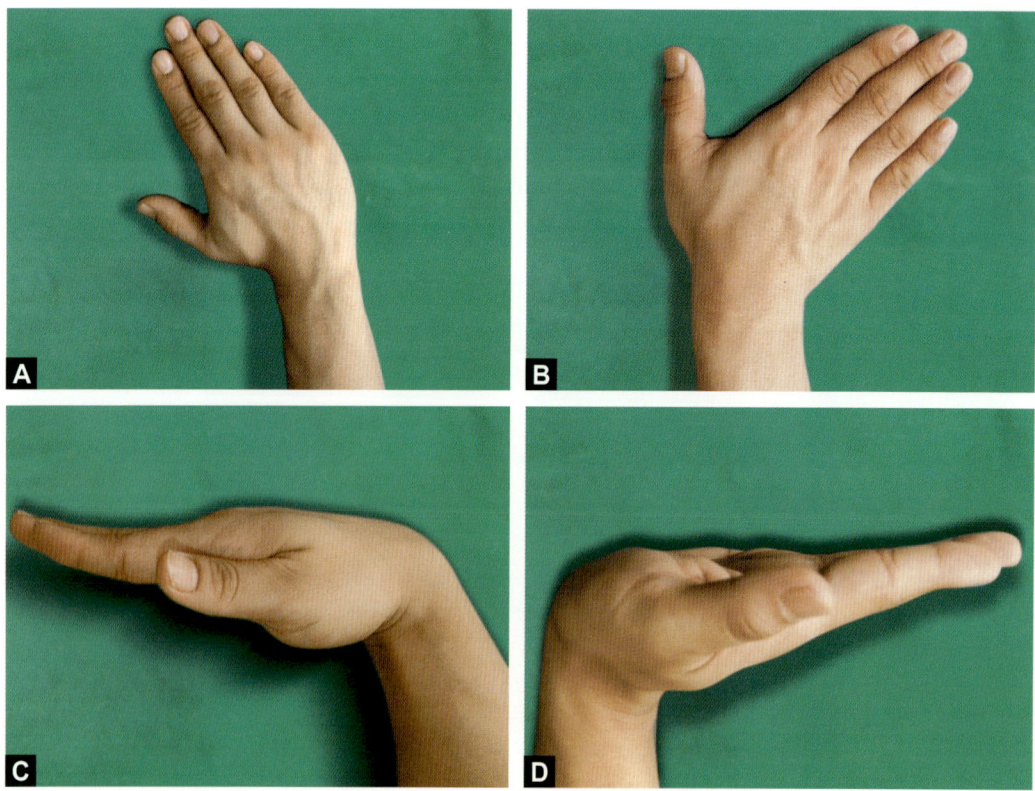

Figs. 6.11A to D: Wrist ROM (A) Radial deviation. (B) Ulnar deviation. (C) Palmar flexion. (D) Dorsiflexion.

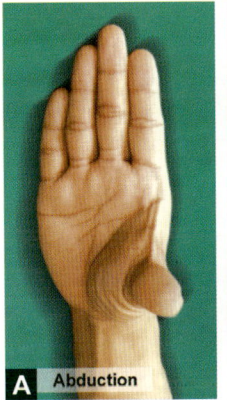 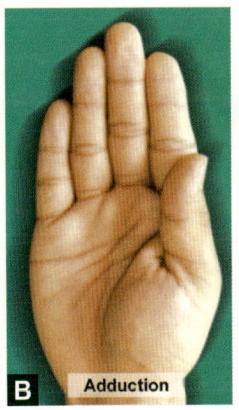 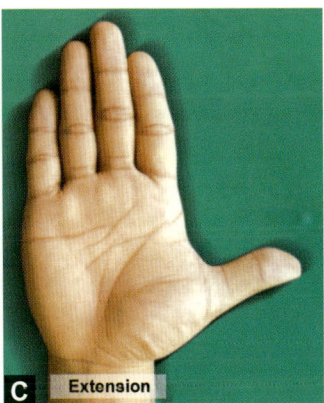 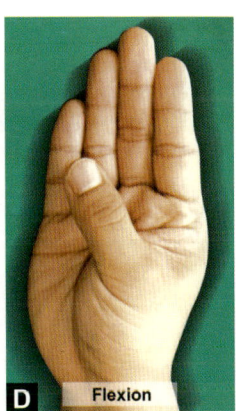

| A Abduction | B Adduction | C Extension | D Flexion |

Figs. 6.12A to D: Thumb movements.

Box 6.3: Normal ROM of joints of thumb and fingers
thumb metacarpophalangeal (MCP) joint.
1. *Flexion*: 0–55°
2. *Hyperextension*: 0–10°
Thumb IP joint
1. *Flexion*: 0–80°
2. *Hyperextension*: 0–15°
Metacarpophalangeal joint of fingers
1. *Flexion*: 0–55°
2. *Hyperextension*: 0–10°
PIP joint of fingers
1. *Flexion*: 0–100°
DIP joint of fingers
1. *Flexion*: 0–80°

Box 6.2: Normal ROM at the wrist.
- *Dorsiflexion*: 0–70°
- *Palmarflexion*: 0–80°
- *Radial deviation*: 0–20°
- *Ulnar deviation*: 0–35°

Note: Wrist joint ulnar deviation is less compared to radial deviation as during abduction of wrist, the radial styloid process, which is longer than ulnar, abuts against scaphoid.

Note: Various movements at the wrist joint occur both at radiocarpal and midcarpal joints.
Wrist palmar flexion: Radiocarpal + midcarpal (more movement here)
Wrist dorsiflexion: Radiocarpal (more movement here) + midcarpal
Wrist ulnar deviation: Radiocarpal (more movement here) + midcarpal
Wrist radial deviation: Midcarpal mostly.

Quadriga effect (Roman four-horse chariot, single charioteer with four reins).
- *Definition*: Active flexion lag in fingers adjacent to a finger whose flexor digitorum profundus (FDP) has been injured/repaired.
- *Etiology*: Due to functional shortening of FDP after injury or repair due to adhesions/overtight repair
- *Pathoanatomy*: If one FDP is tight or poorly functional, others cannot function completely due to mass action of FDP as they share the common belly of tendon.

> **Intrinsic plus hand.**
> - **Deformity**: Flexion at MCP, extension at IP joints (inverse of claw hand)
> - **Etiology**: Rheumatoid arthritis (RA), post-traumatic (after compartment syndrome), neurological injury (post-CVA, Parkinson's, and cerebral palsy)
> - **Pathoanatomy**: Tightness of intrinsic muscle of hand and/weak extrinsic (flexors and extensors)
> - Bunnel–Littler test can be used to differentiate intrinsic and extrinsic tightness

Measurements

1. **Measurement of the length of the upper extremity/forearm:** It is important in those wrist conditions which affect the radius and ulna length (e.g. malunited radius/ulna/both fracture). Measurement of both forearms can be done in a standard fashion from lateral epicondyle to the tip of radial styloid process. Rarely, whole upper limb measurement might be required.

2. **The distance between the two styloid processes** (Fig. 6.13)

   Method: First, a line is drawn over the forearm which represents its midline axis extending from midforearm to the wrist joint (black line). Then, perpendiculars are dropped from two styloid processes (blue and yellow line). The distance between the two perpendiculars represents the distance between the two styloid processes (white arrow).

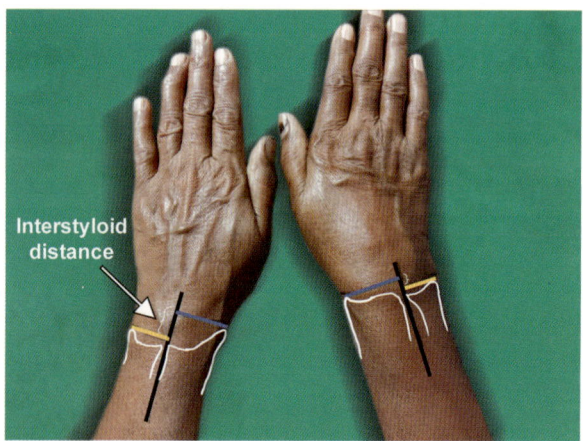

Fig. 6.13: Vertical distance between two styloid processes.

Neurovascular Examination of Upper Limbs

As per the standard protocol.

Special Tests

(A) For carpal tunnel syndrome (CTS) (Figs. 6.14A to C)

1. *Phalen's sign:* The patient is asked to completely palmarflex both his wrists by opposing dorsum of both hands against each other. Development of tingling and/or numbness within 60 seconds in the distribution of median nerve area is indicative of CTS.

2. *Reverse Phalen's sign:* Patient is asked to completely dorsiflex both his wrists by opposing palm of both hands against each other. Development of tingling and/or numbness within 60 seconds in the distribution of median nerve area is indicative of CTS.

3. ***Durkan's test:*** It is the most sensitive test for CTS. The median nerve under the FR is compressed with the thumb of examiner for 60 seconds. Any tingling and numbness within 60 seconds in the area of the median nerve are taken as positive Durkan's test.

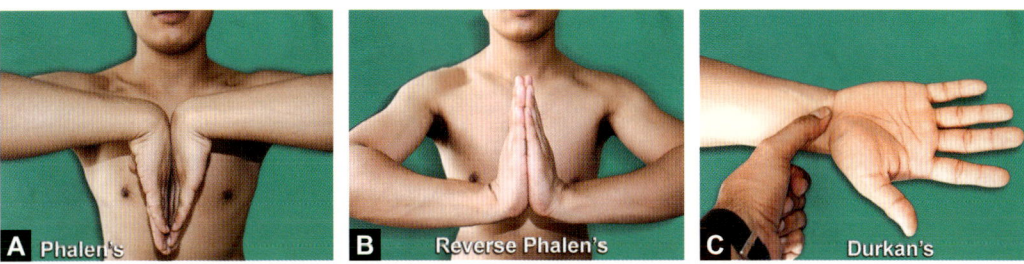

Figs. 6.14A to C: Signs of carpal tunnel syndrome.

(B) For De Quervain's tenosynovitis (texting thumb/blackberry thumb)
- ***Finkelstein test:*** The examiner grasps patient's affected thumb, and deviates it ulnar-wards toward the palm. Now the patient is asked to close the fist. With closed fist and thumb within the palm, the wrist is deviated ulnar-wards (Fig. 6.15). This elicits tenderness over the anatomical snuffbox and area over the radial styloid process in case of De Quervain's tenosynovitis.

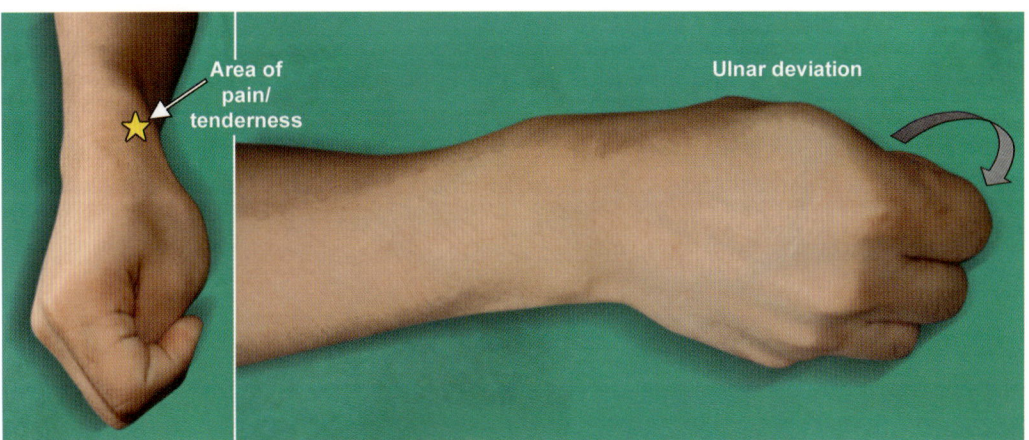

Fig. 6.15: Finkelstein test.

(C) For first carpometacarpal (CMC) joint arthritis
- ***Grind test:*** The patient's thumb is held between the examiner's thumb and index finger, and wrist is held by other hand. Then, axial stress is given along with the rotatory movement of the thumb of the patient. Pain during such maneuver is indicative of first CMC arthritis.

(D) For patency of radial and ulnar artery
- ***Allen's test:***
  ○ Compress both radial and ulnar arteries just proximal to the wrist. Ask the patient to make a fist and open–close it several times. This leads to blanching of the hand.

- ○ Now release only radial artery and watch for hand turning pink due to blood refilling the capillaries of the hand. This confirms the patency of radial artery.
- ○ Now repeat step 1 and release only ulnar artery and watch for hand turning pink. This confirms the patency of ulnar artery.

(E) For radial and ulnar collateral ligament injury of thumb

- *Radial collateral ligament injury of thumb MCP joint:* Hold 1st metacarpal by thumb and index finger of one hand and thumb and index of other hand holds proximal phalanx. Now give ulnar deviation stress to MCP joint of thumb in extension and 30° flexion which could lead to pain and/or abnormal opening on the radial side of the MCP joint suggesting injury to the radial collateral ligament injury of MCP.
- *Ulnar collateral ligament injury of thumb MCP joint (Gamekeeper's thumb):* In the similar way as described above, radial deviation stress to the MCP joint of the thumb in extension and 30° flexion can lead to pain and/or abnormal opening on ulnar side of MCP joint suggesting injury to the ulnar collateral ligament injury of MCP.

(F) For intrinsic stiffness of fingers

- *Bunnel–Littler test:* Keep the MCP in 0° extension and passively flex the PIP and note the ROM (ROM 1). Now flex the MCP and then flex the PIP, and note the ROM (ROM 2). If the ROM 2 of PIP is more than ROM 1, it indicates intrinsic muscle tightness. If ROM 2 < ROM 1, it indicates extrinsic muscle tightness, and if ROM 2 = ROM, it indicates capsular tightness.

(G) For dislocation/subluxation of DRUJ

- **Piano key test:** Ballottement of the ulna.

  Method: The examiner holds the distal end of the radius of the patient between the thumb and index finger of one hand, and the distal end of the ulna is held between the thumb and index finger of other hand. Now, the ulna is subjected to ballottement, up and down, and compare with the normal side (Fig. 6.16). The ballottement should be done in pronation, midprone, and supination.

  Interpretation: An abnormal volar-dorsal movement indicates unstable DRUJ.

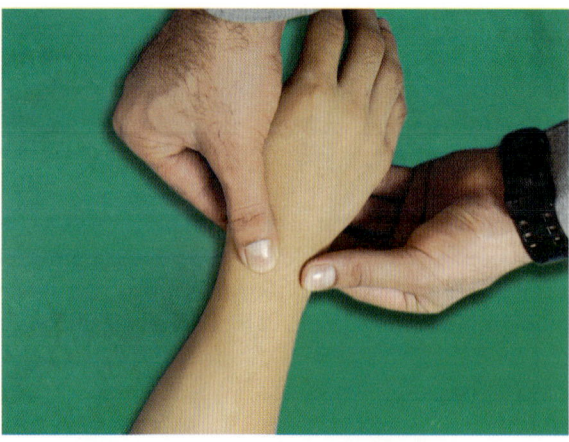

Fig. 6.16: Piano key sign.

(H) For TFCC injury

1. ***Ulnar deviation forearm pronation test:*** The examiner holds the patient's right hand with his right hand and forearm by left hand. Then, the forearm is pronated, and wrist is ulnar deviated. This elicits the pain over ulnar aspect of the wrist if TFCC is injured (Fig. 6.17A).

2. ***Fovea sign:*** Tenderness present over a soft spot, which lies between the ulnar styloid process and FCU, is indicative of TFCC injury (Fig. 6.17B).

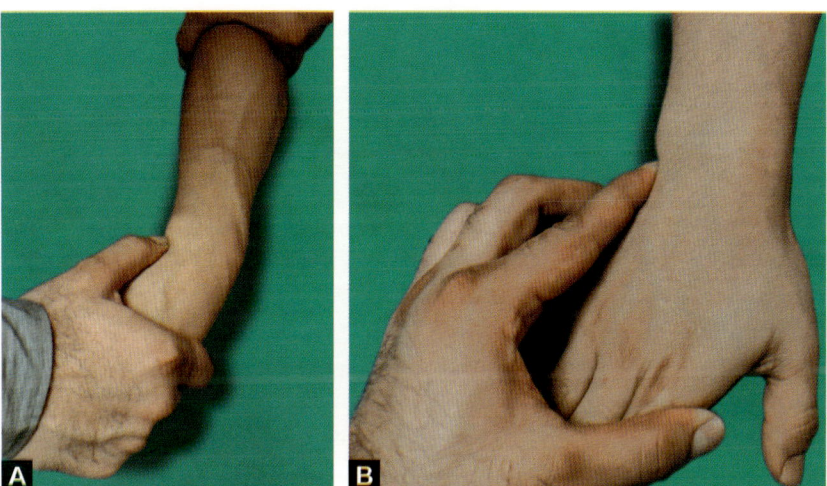

Figs. 6.17A and B: Signs of triangular fibrocartilage complex (TFCC) injury.

(I) Carpal instability

1. ***Kirk–Watson test: For scapholunate (SL) instability***

   Method: For left side injury, keep the left forearm in midprone. Now, examiner hold the left scaphoid of the patient with the left hand from thenar eminence side and right hand holds the metacarpals of the patient. Then bring the wrist in slight ulnar deviation.

   Firm pressure is applied to the palmar tuberosity of the scaphoid with the examiner's thumb in dorsal direction, while the wrist is moved from ulnar-to-radial inclination (*curved arrow*) by the other hand of the examiner (Figs. 6.18A and B). The pressure over the scaphoid tuberosity is released as the wrist is moved completely to radial deviation.

   Interpretation: In normal wrists, the scaphoid cannot flex because of the external pressure by the examiner's thumb. In SL ligament injury, the patient experiences pain when the scaphoid is no longer constrained proximally by SL ligament and subluxes out of the scaphoid fossa (*straight arrow*). A positive test is associated with clunk and pain; when pressure on the scaphoid is removed, it goes back into the position.

   (*Note:* First, clunk without pain can be felt in an individual with ligamentous laxity or even in normal person. Second, the patient can have pain at the dorsum at SL interval due to synovitis or occult ganglion. Third, this test has low sensitivity and specificity.)

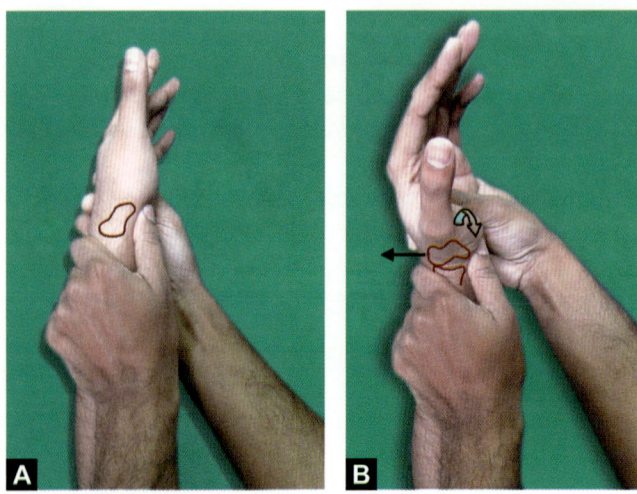

Figs. 6.18A and B: Kirk-Watson test.

2. *Test for Luno-triquetral (LT) ligament injury:*
   (a) Ballottement (Reagan) test
   Method: The lunate is firmly stabilized with the thumb and index finger of one hand of the examiner, while the triquetrum and pisiform are repeatedly displaced dorsally and palmar-wards with the other hand of the examiner (Fig. 6.19).
   Interpretation: A positive result elicits pain, crepitus, and abnormal displacement at the L–T joint. (*Note*: Either lunate or triquetral–pisiform unit can be displaced up and down stabilizing the other one.)

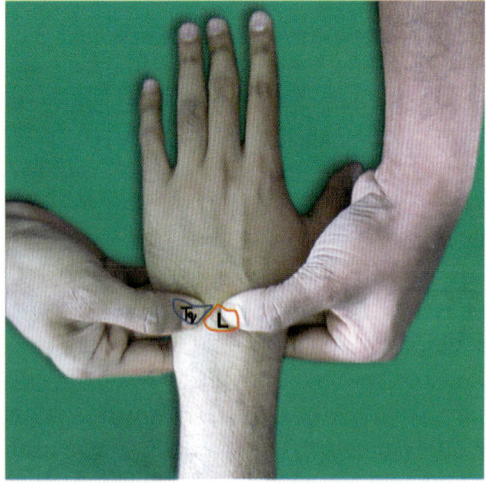

Fig. 6.19: Ballottement test.

(b) Shear test: This is a variation of ballottement test and can be performed by single hand.
Method: The examiner stabilizes the dorsal aspect of the lunate with the index finger and uses the thumb to loads the pisiform–triquetrum complex in a dorsal direction, creating a shear force at the L–T joint (Fig. 6.20).
Interpretation: A positive test causes pain.

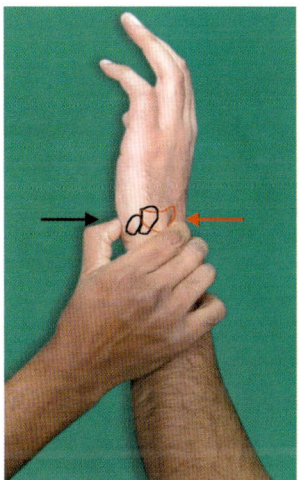

Fig. 6.20: Shear test.

3. ***Test for midcarpal instability:*** Midcarpal instability is due to tear of the dorsal triquetro-hamate ligament or the volar arcuate ligament (triquetral–hamate–capitate ligament).
   Lichtman test
   Method: The examiner holds patient's forearm in pronated position, placing a palmar load over the capitate and then ulnar deviating (curve arrow) the wrist with simultaneous axial load (black arrow) (Figs. 6.21A and B).
   Interpretation: A positive test reproduces a painful clunk, which represents the abrupt change in position of the proximal carpal row from flexion to extension as the head of the capitate engages the lunate and the hamate engages the triquetrum.
   (*Note*: It can be positive in a wrist with ligamentous laxity and it should be ignored if it is not associated with pain.)

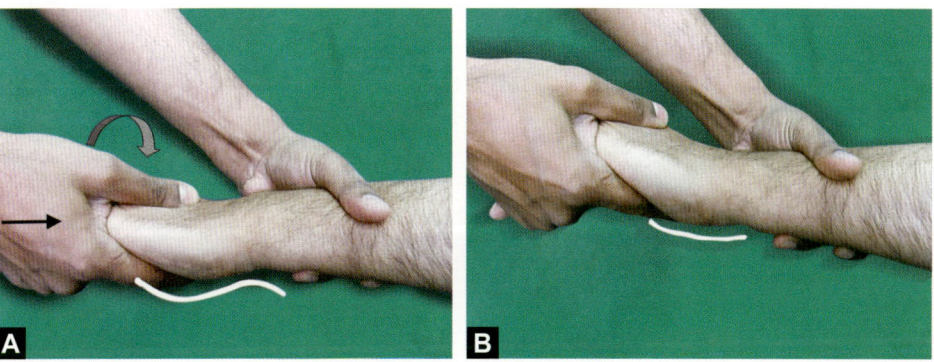

Figs. 6.21A and B: Lichtman test.

4. ***Radiocarpal instability:*** Anteroposterior drawer test and radial glide test are two tests to determine the radiocarpal instability but both are nonspecific tests.

(a) Anteroposterior drawer test:

Method: The examiner translates the wrist in dorso-volar direction while holding the distal forearm in one hand and the metacarpals in the other hand.

Interpretation: Patient will have pain with this maneuver and the examiner can feel the clunk or observe the abnormal translation of the carpus over the distal radius.

(b) Radial glide test:

Method: The examiner translates the wrist (the proximal row) in radial direction while holding the distal forearm in one hand and the metacarpals in the other hand.

Interpretation: This radial shift of the carpus produces pain.

Examination of the Joint Above

- Elbow joint

Lymph Node Examination

- Around the elbow and axillary lymph nodes

Wrist-hand examination proforma

1. **Attitude**
2. **Inspection**
   General findings: *Skin overlying, Swelling, scar, sinus*
   Specifics findings of inspection: *To be looked over wrist and hand (palm and fingers)*
   (a) Wrist
   – Deformity, swelling, DRUJ
   (b) Palm (volar and dorsal)
   – Contractures of palmar fascia, muscle wasting, swelling
   (c) Fingers
   – Deformity, Swelling, nail changes, cascade sign
3. **Palpation**
   - Local rise in temperature
   - Tenderness around wrist (radial to ulnar side, dorsal to volar), wrist joint line tenderness, synovial hypertrophy
   - Tenderness of all other areas of hand, radial and ulnar styloid process relationship
   - Confirmation of palpatory characteristics of swelling, scar, sinus
4. **Movements**: Active and passive for wrist and hand
   - **Wrist:** Dorsiflexion, Palmarflexion, abduction and adduction
   - **MCP and IP joint:** Flexion and extension
   - Crepitus, clicks; if any
5. **Measurements** Limb length, arm-forearm circumference, distance between radial and ulnar styloid process
6. **Neurovascular examination**
7. **Special tests**
   (a) *Carpal Tunnel tests*: Phalen's and reverse Phalen's test, Durkan's test
   (b) *De Quervain's disease*: Finkelstein test
   (c) *1st CMC arthritis*: Grind test
   (d) *Radial and Ulnar artery patency*: Allen's test
   (e) *Radial and Ulnar collateral ligament of thumb test*
   (f) *Intrinsic stiffness of finger*: Bunnel-Littler test
   (g) *DRUJ subluxation/dislocation*: Piano Key test
   (h) *TFCC injury*: Ulnar deviation forearm pronation test, fovea test
   (i) *Carpal Instability*: Scapholunate instability (Kirk-Watson test), Lunotriquetral ligament injury (Ballottement test, Shear test), Midcarpal instability (Litchman test), Radiocarpal instability (anteroposterior drawer and glide test)
8. **Joint above (elbow)**
9. **Lymph node examination**

Common conditions affecting wrist and hand with their salient features

1. **Ganglion**
   - Affects *young patients but can happen in any age, More common in females*
   - *Presents with:* Swelling on the dorsum of the hand, sometimes on volar aspect. Usually of pea-size, which gives a very firm or bony hard feeling on palpation. Often, size shows variation with time, intermittently painful.
   - *Pathologically*: *Not a true cyst*. Many theories; synovial herniation/mucous cyst formation/degeneration of connective tissue and cyst formation.
   - *Clinically*: Swelling with firm or bony hard feeling on palpation (Fig. 6.22).
   - *Diagnosis*: Magnetic resonance imaging (MRI)/ultrasound (USG)
   - *Treatment*:
     - *Conservative/observation*: aspiration and intracystic steroid injection
     - Surgical excision if painful, large or recurrence after aspiration.

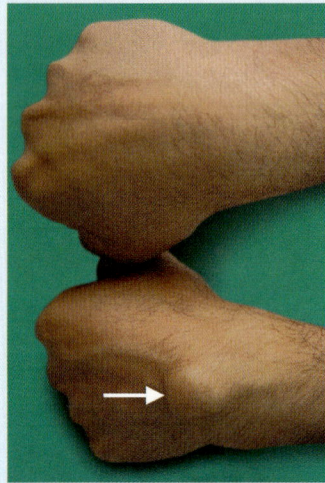

Fig. 6.22: Ganglion over dorsum of the left wrist.

2. **De Quervain's tenosynovitis**
   - *Affects:* Middle-aged
   - *Presents with:* Pain and swelling along the radial border of the wrist over the distal end of radius and/anatomical snuffbox
   - *Pathologically*: *Tenosynovitis of abductor pollicis longus and extensor pollicis brevis* within the region of first extensor compartment.
   - *Clinically*: Tenderness present over the radial border of the wrist, Finkelstein test +
   - *Diagnosis*: MRI/USG
   - *Treatment*:
     - *Conservative*: Nonsteroidal anti-inflammatory drugs (NSAIDs), physiotherapy, local steroid injection, and thumb splint
     - Surgical release of the first extensor compartment.

3. **Malunited Colles' fracture**
   - History of fall on outstretched hand
   - Most common in elderly females and males. Associated osteoporosis
   - *Presents with:* Deformity (manus valgus), pain, restricted ROM
   - *Pathologically*: Malunited distal radius fracture

- *Clinically*:
  - Manus valgus deformity
  - *Altered relation of two styloid processes*: The radial and ulnar styloid processes are at same level or radial styloid moves proximally.
  - Decreased ROM
- *Diagnosis*: X-ray
- *Treatment*:
  - *Conservative*: NSAIDs and physiotherapy
  - *Surgical*: Corrective osteotomy to correct deformity and functional disability, if any.

4. **Complex regional pain syndrome (reflex sympathetic dystrophy/Sudeck's osteodystrophy)**
   - *Affects*: Any age. It can affect any joint but most commonly involves wrist-hand and ankle-foot.
   - Mostly after trauma to the wrist and hand. Sometimes even shoulder becomes painful and stiff. It is known as "*shoulder-hand syndrome.*"
   - *Presents with:* Pain, difficulty in moving fingers and wrist, swelling of hand and wrist, discoloration of fingers, nail changes, and cold hand.
   - *Pathologically:* Idiopathic dysfunction of sympathetic nervous system of the upper limb after the trauma (type 1 CRPS) or after the nerve injury (type 2 CRPS)
   - *Clinically*:
     - *Diffuse tenderness over the hand and fingers*
     - *Gross swelling of the hand and wrist*
     - *Loss of active and passive movements*
     - Hand and finger discoloration
     - Spindle shape fingers, nail changes, altered temperature, abnormal sweating pattern over hand
     - Occasional paresthesia and tingling especially with type 2 CRPS
   - *Diagnosis*: Mostly clinical.
     - *X-ray of affected part*: Patchy osteoporosis
     - *Bone scan*: Increased uptake
     - *NCV*: For type 2 CRPS
   - *Treatment*: *Always* conservative; pain control and physiotherapy are the essence of treatment.
     - *Pain control*: Nonsteroidal anti-inflammatory drugs
     - Pregabalin, carbamazepine
     - Vitamin C, *N*-acetyl cysteine
     - *Physiotherapy*: Gentle active mobilization of the affected part
     - Limb elevation and compression bandage for edema control
     - Local sympathetic ganglion block to improve pain and block the overactive sympathetic outflow to the extremity.

5. **Volkmann's ischemic contracture (VIC)**
   - Sequelae of Volkmann's ischemia (compartment syndrome) of forearm
   - *Presents with*: Flexion contracture of fingers and wrist
   - *Pathologically*: Following ischemia of compartment syndrome of forearm, the flexor muscles of forearm undergo fibrosis leading to shortening of muscle–tendon complex. There is damage to the nerves of forearm too leading to varying sensorimotor symptoms.
   - *Clinically*:
     - Wasting of forearm and hand muscles (Fig. 6.23)
     - Scars of old injury or surgery present over the forearm
     - Cord like firm mass in forearm
     - *Volkmann's sign*: In neutral position of the wrist, the fingers remain in flexed position at MCP and IP joints. This flexion attitude of fingers exaggerates when dorsiflexion is attempted at the wrist. However, partial extension at MCP and IP joints is possible when the wrist is palmar-flexed. This is known as a "bowstringing effect."
     - Neurological deficit in forearm and hand in the median and ulnar nerve distribution.

- **Diagnosis**: Clinical, NCV
- **Treatment**: Occupational therapy, bracing, stretching, muscle sliding surgery (MaxPage procedure), bone shortening, and proximal row carpectomy.

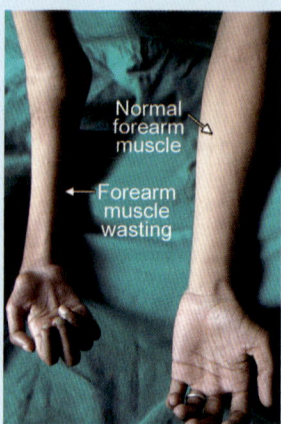

Fig. 6.23: Volkmann's ischemic contracture (VIC) of the right forearm.

6. **Dupuytren's contracture**
   - **Affects**: Middle-age to elderly. Men > female. Seen in alcoholics and smokers, diabetics, and in patients on anti-epileptic medications
   - **Presents with**: Flexion contracture of the ring finger (most commonly) followed by a little finger.
   - **Pathologically**: Contracture of palmar aponeurosis
   - **Clinically**:
     - MCP joint and PIP joint flexion deformity of little and ring finger (most commonly affected)
     - Visible and palpable cord-like palmar aponeurosis (Fig. 6.24) (no wasting of muscles or neurological deficit unlike VIC)
   - **Diagnosis**: Clinical
   - **Treatment**: Mobilization of contracture, local injection of *Clostridium histolyticum* collagenase, needle aponeurotomy, and palmar aponeurectomy

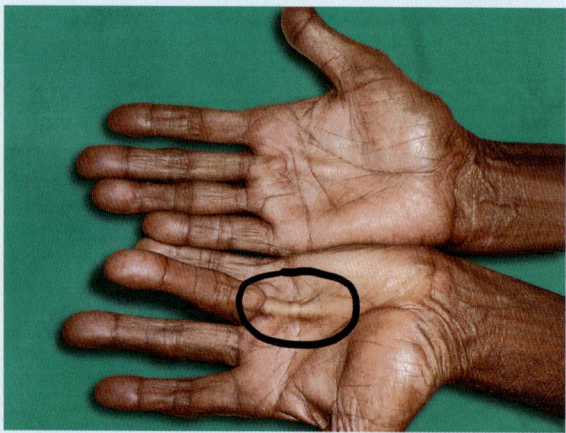

Fig. 6.24: Dupuytren's contracture of the left hand.

7. **Carpal tunnel syndrome**
   - *Affects*: Middle age. Increased risk in hypothyroidism, Diabetes, history of trauma (malunited Colles, Smiths fracture), and pregnancy
   - *Presents with*: Pain around the wrist with associated tingling and numbness over the hand along median nerve distribution area. Pain is often severe in the night.
   - *Pathologically*: Compression of median nerve in carpal tunnel
   - *Clinically*:
     - Phalen's test, Reverse Phalen's test and Durkan's test +
     - Sensory and motor assessment of the median nerve
     - Rarely, wasting of thenar eminence and signs of median nerve weakness are present.
   - *Diagnosis*: X-ray, USG, MRI and NCV
   - *Treatment*: Treat associated condition, conservative, and flexor retinaculum release (open/endoscopic)

   Similar to carpal tunnel syndrome, there is an ulnar tunnel syndrome. The ulnar nerve is compressed in the Guyon's canal above the flexor retinaculum. The clinical features are similar to CTS, but tenderness and sensory motor features are of the ulnar nerve.

8. **Cubital tunnel syndrome**
   - It is ulnar nerve compression neuropathy
   - *Presents with*: Pain and paresthesia over the medial forearm and medial $1^{1/2}$ fingers
   - *Pathologically*: Compression of ulnar nerve within certain areas like two heads of FCU, within arcade of Struthers (hiatus in medial intermuscular septum), between Osborne ligament and MCL, behind medial epicondyle, post-malunion,, cubitus valgus, etc.
   - *Clinically*: Sensory and motor features of ulnar nerve involvement, elbow flexion test positive (deep elbow flexion more than 60 seconds reproduces symptoms over the arm and hand)
   - *Diagnosis*: X-ray, USG, MRI, and NCV
   - *Treatment*: Treat associated condition, conservative, cubital tunnel release (open/endoscopic), and anterior transposition of Ulnar nerve.

9. **Glomus tumor**
   - *Affects*: Young adults.
   - *Presents with*: Paroxysmal pain in the finger with cold intolerance and exquisite tenderness
   - *Pathologically*: Arteriovenous anastomosis incorporating the nerves.
   - *Clinically*:
     - Red- or violet-colored pinhead size tumor under the nail bed
     - Nail ridging is common
     - *Love's pin test*: Pressure with pinhead over nail causes exquisite tenderness
     - *Tourniquet inflation test (Hildreth test)*: Inflating the tourniquet around arm reduces local pain and abolishes tenderness to Love test
   - *Diagnosis*: Clinical, X-ray (phalanx cortical erosion), and MRI
   - *Treatment*: Marginal excision

10. **Compound palmar ganglion**
    - *Affects*: Patients with tuberculosis and RA
    - *Presents with*: Hourglass shape swelling over volar aspect of wrist
    - *Pathologically*: Result of synovitis of flexor tendons (due to TB/RA) under FR
    - *Clinically*: Hourglass shape swelling extending above and below the FR
      - May be associated features of carpal tunnel syndrome
      - Cross fluctuation +
    - *Diagnosis*: Clinical, USG, and MRI
    - *Treatment*: Treat underlying condition and synovectomy

11. **Mallet finger**
    - Persistent flexion deformity of the DIP joint (Fig. 6.25)
    - Due to rupture of extensor tendon slip at the base of distal phalanx

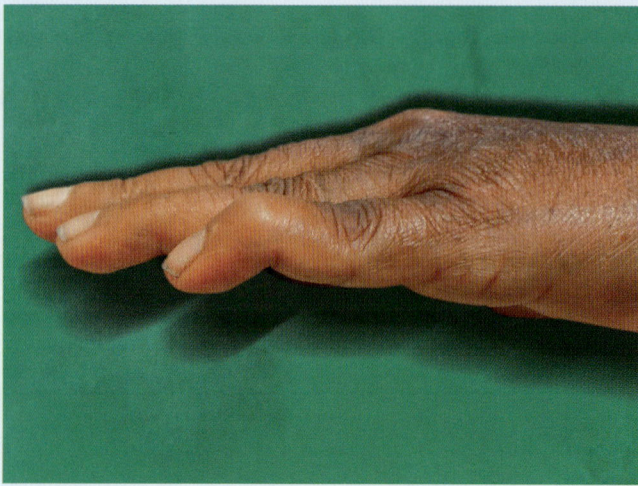

Fig. 6.25: Mallet little finger.

12. Jersey finger
- Reverse of mallet finger, usually at ring finger
- Due to the rupture of FDP tendon

13. Trigger finger
- **Affects**: Middle-aged patients; observed in Rheumatoid Arthritis, Diabetes, Gout
- **Presents with**: Finger extends with effort and with a sudden trigger-like action
- **Pathologically**: Stenosing tenosynovitis of flexor tendon sheath
- **Clinically**: Mostly middle or ring finger
  - The patient is unable to extend his finger with ease. It extends with a sudden release
  - Often, a palpable nodule felt along the flexor sheath of finger
  - A dynamic phenomenon cannot be elicited by passive flexion or extension
- **Diagnosis**: Clinical, USG
- **Treatment**: Observation, local steroid injection, Surgical release of A1 pulley

14. Congenital anomalies
- **Syndactyly**: Webbing of fingers/sideways fused fingers
- **Polydactyly**: Supernumerary fingers
- **Camptodactyly**: Flexion deformity of the finger at PIP joint (usually little finger)
- **Ectrodactyly (split hand)**: Absent fingers
- **Macrodactyly**: Overgrowth of fingers
- **Madelung deformity**: Congenital subluxation of lower end of ulna
- **Radial clubhand**: Radial side tissues (radius bone, thumb, and scaphoid) are less or not developed.

15. Madelung deformity
- **Definition**: A congenital dyschondrosis of distal radius physis leading to disruption of volar and ulnar aspect of physis leading to volar and ulnar tilted distal radial articular surface, volar translation of the hand and wrist, and a dorsally prominent distal ulna
- **Commonly occurs in:** adolescent females, often gymnasts. A hypothesis of occurence is tethering by Vikers ligament (*Vickers ligament is a fibrous band running from the distal radius to the lunate on the volar surface of the wrist (radio-lunate ligament)*)
- **Etiology**: Congenital, post traumatic, dysplastic, rarely infective or metabolic
- **Presents with**: Wrist pain, weakness and deformity, and median nerve symptoms

- – Radial deviation of the hand and flexion deformity of the wrist
- – Bayonet-like deformity of distal radius and dorsal prominence of distal ulna
- – Limited dorsiflexion of wrist and forearm rotation
- Mutation of *SHOX* gene
- *Diagnosis*: X-ray
- *Treatment*: *Conservative, Distal radius corrective osteotomy +/- Distal ulnar shortening osteotomy.*

16. **Radial clubhand**
    - *Definition*: Radial agenesis (total or partial)
    - *Presents with*: Radial deviation of wrist due to partial or total absence of radius with absent radial carpus and or thumb
    - *Syndromes associated*: Associated with TAR syndrome (autosomal recessive, thrombocytopenia, absent radius but thumb present), Holt–Oram syndrome (autosomal dominant with cardiac anomalies), VATER (vertebral anomalies, anal atresia, tracheoesophageal fistula, esophageal atresia, and renal agenesis) anomalies, and VACTERL syndrome (vertebral anomalies, anal atresia, cardiac abnormalities, tracheoesophageal fistula, renal agenesis, and limb defects)

17. **Keinbock's disease**
    - Lunate avascular necrosis (AVN)
    - Often associated with positive ulnar variance

18. **Preiser's disease**
    - Scaphoid AVN

Notes

Clinical Evaluation of the Hip Joint

▍BRIEF ANATOMY AND FUNCTION OF THE HIP JOINT

1. **Basic osteology**
   - It is formed by the acetabulum and the head of the femur.
   - It is the most stable joint due to the structural configuration of the femur and the acetabulum.
2. **Stabilizing structures**
   - The acetabulum margin is lined by the acetabular labrum.
   - Three ligaments: Iliofemoral (ligament of Bigelow), ischiofemoral, and pubofemoral—support the hip joint along with the joint capsule.
3. **Type of joint**
   - The hip joint is a deeply seated ball and socket synovial joint.
4. **Movements**
   - Flexion, extension, abduction, adduction, external, and internal rotation
5. **Important muscles around the hip joint** (Table 7.1).

Table 7.1: Important muscles around the hip joint, their insertion, nerve supply and action.			
Muscle	**Insertion**	**Nerve supply**	**Principal action**
Iliopsoas	Lesser trochanter	Femoral nerve and direct branch from lumbar plexus	Hip flexor
Gluteus maximus	Gluteal tuberosity of femur	Inferior gluteal nerve	Extensor
Gluteus medius, Gluteus minimus	Lateral, anterior, and superior surfaces of greater trochanter (GT)	Superior gluteal nerve	Abductor
Adductor longus, brevis, magnus, and gracilis	Medial aspect of femur	Obturator nerve	Adductor
Anterior fibers of gluteus medius and minimus, tensor fascia lata	Greater trochanter	Superior gluteal nerve	Internal rotator
Piriformis, gemelli, quadratus femoris, and obturator externus	Piriformis fossa, Posterior aspect of the greater trochanter	Muscular branches of Sciatic nerve	External rotator

Common conditions affecting hip joint.

- *Congenital*: Developmental dysplasia of hip (DDH)
- *Developmental*: Slipped capital femoral epiphysis (SCFE)
- *Idiopathic*: Avascular necrosis (AVN) of the head of the femur, Perthes disease
- *Traumatic*: AVN, 2° osteoarthritis, fractures, dislocation, labral tears
- *Infective*: Tom Smith arthritis, Tubercular arthritis, pyogenic arthritis
- *Degenerative*: Primary hip osteoarthritis, femoro-acetabular impingement (FAI)
- *Inflammatory*: Rheumatoid arthritis (RA), Ankylosing spondylitis (AS)
- *Hematological*: Sickle cell anemia causing AVN

Relevance of age and gender in the diagnosis of hip conditions.

Age
- *0–5 years*: Developmental dysplasia of hip (DDH), Septic arthritis, Tom Smith arthritis
- *5–10 years*: Infections, Perthes disease
- *10–15 years*: Slipped capital femoral epiphysis (SCFE), infections, Perthes disease, Juvenile Rheumatoid arthritis
- *20–40 years*: 2° arthritis, femoro-acetabular impingement (FAI), Labral tears, Ankylosing spondylitis (AS), Rheumatoid arthritis (RA), Avascular necrosis (AVN)
- *Over 40 years*: Primary osteoarthritis of the hip, FAI, AVN, AS sequelae causing 2° hip osteoarthritis
- *Any age*: Tuberculosis

Gender
- *Male*: Perthes disease, AS
- *Female*: DDH, RA and postpartum AVN

■ HISTORY AND ITS EVALUATION

Chief Complaints

Patients with hip pathology come up with certain specific complaints.
- Pain
- Morning stiffness
- Deformity
- Limp
- Limb length discrepancy
- Locking, clicks, rarely instability
- Systemic symptoms

> One must always ask two questions in the beginning before the chief complaint is elaborated.
> A. How did the problem(s) start, i.e. Insidious onset/traumatic in origin/any other preceding event?
> B. Were you (patient) perfectly all right before this started or did you have this problem in the past and the complaint has exacerbated now?

1. **Pain**
   - It must be evaluated in detail for site (uni/bilateral), onset, duration, progression, severity, character, radiation, timing, and diurnal variation (if any) with or without a functional disability.
   - Traumatic or nontraumatic in origin.
   - Bilateral involvement is seen in systemic conditions like rheumatoid arthritis (RA) and ankylosing spondylitis (AS). Avascular necrosis (AVN) is often bilateral due to its several systemic etiologies.
   - *Referred pain*: Often, the pain due to hip pathology is referred to the knee due to similar nerve supply of both joints.
   - *Night cry*: History of night cry or severe pain in the night suggests tuberculosis (TB) or even other inflammatory arthritis.
   - *Aggravating and relieving factors*: Pain due to osteoarthritis of the hip is more with activity and at the end of the day, whereas pain due to inflammatory arthritis is more at night or rest and improves with activity.
   - *Remission and exacerbation*: Denotes inflammatory arthritis.
2. **Morning stiffness**
   It may indicate inflammatory lesion in the hip (RA and AS).
3. **Deformity**
   Questions on onset, duration, progression, associated symptoms, and any history of trauma or infection to be asked.
4. **Limp**
   - It must be evaluated with pain. Limp could be painless or painful.
   - Limp could be due to pain, stiffness, short limb, weak abductor mechanism of hip, DDH, etc.
5. **Limb length discrepancy**
   Onset (after trauma/infection/others), duration, progression
6. **Locking, clicks, and instability:** History of locking or clicks may indicate labral tear or loose body. Instability is quite rare in hip conditions but could be a rare complication after dislocation.

7. **Systemic features**
   - Fever, loss of weight, and loss of appetite are important in the case of TB. Systemic features are also sometimes noted in inflammatory arthritis.
   - History of high-grade fever suggests acute infection, whereas history of low-grade fever and evening rise in temperature is suggestive of chronic infections like TB.
   - It is also important to clinically investigate the primary site of TB as *musculoskeletal TB is always secondary to primary elsewhere*. History of contact with TB is also important in suspected cases.

8. **Current disability**
   - Enquiry to be made as to how the current problem has affected the activities of daily living, occupation, sports, etc. For example, the disability to sit cross-legged, or to squat must be enquired in hip joint pathology. Difficulty in squatting suggests restriction of extreme hip flexion, while difficulty in sitting cross-legged is suggestive of the restriction of the flexion, abduction, and external rotation of the hip joint.

9. **Use of walking aids**
   - Use of a walking aid may suggest a painful or unstable hip

10. **Past history**
    - History of trauma and surgery/treatment should be evaluated in detail. Fracture neck femur of the hip can cause AVN or nonunion, whereas intertrochanteric femur can cause malunion. History of dislocation can predispose to AVN of the femur head. Chronic gout and sickle cell anemia can cause AVN of the hip.
    - Childhood history of DDH, Perthes disease, and SCFE can predispose to 2° OA of the hip. Here patient can complain about pain over the hip and limp during childhood along with/without treatment history.
    - Past history of TB, diabetes mellitus (DM), etc.

11. **Family history**
    - The family history of DDH, TB, spondyloarthropathy, gout, rheumatoid arthritis, and hemoglobinopathies (sickle cell anaemia) is important.

12. **Treatment history**
    - The treatment for any systemic disease involving prolonged steroid intake can cause AVN of the hip. Prolonged gout can cause AVN of the hip.

13. **Personal history**
    - Habits of chronic alcohol intake can cause AVN of the hip. Others like smoking can cause nonunion of fractures.

14. **Menstrual history, allergies, etc.**

CLINICAL EVALUATION

General and Systemic Examination

Standard general and systemic examination must be performed as many hip disorders are a part of systemic disorder (e.g. RA, sickle cell anemia, TB, AS, etc.).

- Anemia, cachexia would be indicative of poor nutritive status, which favors the diagnosis of TB. Lymph node examination is important in suspected cases of infection.

- Stature should be noted to rule out the generalized skeletal disorder.
- Chest expansion should be measured to rule out ankylosing spondylitis. (Normal chest expansion is 4–5 cm; reduced in AS).
- Head-to-toe assessment of eye (blue sclera, uveitis), pinna (blackish discoloration, low set), face (malar rash), hair line, neck, nails (psoriasis), etc. can give a clue about hip disease of systemic origin.

Local Examination

After appropriate consent, privacy and chaperone, the patient should be suitably undressed, but private parts should be adequately covered. A female attender is a must in case a female patient has to be examined. ***The clinical examination of the hip should always be performed on a hard bed.***

Gait

It must be noted if the patient can walk. There are various types of gait such as antalgic gait, Trendelenburg gait, waddling gait, short-limb gait, gluteus maximus, high-stepping gait, in-toeing or out-toeing gait.

> **Types of gait in hip pathologies.**
> - ***Antalgic gait***: Stance phase of the affected side is reduced, and patient lurches to the affected side.
> - ***Trendelenburg gait***: The patient lurches to the affected side with normal stance phase.
> - ***Short-limb gait***: When the affected side shoulder, trunk, pelvis dip with ipsilateral hip, knee extended, ankle plantar flexed with contralateral hip and knee are flexed. The patient often walks with equinus at the ankle to compensate for shortening.
> - ***Gluteus maximus gait***: The patient walks with backward lurching.
> - ***Stiff-hip gait***: A stiff hip produces a characteristic pelvis swinging with circumduction of the leg to clear ground.
> - ***High-stepping gait***: Patients with foot drop with ipsilateral hip and knee hyperflexion than normal side.

Attitude

Described in supine position (Fig. 7.1).

Inspection

- It should be done in both standing followed by supine positions and, in a sequence *"proximal-to-distal not to miss any landmark/finding." Always examine on a hard bed.*

General findings
- Swelling, scar, sinus anywhere should be described as per the standard descriptions.

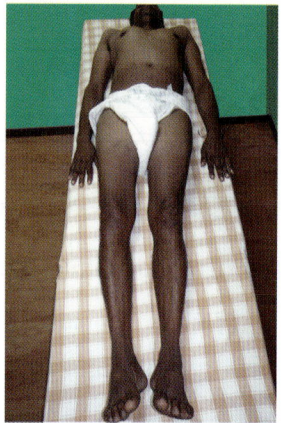

Fig. 7.1: Lower limb attitude.

Specific findings

Inspection in Standing

(A) From front (Fig. 7.2)

1. ***Head position,*** any neck tilt
2. ***Level of both shoulders, Shape of chest wall.***
3. ***Position of the anterior superior iliac spine (ASIS)*** (lower/higher/same level) must be noted.
4. ***Rotational deformity of lower limb (external/internal rotation):*** Whether the lower limb appears externally or internally rotated or is in normal position, should be noted for in this triangle.
5. ***Scarpa's triangle:*** Scar/sinus/swellings should be noted.
6. ***Level of greater trochanter (GT):*** Two GT levels must be compared. Easy in thin patient but may not be possible in obese individuals.
7. ***Thigh folds:*** Asymmetric or prominent in case of unilateral DDH
8. ***Thigh and calf muscle wasting:*** Indicative of a chronic condition.
9. ***Patella orientation:*** In standing, the patella always faces slightly laterally. Excess lateral facing of the patella with respect to normal side indicates external rotation deformity of the limb.

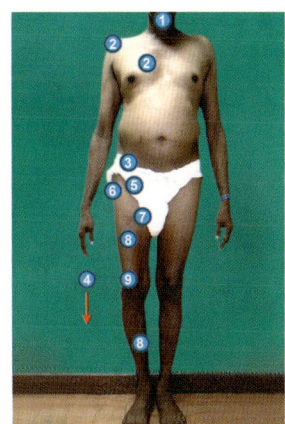

Fig. 7.2: Inspection from front (point 4 with arrow suggests rotational alignment)

> **Lower level of ASIS of index side:** May indicate abduction deformity at the hip
> **Higher level of ASIS of index side:** May indicate adduction deformity at the hip

> **Scarpa's (femoral) triangle:** It is a triangle in the upper part of the thigh bounded superiorly by the inguinal ligament, laterally by the lateral border of the sartorius and medially by the medial border of the adductor longus. The floor is formed laterally by the iliopsoas and medially by the pectineus.
> **Contents (from lateral to medial):** Femoral nerve, artery and vein, lymph nodes

(B) From side

1. ***Lumbar lordosis:*** Best examined in supine position. Also lo racic kyphosis..
2. ***Flexed attitude of hip and knee, level of heel***
3. ***Trochanteric region***

(C) From back (Fig. 7.3)

1. ***Neck position, hair line***
2. ***Level of scapula, any rib hump***
3. ***Spine:*** Look for deformities like scoliosis. It could be functional/structural. Functional scoliosis is differentiated from structural scoliosis by examining the spine in standing and sitting positions and bending forward.
   - Functional scoliosis: It disappears in sitting erect position, while it appears in standing position to compensate for limb length discrepancy or spasm.

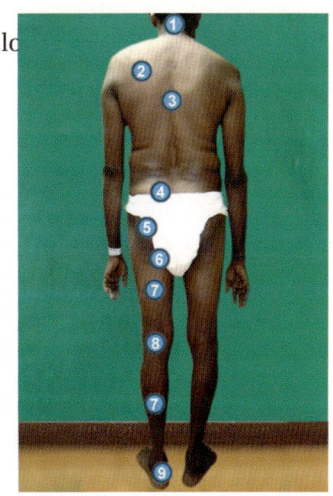

Fig. 7.3: Inspection from back.

- Fixed structural scoliosis does not disappear on sitting or bending forward.
  Observe for ***any signs of spina bifida (occulta/aperta)***
4. ***Level of Posterior superior iliac spine (PSIS,*** "Dimple of Venus")
5. ***Gluteal muscle wasting:*** Underlying gluteal wasting indicates long-standing hip pathology.
6. ***Gluteal folds:*** Position and symmetry of gluteal folds give an idea of unilateral/bilateral hip pathology.
7. ***Thigh and calf wasting***
8. ***Popliteal fossa:*** Look for any swelling
9. ***Heel status:*** Flat on ground/equinus/calcaneus.

> **Abnormal gluteal folds are seen in!**
> - Developmental dysplasia of hip (DDH), gluteal atrophy
> - Gluteus maximus contracture
> - Fixed pelvic obliquity

Inspection in Supine Position

(A) From front: *The findings are similar to those as in standing. However, limb length discrepancy is easily noted in supine position by comparing both heel/malleolus levels.*

1. ***Level of both ASIS:*** Lower/higher/same
2. ***Rotational deformities of lower limb:*** In a normally aligned lower limb, the patella faces slightly laterally and upwards. Further, if one draws an imaginary line from the center of the patella to the shaft of tibia, the line passes through the second toe. This is a normal alignment. With the tibia in the external or internal rotation, the line passes either medial or lateral to the second toe giving an idea about the rotational deformity (Fig. 7.4).
3. ***Scarpa's triangle***
4. ***Level of greater trochanter (GT)***
5. ***Thigh folds***
6. ***Thigh and calf muscle wasting***
7. ***Patella orientation***
8. ***Limb length discrepancy:*** Assessed by checking the level of both ASIS, lower pole of the patella, medial malleolus or the heel.

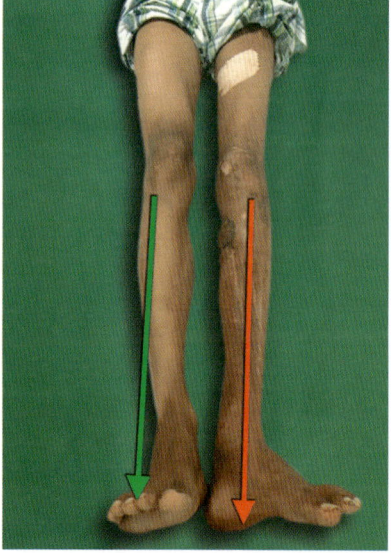

Fig. 7.4: Normal rotational alignment of right side (green arrow) and abnormal external rotation of left lower limb (red arrow).

(B) From side:

1. ***Lumbar lordosis:*** It is best examined from the side, in supine position.
   In a normal person in the supine position, there is no space between the couch and the normal lordotic lumbar spine when the examiner brings his eyeline parallel to the lumbar spine and the couch. However, in case of exaggerated lumbar lordosis, there is enough space so that the examiner can view the other side or can insinuate his hand between the lumbar spine and the couch (Fig. 7.5).
   "Exaggerated lumbar lordosis is indicative of fixed flexion deformity of the hip in most cases."

2. *Flexed attitude of hip and knee*

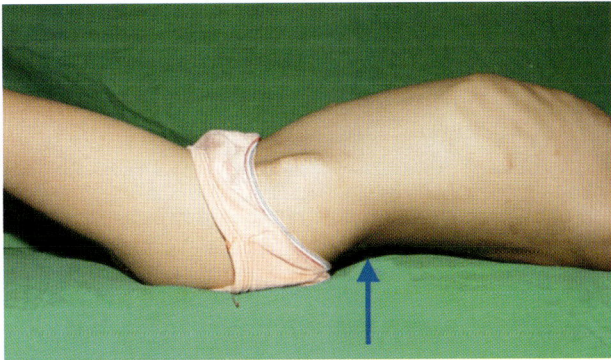

Fig. 7.5: Exaggerated lumbar lordosis (blue arrow).

Palpation

(A) From front:

1. *Local temperature*: It should be felt for, in anterior, lateral, and posterior aspects of the hip joint.
2. *Level of both ASIS*: ASIS is the first bony prominence palpated at the lateral end of the inguinal ligament while examiner runs his thumb along the inguinal ligament. Confirm its level; high, low or same as compared to the normal side.
3. *Tenderness*: Over the anterior and posterior hip joint line, GT, pubic tubercle, symphysis pubisand other bony and soft tissue landmarks.
   (i) *Method to palpate anterior hip joint line*: The anterior hip joint line is located 2–3 cm below and lateral to the mid-inguinal point (the point between the ASIS and pubic symphysis) (Fig. 7.6).
   (ii) *Method to palpate posterior hip joint line*: The posterior hip joint line lies at the lateral 1/3rd – medial 2/3rd junction of the line joining the PSIS and the tip of the trochanter.

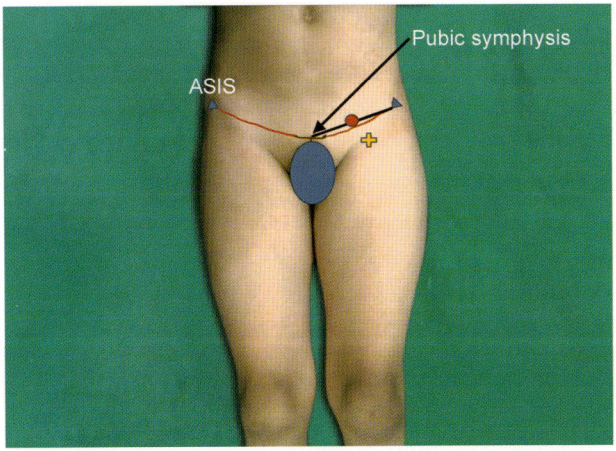

Fig. 7.6: Location of anterior hip joint line (yellow cross). Red circle indicates mid inguinal point.

4. *Palpation of greater trochanter*: *Compare two sides*
- *Level*: High or low- compare the level of tip of GT bilaterally
- Broadening, if any: place the index finger at the tip, thumb at anterior, and middle finger at the posterior border of GT respectively. This gives a measure of broadening of GT.
- Surface smooth or irregular
- Tenderness.

> **Method to elicit tenderness over the hip and greater trochanter (GT).**
> 1. **Direct tenderness**: Palpate the joint lines or GT directly for tenderness.
> 2. **Indirect bi-trochanteric compression test**: Examiner keeps his hands over the GT and a medially directly gentle thrust is given. The tenderness is elicited if there is any pathology at the trochanter, neck, and acetabulum.

(B) From side:
1. *Lumbar lordosis*: Normally, the lumbar spine touches the couch, and the examiner cannot insinuate his hand underneath the lumbar spine. However, in case of exaggerated lumbar lordosis, the examiner will be able to pass his hand through the gap between the lumbar spine and couch.

(C) From back:
1. *Palpate the spine* for any tenderness, defect in spinous process, step in the midline etc.
2. *Tenderness over other areas*: Over PSIS, SIJ, gluteal region, and ischial tuberosity (IT).
3. *Palpate for any abnormal mass or swelling in the gluteal region* (dislocated head of femur).

> The ischial tuberosity (IT) is a bony prominence which is mid-way between the lower sacrum and the tip of GT. The IT is palpated with the patient in lateral position and the trochanteric region facing upwards. It can be made prominent if the patient is asked to flex his knee against resistance as this makes hamstring taut which originates from the IT.

(D) Assessment of deformity:

> Sagittal, coronal, and axial plane (rotation) deformities should be examined before checking the range of motion of the hip joint.
> *Sagittal and coronal plane deformities are concealed deformities while rotational deformities are revealed deformities.*
> Revealing hidden deformities should be done by obliteration of lumbar lordosis (in sagittal plane) or squaring the pelvis (in coronal plane).

1. **Deformity in sagittal plane:** Fixed flexion deformity (FFD) of the hip (unilateral/bilateral) is the deformity in sagittal plane. It's presence is indirectly indicated by "exaggerated lumbar lordosis".
   Unilateral FFD assessment is done by Thomas hip flexion text whereas bilateral FFD assessment is performed by supine method/Staheli method.

Test for Unilateral Flexion Deformity: Thomas Hip Flexion Test

Method: The patient lies supine over a hard couch with both lower limbs parallel to each other. In an exaggerated lordosis of the lumbar spine, the examiner can insinuate his hand between the spine and the couch. Keeping his hand under the exaggerated lordotic lumbar spine, the unaffected hip is gradually flexed keeping the knee in flexion till the lumbar lordosis is obliterated. Once taken out, the hand cannot be insinuated again between the couch and the lumbar spine. At the same time, the index hip goes in for flexion. Now ask the patient to hold the unaffected flexed knee and measure the flexion of the affected hip on the horizontal plane (Figs. 7.7A and B).

Test for bilateral hip fixed flexion deformity (FFD)

There are two methods to detect hip FFD.

(i) ***Supine method***: The patient lies supine on the couch with his/her leg and foot brought by the edge of the couch. Then, the hips are flexed one by one to obliterate the lumbar lordosis and reveal the FFD of the other side (Figs. 7.8A and B).

(ii) ***Staheli prone extension method***: The patient lies prone on the couch with his/her hips and legs left dangling from the edge of the couch. Then, one hand is kept over the sacrum and gradually one hip at a time is extended till pelvic motion is detected. The angle between the thigh and the horizontal is the amount of FFD at the hip. The same is repeated for the other hip to detect FFD.

> One may find difficulty in performing the Thomas hip flexion test in obese patients and patients with knee stiffness/ankylosis whose knees cannot be flexed.

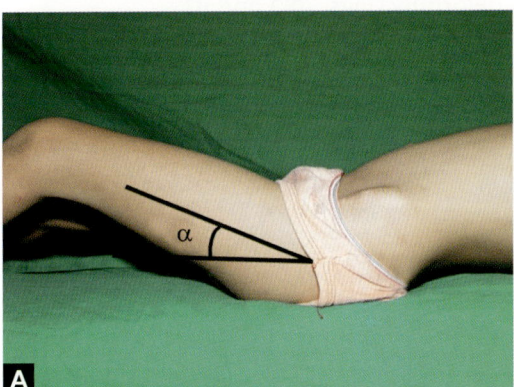
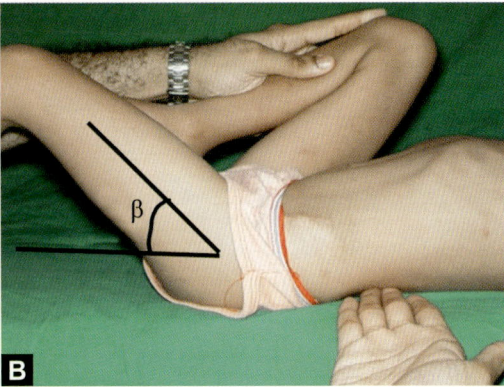

Figs. 7.7A and B: Thomas hip flexion test for unilateral fixed flexion deformity of the hip.

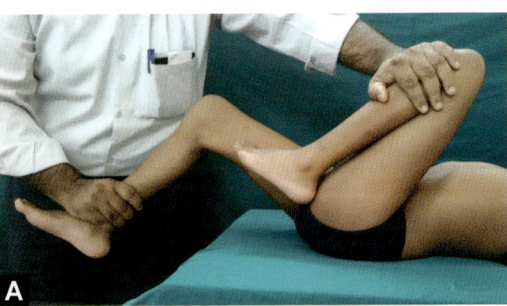
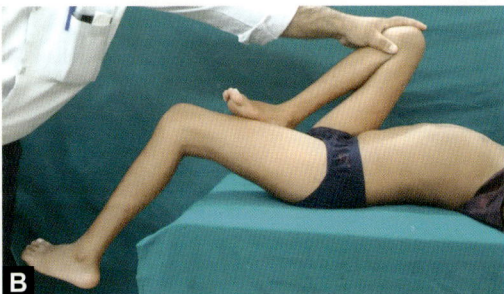

Figs. 7.8A and B: Method to detect bilateral fixed flexion deformity of the hip.

2. **Deformity in coronal plane:** Adduction or abduction deformity is the deformity in coronal plane. It's presence is indirectly indicated by uneven levels of both ASIS.

- **When the index side ASIS is lower than the normal side,** one must suspect *abduction deformity* of the index hip joint.
- *If the index side is higher than the normal side,* one must suspect *adduction deformity* of the index hip joint.

Coronal plane deformity (adduction/abduction) assessment is done in two ways:
  (a) **If pelvis can be squared:** One must square the pelvis (both ASIS in the same line/plane is called squaring of the pelvis) to reveal the amount of coronal plane deformity
  (b) **If pelvis cannot be squared:** Use *Kothari's parallelogram method.*

(a) Method to Square the Pelvis and Assess the Coronal Plane Deformities

  (i) *When ASIS of the index side is lower:* The patient lies supine over the couch. Mark both the ASIS. For the right side, the thumb and middle finger of the left hand is to be kept over index side ASIS and the normal side ASIS, respectively. Then, hold the leg of the index side with the right hand and start *abducting the index hip which starts elevating the index side ASIS.* Stop abducting the index hip when both ASIS appear at the same level through an interspinous line (line joining both ASIS). This reveals the abduction deformity at the index hip joint. The angle between the abducted limb and the midline (α) is the abduction deformity (Figs. 7.9A and B).

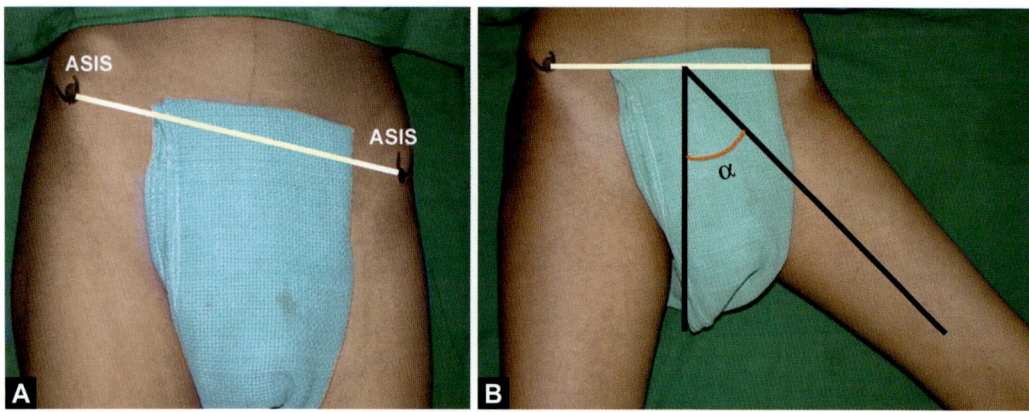

Figs. 7.9A and B: (A) Left side anterior superior iliac spine (ASIS) is at lower level. (B) Both ASIS at same level after squaring pelvis.

  (ii) *When ASIS of index side is higher:* The patient lies supine over the couch. Mark both ASIS and keep the thumb and middle finger over the index side ASIS and the normal side ASIS, respectively. *Then, gently adduct the index hip which lowers the index side ASIS.* Stop adducting index hip when both ASIS are at the same level. This reveals the adduction deformity at the index hip joint. The angle between the adducted limb and the midline is the abduction deformity.

(b) Method to assess the coronal plane deformity if pelvis cannot be squared: *Kothari's parallelogram method*

Method: The patient lies supine on a couch. The pelvis is not squared However, limbs are kept parallel to each other. Now, a midline axis is drawn. Now, another line is drawn joining the two ASIS.

When can pelvis not be squared?
• Fixed pelvic deformities, bilateral fixed coronal plane deformities
• Scoliosis, post-traumatic malunited pelvis
• Ankylosing spondylitis

Further, a perpendicular is dropped from the ASIS to the midline axis.

The angle (α) between the line joining both ASIS and perpendicular over midline axis gives an estimate of adduction or abduction deformity (Fig. 7.10).

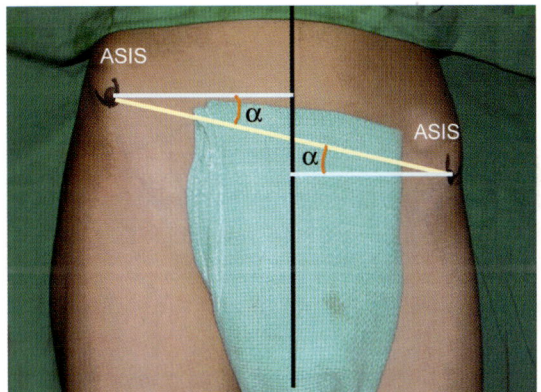

Fig. 7.10: Kothari method of deformity assessment.

3. **Deformity in the axial plane (rotational deformity):** *Rotational deformities* (internal and external rotation) are *revealed deformities*. They are not hidden with the movements of the pelvis or the spine. If the patient keeps the limb in internal or external rotation position in a supine or prone position, it is a rotational deformity. It can be detected with the patient in supine or prone position.

Certain deformities may give a clue to the pathology/diagnosis
• Flexion, adduction, external rotation—1° osteoarthritis
• Flexion, adduction, internal rotation—2° osteoarthritis

Movement

Always check the deformities before commenting upon the range of motion (ROM).

- **The ROM should be checked in all planes**—flexion, extension, abduction, adduction, internal rotation, and external rotation, both active and passive.
- It should also be described with respect to associated pain/spasm.
- If the joint has a deformity, the ROM must be described with fixed deformity and further movements. E.g. 20° flexion deformity with further flexion upto 80°;. Then the ROM of flexion is 20°–80°.

- The rotation should be checked with the hip in flexion and extension. Normally, the rotations are 5°–10° more with a flexed hip compared to an extended hip. However, if the rotation ROM varies more than 20° in flexion than extension, it is described as differential rotation. In AVN of the hip, the ROM of internal rotation increases in a flexed hip compared to an extended hip. This *positive differential rotation is also called sectoral sign.* It describes the involvement of the anterolateral part of the femoral head in AVN.
- *Exaggeration of all ROM* is seen in *Tom Smith arthritis or dysplastic hip.* Occasionally, collagen disorders such as Ehler's Danlos syndrome can cause hyperlaxity presenting similarly. Selective exaggeration of extension, adduction, and external rotation is seen in slipped capital femoral epiphysis.
- Method to check hip ROM (for right side) (Figs. 7.11 to 7.13).

(A) Hip flexion: The hip flexion ROM is assessed with the knee in flexion.
(Note: During the flexion of the hip, one can also assess the axis deviation which is described below.)
(B) Hip extension: This can be tested in a lateral position till movement of pelvis is detected and in a prone position, with the knee in flexion.
(C) Abduction: The examiner holds the right leg near the ankle by his right hand while his left-hand thumb and the middle finger are kept over the ASIS to detect any pelvic movement.

Now, the hip is gently abducted till the ASIS movement is first detected. The angle between the midline and the abducted limb gives a measure of the abduction.

> **How to measure angle with a goniometer?**
> Place one of the arms of the goniometer parallel to the abducted limb whereas the other arm of the goniometer is kept parallel to the imaginary midline of the body. The angle between the two arms of the goniometer is the angle of abduction (Fig. 7.14). *[For further understanding about goniometer and ROM measurement, read chapter 1].*

(D) Adduction: The examiner holds the leg by the right hand while the left-hand thumb and the middle finger are kept over the ASIS to detect any pelvic movement.

Now, the hip is gently adducted till the ASIS movement is first detected. That is the adduction ROM. Normally, the adducted thigh can cross the proximal-third/middle-third of other thigh in the adducted position. The angle between the midline and the adducted limb gives a measure of adduction.
(E) External and internal rotation with the knee flexed: With the patient in supine position, the hip and knee are flexed to 90°. Then, the examiner holds the right leg by the right hand while the left-hand thumb and the middle finger are kept over the ASIS to detect any pelvic movement. Now the hip is externally and internally rotated to assess the rotations just when the ASIS moves. This gives the rotation ROM of the hip. The angle between the imaginary vertical axis passing via the pelvis and the rotated leg gives the estimate of rotation.

The *rotational ROM assessment can also be done in prone position which may be easy as it fixes the pelvis.*

(F) External and internal rotation with hip and knee extended: Lift both the legs at the level of the ankle by 2–3" above the couch.

This locks the knee. Now externally rotate or internally rotate to note the ROM at the hip.

- **Axis deviation, if any, should be noted:**

Method: Keeping the knee flexed, the index hip is gradually flexed. Normally, when the hip is flexed with a flexed knee, the knee points toward the same or the opposite shoulder. However, when a sector of the head is deformed, or irregular, the knee sways away from the midline (Fig. 7.15). Classically, it is observed in SCFE.

- **Associated crepitus should be noted** which indicates an arthritic hip joint, or rarely loose body in the joint.

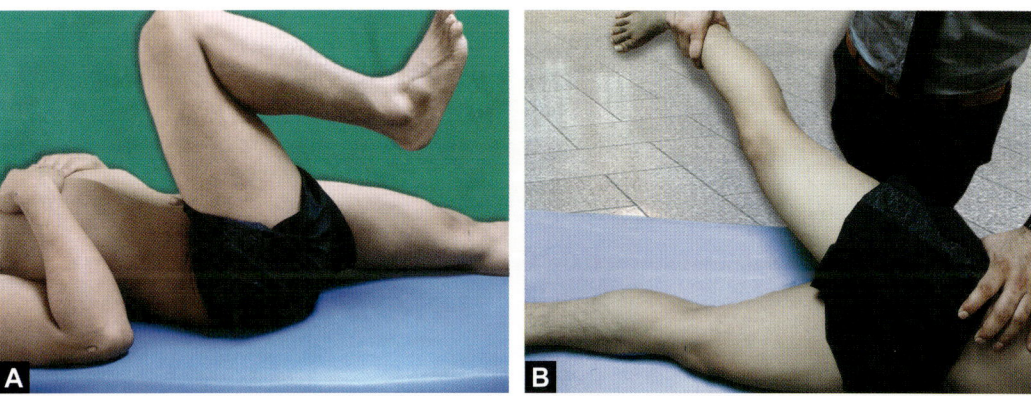

Figs. 7.11A and B: Hip movement: flexion and extension.

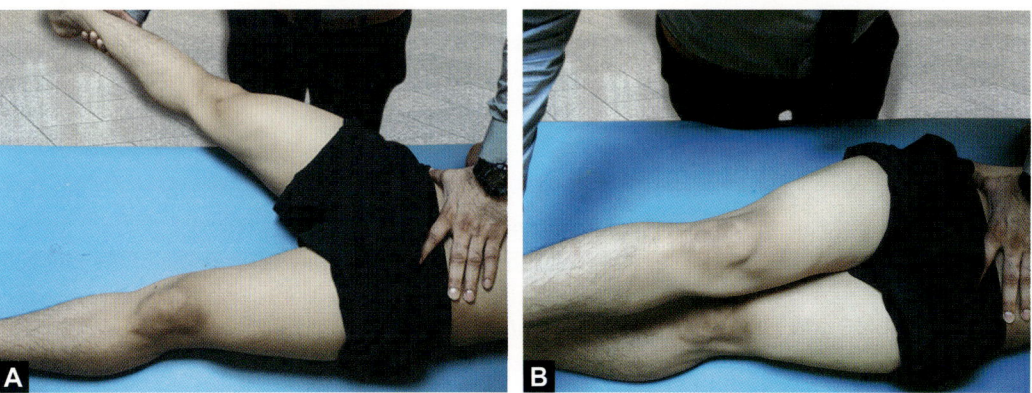

Figs. 7.12A and B: Hip movement: abduction and adduction.

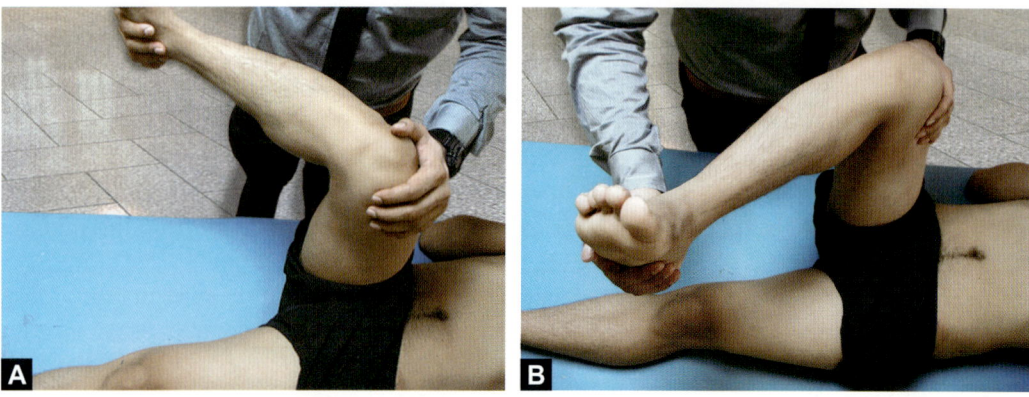

Figs. 7.13A and B: (A and B) Hip movement; external and internal rotation in 90° flexion of hip.

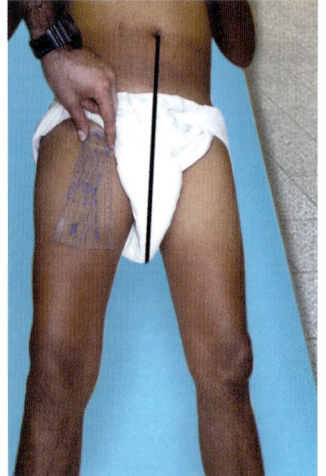

Fig. 7.14: Range of movement (ROM) measurement with a goniometer.

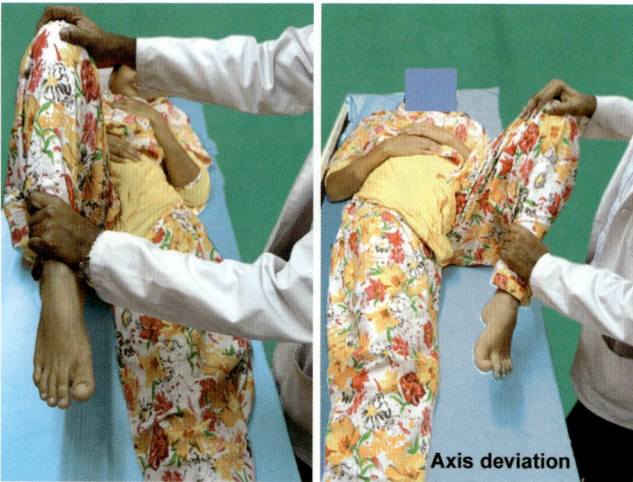

Fig. 7.15: Axis deviation of the left hip.

Measurement and Various Lines

(A) **Limb length measurement–Apparent and True**

   1. *Apparent limb length:* The lower limbs should be kept parallel *(squaring of the pelvis is not required)* to measure the apparent limb length discrepancy.

   Method: It should be measured from *Xiphisternum* to the tip of the medial malleolus on both sides (Fig. 7.16).

   2. *True limb length:* It should be measured *only after squaring the pelvis.*

   Method: After squaring the pelvis, place both limbs in identical position. Then, measure the *distance between the ASIS and the medial joint line of knee* and between the *medial joint line and the tip of the medial malleolus* (Figs. 7.17A and B). This gives a measure of total length of the limb and segmental length of the thigh and leg. It also reveals the exact location (thigh/leg/both) of limb length discrepancy.

> *Without coronal plane deformity (abduction/adduction),*
> *the apparent and true length will be equal.*

Example of 'squaring the pelvis' and measuring the limb length.

- *If there is a 20° adduction deformity* on the left side, the left ASIS will be at a higher level than the right. To square the pelvis, the left limb is adducted by 20°. This brings 'ASIS of affected side' at the level of 'ASIS of normal side'. After squaring the pelvis, the right limb should also be kept in 20° adduction. Now, sequentially measure the true length of the limb keeping both limbs in 20° adduction.
- *If there is 30° abduction deformity* on the right side, the right ASIS will be lower than left. To square the pelvis, the right lower limb is abducted by 30°. This brings 'ASIS of affected side' at the level of 'ASIS of normal side'. After squaring the pelvis, the left hip should also be kept in 30° abduction. Now, sequentially measure the true length of the limb keeping both limbs in 30° abduction.

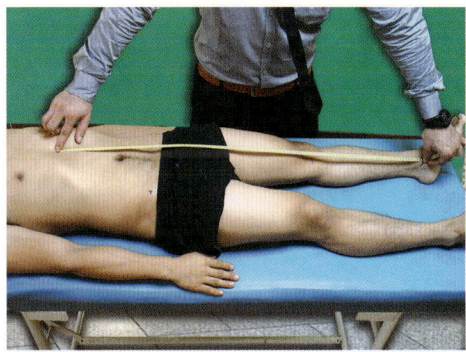

Fig. 7.16: Technique to measure apparent length of lower limb.

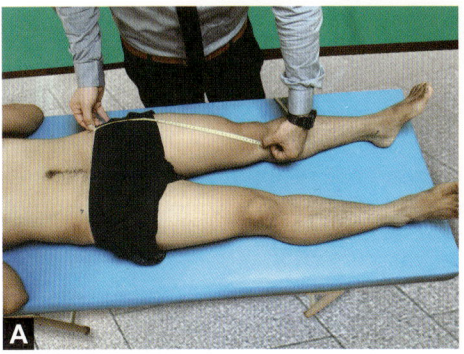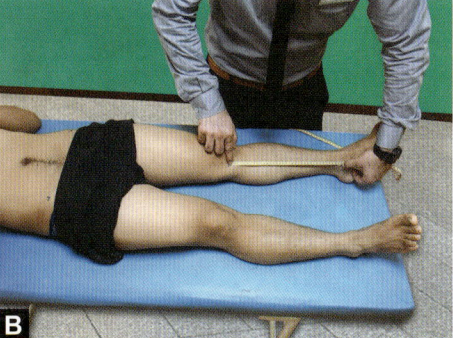

Figs. 7.17A and B: Technique to measure the true length of lower limb after squaring the pelvis.

3. **Bryant triangle measurement:** This is done to ascertain whether shortening in the limb is supratrochanteric or infratrochanteric (Fig. 7.18).

   Method: The patient lies *supine* with the *pelvis squared* and the *limbs in identical* position. Then, the ASIS and the tip of the greater trochanter (TGT) are marked on both sides and the

ASIS and the TGT are joined by a straight line (black). Next, a plumb line is drawn from the ASIS toward the floor (orange). Further, a perpendicular line (x) is dropped from the TGT to the plumb line (blue). The length of the perpendicular line (x1) is measured. A similar triangle is drawn on the normal side too with x2 length of the base of triangle.

How to palpate the tip of GT?

The examiner places his fingers over the lateral aspect of the proximal shaft of the femur and continues to palpate proximally eventually crossing the most proximal part of the GT. Subsequently the hand abruptly dips in the soft spot. The bony hard point just proximal to the soft spot is the tip of the GT.

Interpretation:
- *Supratrochanteric shortening*: The discrepancy in limb length will be equal to x2–x1.
- *Infratrochanteric shortening*: There will be no discrepancy in x1 and x2.

Fallacy of Bryant's triangle measurement:
It is valid only in a squared pelvis and in a unilateral pathology of the hip joint.

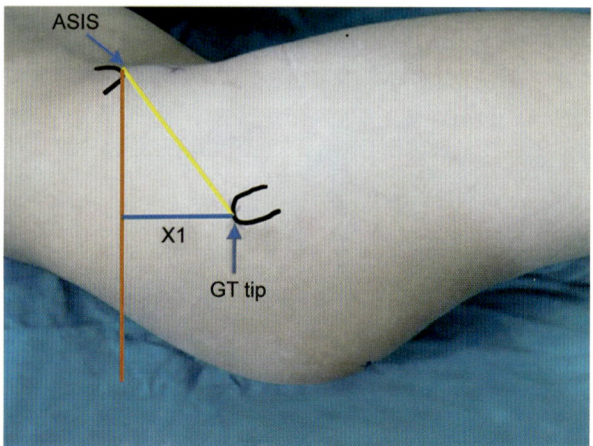

Fig. 7.18: Measurement of Bryant's triangle.

4. **Wasting of thigh and calf muscles:** The circumference of thigh (15 cm proximal to superior pole of patella) and calf (at maximum girth of calf) should be measured in every case (Fig. 7.19).
5. **Craig test: Angle of Hip anteversion**
   Method: The patient is made to lie prone and the knee is flexed to 90°. The examiner keeps his hand over the GT and internally rotates the hip till the GT becomes most prominent laterally. The angle between the leg and the vertical is the "angle of hip anteversion."
6. **Galeazzi test/Allis sign:** To assess the component of limb length discrepancy (LLD)
   Method: The patient lies supine with both hips flexed at 45° and knee at 90°. Now watch the level of the knee from front or side and parallelism of tibia and femur (Fig. 7.20).
   Interpretation: Normally if there is no LLD, the levels of both the knees are the same. However, if there is a LLD, the index knee will be at a lower level (blue arrow). Further, *If knee at different level with, parallel tibia*: Length discrepancy is in the tibia

If knee at different level with, parallel femur: Length discrepancy is in the femur

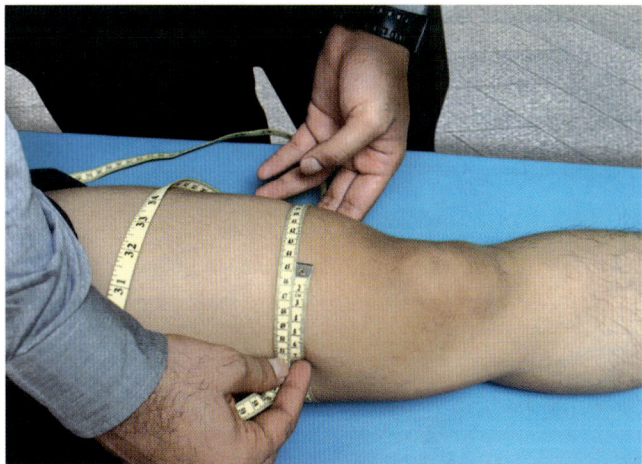

Fig. 7.19: Measurement of thigh wasting.

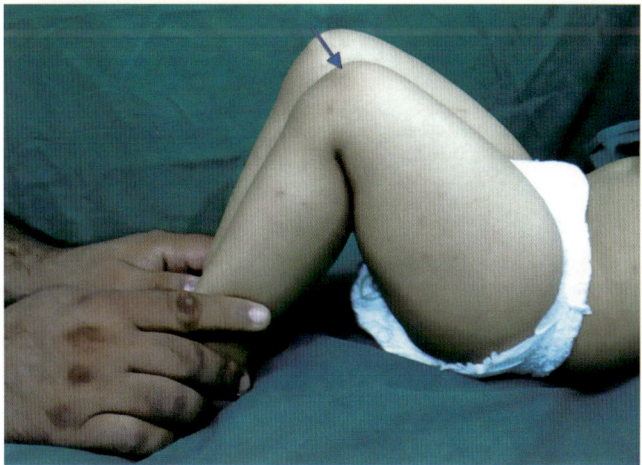

Fig. 7.20: Galeazzi test.

Three measurements to assess the proximal migration of GT;
Nelaton's, Shoemaker's, and Chiene's line

(B) Nelaton's line: To confirm the superior or inferior migration of GT.
   Method: The patient lies lateral on the sound side with index side of the hip facing up keeping the knee slightly flexed [flexed hip makes Ischial tuberosity (IT) prominent]. The ASIS and IT is marked and joined by a straight line (Fig. 7.21).
   Interpretation: Normally, the ASIS-IT line must touch the tip of GT. The tip of the proximally migrated GT will be above this line.
(C) Shoemaker's line: To confirm the superior migration of GT.
   Method: The patient lies supine on a couch. Both the ASIS and the GT tip are marked and joined by a straight line and advanced toward the umbilicus (Fig. 7.22).

Interpretation: Normally, the two lines (between GT and ASIS) must intersect in the midline. Any upward displacement of the index side GT will lead to the intersection of the two lines on the opposite side of midline.

(D) Chiene's line: Normally, the lines joining the two ASIS and tip of GT are parallel to each other (Fig. 7.23). However, if GT on the index side is proximally migrated, the lines converge on the index side.

(E) Morris' bitrochanteric line: The distance between the tip of GT and the pubic symphysis is equal on both sides (Fig. 7.24). However, in case of central fracture dislocation or protrusio acetabuli, the hip migrates medially, and the distance becomes unequal.

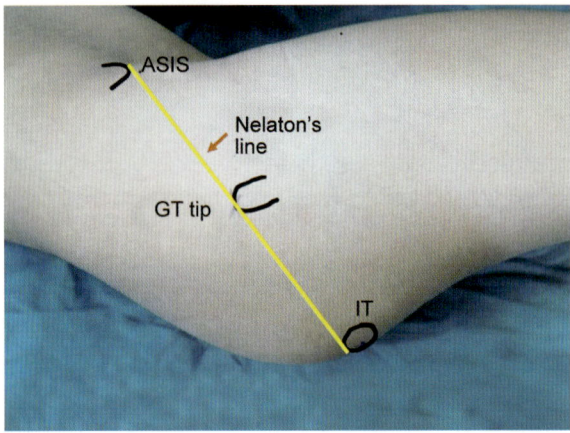

Fig. 7.21: Nelaton's line.

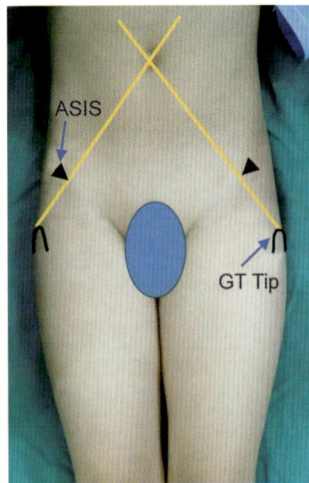

Fig. 7.22: Shoemaker's line.

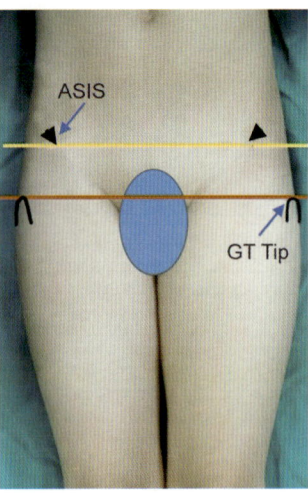

Fig. 7.23: Chiene's line.

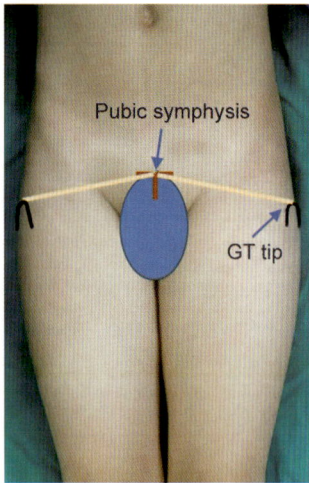

Fig. 7.24: Morris' bitrochanteric line.

Special Tests

1. **Telescopy test (Dupuytren's test):** It is performed when the lever arm of the hip (neck) is suspected to be broken (fracture neck femur), or the fulcrum is disturbed (dislocated head).

   Method: With patient in supine position, the hip and knee joints are flexed to 90° and the hip is adducted by 10°. For the left side, the examiner keeps the right thumb over the ASIS to stabilize the pelvis while the other fingers of the right hand are kept over the tip of GT to feel the excursion of the femur. The left hand holds the knee to give a push (red arrow) and pull (black arrow) along the line of the femur. Now the gentle push–pull force is applied along the long axis of femur via the knee, and the trochanteric excursion is felt (Fig. 7.25).

   Interpretation: Normally excursion (movements) of the GT is less than 1 cm. In telescopy positive cases, an excursion upto 4–5 cm is felt.

   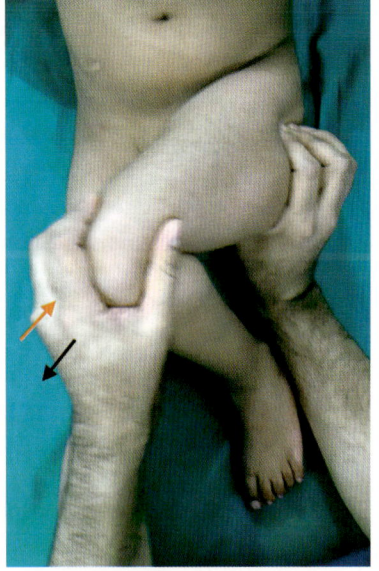

   Fig. 7.25: Telescopy test.

   > *Note:* One should never perform telescopy test in acute fracture/dislocation

   > **Positive telescopy test.**
   > - Nonunion femoral neck fracture or intertrochanteric fracture
   > - Chronic posterior dislocation of the hip
   > - Developmental dysplasia of the hip

2. **Trendelenburg test:** It is performed to assess the integrity of the abductor mechanism of the hip. (*Read description of Trendelenburg at the end of the chapter.*)

   Prerequisites for the Trendelenburg test:
   - Patient should be able to stand on the affected side for at least 30 seconds.
   - Atleast 15° free adduction should be possible on the index side.

   Method: With patient standing, the examiner stands behind the patient. Both PSIS are exposed. The patient is asked to stand on the normal side (N) with the affected side (A) foot off the ground keeping the affected hip extended. The PSIS on the affected side should move upwards or at least stay at the same level (normal). Then, ask the patient to stand on the affected side keeping the normal side foot off the ground (with normal hip extended) (Figs. 7.26A and B).

   Interpretation: The test is positive if the PSIS of the normal side goes down while weight bearing on the affected side for 30 seconds.

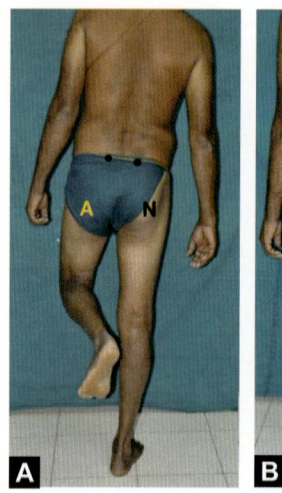
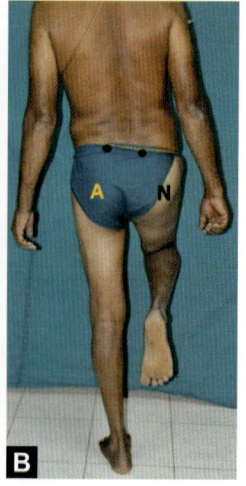

Figs. 7.26A and B: Trendelenburg test
(A: Affected hip; N: Normal hip).

Positive Trendelenburg test.
- Posterior dislocation of the hip
- Developmental dysplasia of the hip
- Fracture neck of the femur/nonunion
- Paralysis of hip abductors
- Developmental coxa vara
- Greater trochanter overgrowth

Kneeling method or Assisted Trendelenburg test:
The examiner kneels in front of the patient, places his thumb over both ASIS of the patient, and asks the patient to place both his hands over the examiner's shoulder. Now the examiner asks the patient to stand over his normal leg. With the patient exerting equal pressure over both shoulders of the examiner, there will be no drooping of pelvis. Next, ask patient to stand over his affected/index leg (Fig. 7.27). A positive test will be indicated by drooping of the pelvis and the patient exerting more pressure over the examiner's opposite shoulder by his hand when the patient is standing over the affected leg.

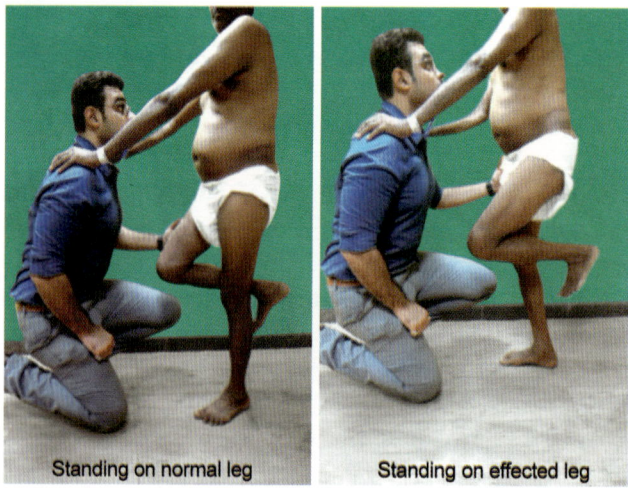

Fig. 7.27: Assisted Trendelenburg test.

False positive Trendelenburg test: Fixed adduction deformity of the index hip, quadratus lumborum palsy, painful condition of the hip and the knee.
False negative Trendelenburg test: Fixed abduction deformity of the index hip, an arthrodesed hip.

3. **Vascular sign of Narath:** It is performed to assess whether the hip is dislocated or not.
   Method: The patient lies supine on a couch. The femoral artery is palpated against the head of the femur at the mid-inguinal point (midpoint of the symphysis pubis and the ASIS).
   Interpretation: In a normal hip, a normal pulsation of the femoral artery is well palpable whereas in a dislocated or subluxated head, it is feeble or not felt.
   It might be difficult to assess in obese patients.

4. **Test for developmental dysplasia of hip (DDH)**
   (i) Barlow test: To detect DDH, especially whether the *hip is dislocatable* or not.
   Method: With the hips and knees flexed, the examiner holds the thigh with his hand. The thumb is placed on the medial aspect of the thigh whereas the index and middle fingers are placed over the GT. The hip is adducted with gentle downward pressure along the long axis of the femur; simultaneously lateral pressure is exerted by the thumb on the medial aspect of the thigh (Fig. 7.28).
   Interpretation: The test is positive if the femoral head can be pushed out of the acetabulum.

   (ii) Ortolani test: To detect DDH, especially whether the *hip is relocatable or reducible* or not.
   Method: With the hips and knees flexed, the examiner holds both thighs with his hands. The thumb is placed on the medial aspect of the thigh, whereas the index and middle fingers are placed over the GT. The hip is abducted with gentle traction, and simultaneously the trochanter is gently levered upward and forward (Fig. 7.29).
   Interpretation: The test is positive if the femoral head reduces into the acetabulum with a "click."

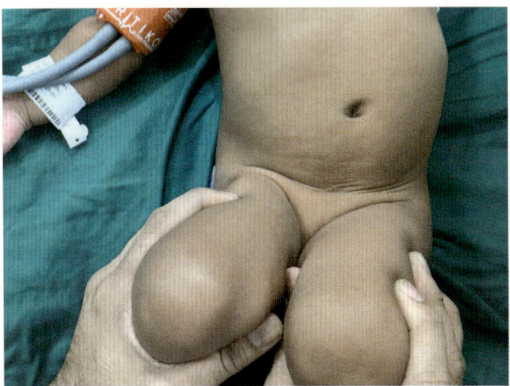 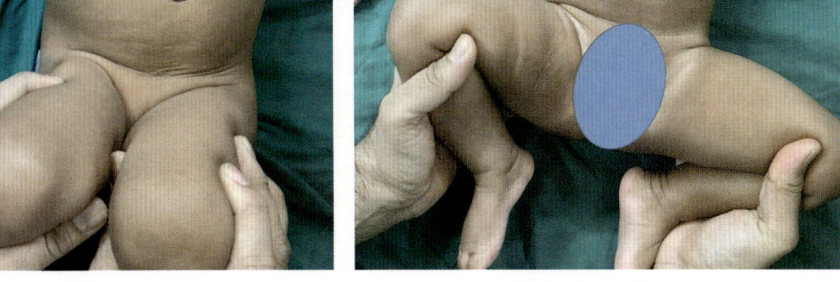

Fig. 7.28: Barlow test.   **Fig. 7.29:** Ortolani test.

5. **Tests for muscle contracture:** Contracture is quite frequent in two muscles around the hip; Rectus femoris (Ely's test) and Iliotibial (IT) band (Ober's test)
   (i) Ely's test: For rectus femoris contracture
   Method: The patient is made to lie prone on the couch. With hip in extension, the knee is gradually flexed to 90° (Fig. 7.30).

Interpretation: As the knee is flexed, the hip appears to flex gradually in case of rectus femoris contracture.

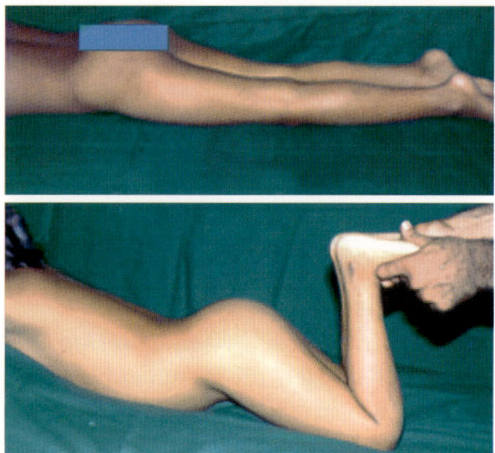

Fig. 7.30: Ely's test.

(ii) Ober's test: *For IT band contracture*
Method: *The patient lies in a lateral position with the index side up. The hip and the knee of the unaffected side are flexed t*o 90°. Then, the hip of the index side is abducted, externally rotated and extended, and gently dropped.
Interpretation: In a patient having a normal IT band without contracture, the limb drops down and rests on the couch. However, if there is an IT band contracture, the limb remains held in abduction after dropping to an extent.

(iii) Test for piriformis tightness (in piriformis syndrome)
Method: The patient lies in a lateral position with the index side up. The hip and the knee of the index side are flexed to 90°. Then, the index hip is adducted and internally rotated.
Interpretation: In a patient with tight pyriformis muscle, this maneuver produces pain in the gluteal region overlying the pyriformis area.

6. **Tests for hip impingement:** Usually, there is pain, loss of rotation and flexion movement with occasional locking/clicks.
(i) *Anterior impingement FADDIR (flexion, adduction, internal rotation) test*
Method and interpretation: The patient lies supine. The index hip is flexed to 90° adducted and internally rotated. This produces pain in the anterior part of hip/groin indicative of anterior impingement.

(ii) *Posterior impingement test (Extension, abduction, external rotation)*
Method and interpretation: The patient lies supine and the index hip is flexed to 90°. Now gradually abduct, externally rotate, and extend the hip. This produces pain in the posterior part of hip indicative of posterior impingement.

(iii) *FABER (flexion, abduction, external rotation) test*
Method and interpretation: The patient lies supine. The index hip is brought into flexion, abduction, and external rotation (figure of four position). Then, a downward force is applied to the medial aspect of the knee forcing the hip into further abduction and

extension. This produces pain over the hip joint. (The same test is applicable for SI joint pathology where pain is felt over the SI joint.)

Neurovascular Examination

As per the standard protocol.

Examination of Joints Above and Below

Ipsilateral knee, ankle, opposite side hip, knee, ankle, and spine with the SI joint should be examined.

Lymph Node Examination

Important in infective and tumor conditions.

▍A NOTE ON TRENDELENBURG TEST

The Trendelenburg test is performed to assess the integrity of abductor mechanism of the hip. So the question is "What is abductor mechanism of the hip?" "Is it merely about the abductor muscle of the hip?"

No, the hip abductor mechanism is not merely abductor muscle function but is a class one lever mechanism comprising of the fulcrum, the lever arm, and forces on either end (Fig. 7.31). This "intact" lever mechanism involves balancing the weight of the body which passes via the pelvis without letting the pelvis drop while the leg is off the ground (swing phase).

The mechanism comprises of:
- *Fulcrum:* Acetabulum
- *Lever arm:* Head, neck, and trochanter
- *Force:* Generated in hip abductors (gluteus medius and gluteus minimus)
- **Load (weight) of the body**

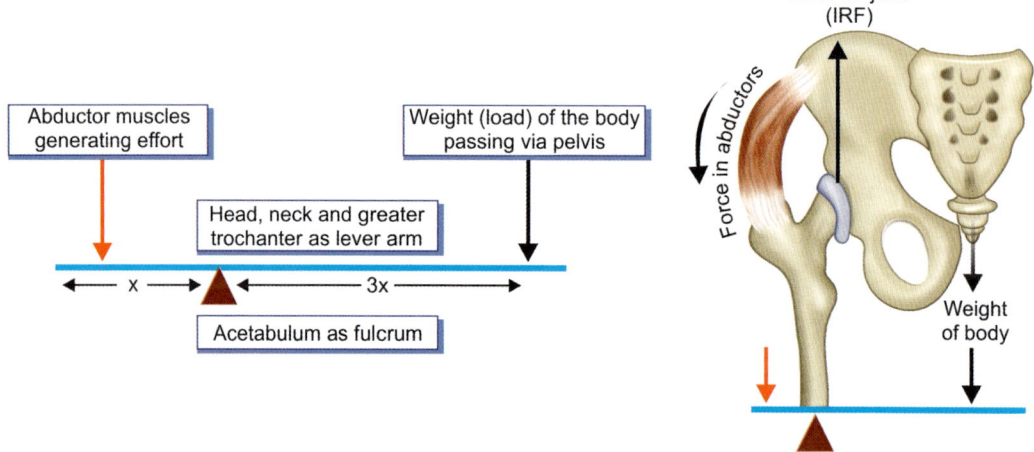

Fig. 7.31: Acetabulum as fulcrum.

The normal response of abductor mechanism: When one of the legs is off the ground (swing side), the pelvis on the same side 'tends' to drop due to the effect of gravity on the unsupported side of the hip. However, the pelvis is balanced and lifted up by the "intact abductor mechanism" of the opposite side (stance side) (Fig. 7.32).

Abnormal response of abductor mechanism: In case of a faulty "abductor mechanism of the stance side," the pelvis on the swing side tends to drop.

This is known a *'positive Trendelenburg test'.*

However, while walking, the body responds by tilting/lurching to the stance side/affected side using the trunk muscle, and the drooping pelvis goes up again. This is known as the Trendelenburg gait with pelvis 'rocking up and down' with trunk lurching to affected side.

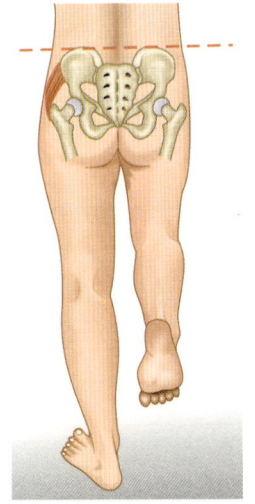 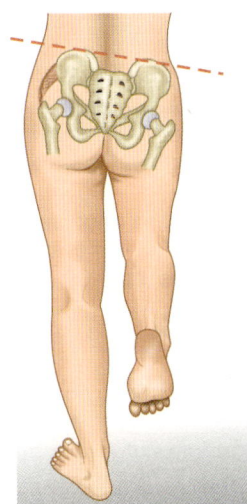

Normal response: Unsupported side pelvis moves upward

Abnormal response: Unsupported side pelvis drops downward

Fig. 7.32: Normal and abnormal responses of abductor mechanism.

The abnormal response (positive Trendelenburg) can happen due to:

1. ***Fulcrum issues:*** *Lever is not on the fulcrum in* the dislocated hip (congenital/traumatic), central fracture dislocations.
2. ***Broken or altered length of lever:*** Fracture neck femur, intertrochanteric femur fracture, slipped capital femoral epiphysis.
3. ***Ineffective force generation in abductors due to:***
   - *Neuromuscular affections of abductors:* Superior gluteal nerve injury/affections leading to palsy of abductors and myopathies affecting muscles.
   - *Postsurgery weakness of abductors:* Any surgery that could damage the abductors during exposure of the pelvis or the hip can affect the function of abductors.
   - *Altered length of abductors in coxa vara or coxa valga:* In cases with coxa vara/valga, the length of the abductor decreases or increases respectively, which alters muscle contraction function. Also, the abductor lever arm increases or decreases in vara or valga, respectively. Together, this affects the normal functioning of abductor mechanism.

Use of cane in hip diseases: To balance the faulty abductor mechanism with the falling pelvis on the opposite side, the body tends to lurch on the same side. However, this is an energy-consuming mechanism. Also, in painful hip conditions, there is a need for an alternative mechanism that can reduce the joint reaction force (JRF).

This can be accomplished by using a cane on the unaffected side. When the cane touches the ground with minimal force, this produces a vertical force, which adds up to the forces generated in the abductor mechanism. This reduces the JRF by almost 50% where a mere 15% of the body weight is applied to the ground with a cane. The cane can produce more ground reaction force (which assists in the reduction of JRF) with little weight application as the lever arm of the cane is longer (more mechanical advantage).

Hip examination proforma

1. **Gait**
2. **Attitude**
3. **Inspection (standing, supine)**
   - **General findings:** *Skin overlying, swelling, scar, sinus*
   - **Specifics findings in inspection on standing**
     (a) *From front*
       - Head position, shoulder level, shape of chest, position of ASIS, rotational deformity (if any), Scarpa's triangle, GT level, thigh fold, patella orientation, thigh and calf muscle wasting
     (b) *From side*
       - Lumbar lordosis, flexed attitude of hip and knee, trochanteric region
     (c) *From back*
       - Level of scapula, rib hump, spine (overlying skin, deformity, swelling), PSIS level, gluteal wasting, gluteal fold, thigh and calf wasting, popliteal fossa and heel status
   - **Specifics findings of inspection in supine position**
     (a) *From front*
       - ASIS level, rotational deformity, Scarpa's triangle, GT level, Thigh fold, Thigh and calf muscle wasting, patella orientation, limb length discrepancy
     (b) *From side*
       - Lumbar lordosis, flexed attitude of hip and knee (if any)
4. **Palpation**
   (a) *From front*
     - Local rise in temperature
     - Tenderness: Soft tissue and bony landmarks, hip joint line, GT (level, broadening, surface, tenderness)
   (b) *From side*
     - Lumbar lordosis
   (c) *From back*
     - Spine, SIJ, PSIS, gluteal region, ischial tuberosity
   (d) *Deformity assessment*
     - **Sagittal plane deformity:** Hip flexion deformity (uni- or bilateral)
       - Thomas hip flexion test, Staheli test, supine method
     - **Coronal plane deformity:** Abduction/adduction deformity
     - **Rotational deformity**
   (e) *Confirmation of palpatory characteristics of swelling, scar, sinus*
5. **Movements**: Active and passive
   - Flexion, extension, abduction, adduction, external and internal rotation
   - Crepitus, clicks; if any
6. **Measurements and various 'lines':** Limb length (apparent and true), thigh-calf circumference, Bryant's triangle, Galeazzi sign, Craig test (for hip anteversion angle), Nelaton's, Shoemaker's, Cheine's and Morris' Bitrochanteric line.
7. **Neurovascular examination**
8. **Special tests**
   (a) *Telescopy test, Trendelenburg test, Vascular sign of Narath*
   (b) *Test for DDH*: Barlow and Ortolani test
   (c) *Tests for Muscle contracture*: Ely's and Ober's test
   (d) *Test for Piriformis tightness*
   (e) *Test for Hip impingement*: FADDIR (anterior impingement), posterior impingement test and FABER
9. **Joint above (Spine) and below (knee, ankle), contralateral hip, knee and ankle**
10. **Lymph node examination**

**Common conditions affecting hip with their
salient features**

1. **Developmental dysplasia of the hip**
   - *Affects*: First born, female, left side
   - *Pathology*: Dysplasia of the acetabulum and head of the femur
   - *Clinical features*: Present at birth, walking age/may present later
     - Painless limp
     - Abduction restricted whereas both rotations are exaggerated
     - Supratrochanteric shortening
     - Trendelenburg and telescopy positive
     - *Vascular sign of Narath*: Positive
     - Barlow's and Ortolani ± (depending upon age)
   - *Diagnosis*: X–ray— Hilgenreiner's and Perkins line, acetabular angle, USG
   - *Treatment*: Closed reduction, bracing, open reduction, varus derotation osteotomy, pelvic osteotomy
2. **Developmental coxa vara (decrease in neck-shaft angle)**
   - *Affects*: Present at walking age/may present later
   - *Presents with*: Painless limp
   - *Pathologically*: Abnormal development of proximal femoral cartilaginous physis, defective ossification of adjacent metaphysis, separate triangular fragment at the inferior-medial part of neck.
   - *Clinically*:
     - *Vascular sign of Narath*: Negative
     - Abduction restricted while adduction is increased, internal rotation less than external rotation
     - Supratrochanteric shortening
     - Trendelenburg positive
     - Telescopy negative
   - *Diagnosis*: X-ray (neck shaft angle <125°)
   - *Treatment*: Observation, corrective valgus derotation osteotomy
3. **Tom Smith arthritis:**
   - *Affects*: Neonates and infants whose femoral epiphyseal cartilage has not yet formed
   - *Presents with*: Painless limp, h/o neonatal infection, or NICU admission
     - Present at walking age/may present later
   - *Pathologically*: Destroyed femoral head due to septic arthritis during infancy (typically within 9 months of age).
   - *Clinically*:
     - Vascular sign of Narath: Positive
     - All movements are exaggerated
     - Trendelenburg and telescopy: Positive
     - Supratrochanteric shortening: Positive
   - *Diagnosis*: X-ray
   - *Treatment*: Pelvic support osteotomy, arthrodesis, THR
4. **Tuberculosis of the hip:**
   - *Affects*: Any age
   - *Presents with*: Painful limp, pain in the hip, deformity, h/o contact with patients suffering from TB ±
   - *Pathologically*: TB of the hip; stage of synovitis/arthritis/deformity
   - *Clinically*: Deformity according to the stage
     Stage of synovitis: Flexion, abduction, external rotation; apparent lengthening
     Stage of arthritis: Flexion, adduction, internal rotation; apparent shortening

Stage of advanced arthritis: Flexion, abduction, external rotation; true shortening. There may be dislocation, subluxation, gross destruction of head of femur, protrusio, etc. in this age:
  - Thigh muscle wasting ++
  - Restriction of abduction and internal rotation
  - Supratrochanteric shortening (depends on stage)
  - *Vascular sign of Narath: Negative;* **Trendelenburg sign:** *caution while testing due to fixed deformities;* **Telescopy:** *Negative (even in case of subluxation due to fibrosis)*
- *Diagnosis*: X-ray, biopsy, other tests for TB
- *Treatment*: ATT, according to pathological stage (synovectomy, arthrodesis, joint replacement)

5. **Transient synovitis of hip:**
    - *Affects*: Age 4–10 years
    - *Presents with*: Dull aching hip pain
    - *Pathologically*: Synovitis of the hip
    - *Clinically*:
      - Flexion, abduction, external rotation attitude
      - Usually no fixed deformity, occasionally abduction deformity
      - *Restricted terminal range of motion in all planes (extreme movements)*
      - No true shortening/lengthening
      - *Trendelenburg and Telescopic sign*: Negative
      - *Vascular sign of Narath*: Negative
    - *Diagnosis*: Clinical, X-ray, MRI
    - *Treatment*: Conservative, rest, traction, NSAID

6. *Acute septic arthritis*:
    - *Affects*: Mostly neonates/children
    - *Presents with*: *Pseudoparalysis*, throbbing hip pain, fever, refusal to feed
    - *Pathologically*: Acute septic arthritis of hip, *Staph. aureus* being most common organism
    - *Clinically*:
      - Flexion, abduction, external rotation attitude
      - *Severe tenderness over the hip joint*
      - *All range of motion grossly restricted and very painful*
      - *Vascular sign of Narath*: Negative
      - No true shortening/lengthening
      - *Trendelenburg and Telescopic sign*: Negative (Should not be tested due to severe pain)
    - *Diagnosis*: Hip aspiration, USG
    - *Treatment*: Arthrotomy and drainage, IV antibiotics

7. *Perthes disease (Legg–Calve–Perthes disease, pseudo-coxalgia)*
    - *Affects*: Age 5–11 years, Common in South West region of India
    - *Presents with*: Painful limp, mechanical hip pain, occasionally presents with knee pain (radiation)
    - *Pathologically*: Idiopathic avascular necrosis of the hip followed by revascularization and reformation–remodeling of the head of femur.
    - *Clinically*:
      - *Abduction and internal rotation restricted*, occasionally all ROM restricted
      - *Vascular sign of Narath*: Negative
      - *Supratrochanteric shortening*: Later stage
      - Axis deviation present in late cases (deformed head of femur).
      - *Trendelenburg sign positive;* **Telescopic sign:** Negative
    - *Diagnosis*: X-ray
    - *Treatment*: Bracing, varus derotation osteotomy, pelvic osteotomy (containment surgery)

8. **Slipped capital femoral epiphysis (adolescent coxa vara)**
   - *Affects*: *Obese adolescents;* may be associated with endocrinal abnormality (hypothyroidism, growth hormone treatment)
   - *Presents with*: Painful limp, mechanical hip pain, occasionally presents with knee pain (radiation)
   - *Pathologically*: Disease of proximal femoral physis leading to slip of the femoral metaphysis with respect to the femoral epiphysis
   - *Clinically*:
     - *Adduction and external rotation deformity*
     - Flexion, abduction, and internal rotation restricted. Occasionally, all ROM restricted (in chondrolysis).
     - *Axis deviation*: Present
     - *Supratrochanteric shortening*: Later stage
     - *Trendelenburg sign positive; Telescopic sign:* Negative
     - *Vascular sign of Narath*: Negative
   - *Diagnosis*: X-ray, endocrine workup
   - *Treatment*: Observation, in situ pinning of the femoral epiphysis, proximal femur osteotomy
9. **Nonunion neck femur:**
   - *Affects*: Adult patients, H/o trauma—significant in younger patients, trivial in older patients, associated osteoporosis, treated or untreated trauma
   - *Presents with*: Difficulty in walking or weight bearing
   - *Pathology*: Nonunion of the fracture neck of femur
   - *Clinical features*:
     - Active SLR not possible
     - External rotation deformity
     - *Passive range of motion*: Normal
     - Supratrochanteric shortening +
     - *Vascular sign of Narath*: Negative
     - *Trendelenburg and Telescopic sign*: Positive
   - *Diagnosis*: X-ray
   - *Treatment*: **Young patients**: Open reduction and internal fixation (± valgus osteotomy ± graft), replacement arthroplasty
10. **Malunion of intertrochanteric fracture**:
    - *Affects*: Elderly patients
    - *Presents with*: Painless limp with short limb, h/o trauma, treated or untreated trochanteric fracture
    - *Pathologically*: Malunited intertrochanteric fracture
    - *Clinically*:
      - External rotation deformity
      - Active SLR possible
      - Broadening and irregularity of GT +, proximally migrated greater trochanter
      - *Vascular sign of Narath*: Negative
      - Supratrochanteric and infratrochanteric shortening +
      - *Trendelenburg sign positive, Telescopic sign* negative
    - *Diagnosis*: X-ray—malunited IT fracture with coxa vara
    - *Treatment*: Mostly conservative, corrective osteotomy
11. **Osteoarthritis hip**
    - *Affects*: Age after 50 years
    - *Presents with*: Mechanical hip pain
    - *Pathologically*: Primary hip osteoarthritis

- **Clinically:**
  - **Deformity:** Flexion, adduction, external rotation
  - All ROM restriction, painful
  - **Vascular sign of Narath:** Negative
  - **Supratrochanteric shortening:** Minimal or none
  - **Trendelenburg and Telescopic sign:** Negative
- **Diagnosis:** X-ray
- **Treatment:** Total hip replacement

12. **Avascular necrosis of the hip:**
  - **Affects:** Mostly young adults
  - **Presents with:** Painful limp, mechanical pain at the hip, h/o trauma (hip dislocation, fracture neck femur), chronic alcoholism, steroid intake, chronic gout, Caisson's disease, Goucher's disease, sickle cell anemia.
  - **Pathologically:** Due to the above said etiology(s), avascularity of the subchondral bone leads to necrosis and collapse of the subchondral bone followed by damage to the overlying cartilage leading to 2° hip osteoarthritis.
  - **Clinically:**
    - Hip joint tender
    - Painful ROM (active and passive), limited abduction and internal rotation
    - Axis deviation present due to sectoral damage to the femoral head
    - Vascular sign of Narath: Negative
    - Telescopy negative
    - Slight shortening of the limb
  - **Diagnosis:** X-ray, MRI
  - **Treatment:** Core decompression, hip replacement

Notes

Clinical Evaluation of the Knee Joint

BRIEF ANATOMY AND FUNCTION OF THE KNEE JOINT

1. Basic osteology

- The knee joint is formed by the lower end of the femur, the upper end of the tibia and the patella (Figs. 8.1 and 8.2). So, it is a combination of two joints named:
    - i. Tibiofemoral joint
    - ii. Patellofemoral joint
- *Tibial condyles* are relatively flat and femoral condyles are rounded. This *makes articulation quite shallow*. Menisci deepen the tibial condyle and provide further stability.
- The patella tracks over the femoral trochlea in flexion-extension.
- The osseous geometry of the trochlea, patella, various muscles around patella and intact medial patellofemoral ligament (MPFL) keeps the patella in the trochlear groove and prevents dislocation.

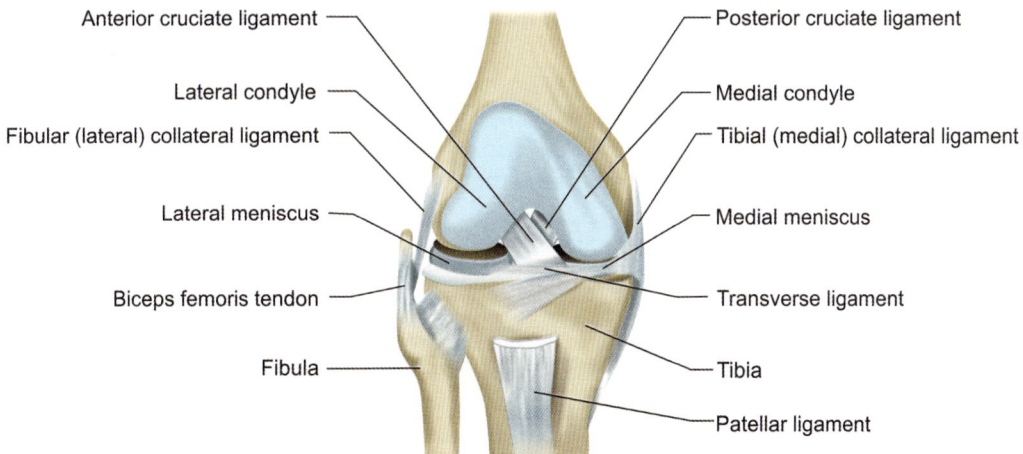

Fig. 8.1: Anatomy of the knee joint.

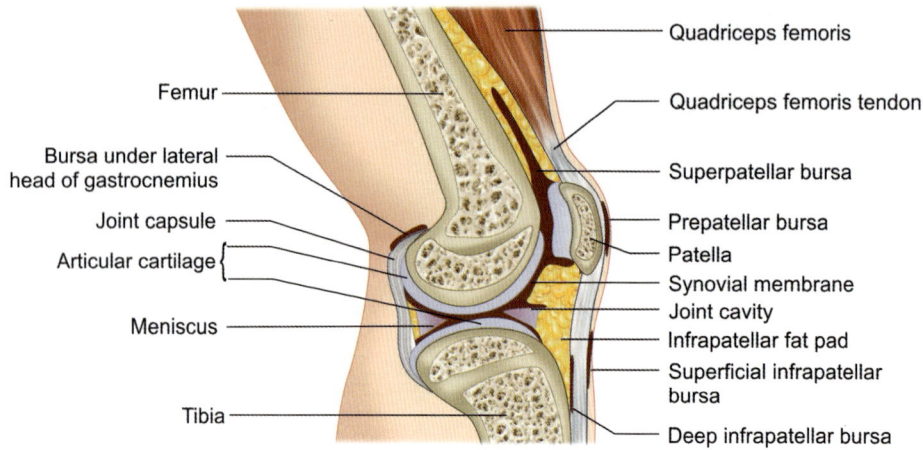

Fig. 8.2: Sagittal anatomy of the knee joint.

2. **Stabilizing ligaments**
   - *Two menisci:* Medial and lateral; *Two cruciates:* Anterior and posterior; *Two collaterals:* Medial and lateral.
   - *Menisci* are crescent-shape fibrocartilaginous structures attached on to the periphery of the tibial condyle. Menisci are *shock absorbers, deepen the articular surface and provide stability* to the knee.
   - *Anterior cruciate ligament (ACL)* is distally attached to the tibia, just anterior to the intercondyloid eminence of the tibia and proximally on to the medial wall of the lateral femoral condyle.
     Function: It prevents the excess anterior translation of the tibia over the femur.
   - *Posterior cruciate ligament (PCL)* is attached proximally on to the lateral wall of the medial femoral condyle (MFC) and distally to the posterior tibia 1–1.5 cm below the plateau in the midline.
     Function: It prevents the excessive posterior translation of the tibia over the femur. It also helps in screw home mechanism of the knee.
   - *Medial collateral ligament (MCL)* is proximally attached on to the MFC just below the medial epicondyle and distally over the proximal medial tibia under the pes anserinus.
     Function: It provides valgus stability to the knee joint especially in 30–90° flexion of the knee (cf. *posteromedial corner structures which provide stability in extended knee*).
   - *Lateral collateral ligament (LCL)* is proximally attached on the lateral epicondyle and distally over the anterolateral part of fibular head.
     Function: It provides varus stability to the knee joint between 5–30° of flexion.
   - *Posteromedial corner of the knee:* Posterior oblique ligament, posterior capsule, posterior horn of medial meniscus (MM), Semimembranosus tendon.
     Function: Valgus stability in extension (alongside cruciates) and internal rotation stability.
   - *Posterolateral corner of the knee (PLC):*
     Static structures: Lateral collateral ligament, popliteus tendon, popliteofibular ligament, fabellofibular & arcuate ligament, lateral capsule.
     Dynamic structures: IT band, biceps femoris, popliteus muscle.
     Function: It resists varus, external rotation and posterior translation forces on the knee.

- *Medial patellofemoral ligament (MPFL)* stabilises the patella into the trochlear groove when the knee flexes between 0–30°.

3. **Type of joint**

   The knee joint is a modified hinge-type bicondylar synovial joint.

4. **Movements:** Predominantly flexion-extension. However, a small degree of rotations too happen.

5. **Other facts**
   - *Normal alignment* for the knee is 4–7° of valgus.
   - *Normal Q angle*: 14–17°
   - Patella *increases the lever arm of the quadriceps* and hence, enhances the power of quadriceps.
   - Physiological locking or 'screw home' of the knee joint is internal rotation of femoral condyles over tibial plateau during terminal extension. Unlocking is performed by Popliteus by laterally rotating the femur over tibial plateau. Both locking and unlocking occur with foot fixed on the ground (closed chain contact).
   - *Vasculature of the knee*: Anastomosis around the knee
   - *Nerve supply to the knee*: Femoral, common peroneal and tibial
   - *Major bursae*: Prepatellar, Infrapatellar, Suprapatellar, Pes Anserine and Semimembranosus bursa

6. **Muscles around knee joint** (Table 8.1).

Table 8.1: Muscles around knee joint, their insertion, nerve supply and action.

Muscles	*Insertion*	*Nerve supply*	*Action*
Quadriceps (rectus femoris, vastus lateralis, vastus intermedius and vastus medialis)	Over the superior pole, medial and lateral border of patella	Femoral nerve	Knee extension. Vastus medialis obliqus (VMO) is also responsible for terminal extension of the knee.
Hamstrings (biceps femoris, semitendinosus, semimembranosus)	Over tibia and fibula (Biceps femoris)	Sciatic nerve	Knee flexion

Common conditions affecting the knee joint.

1. **Congenital**
   (a) Congenital dislocation of knee
   (b) Discoid meniscus
2. **Traumatic**
   (a) Ligament injuries: ACL, PCL, MCL, LCL
   (b) *Recurrent dislocation patella (RDP)*: Medial patellofemoral ligament tear
   (c) Post-traumatic: Stiffness, arthritis, deformity
   (d) Meniscal tears
3. **Infections:** Tuberculosis of knee, pyogenic arthritis
4. **Inflammatory:** Rheumatoid arthritis, Reiter's arthritis
5. **Metabolic:** Gout and pseudogout arthritis, Rickets
6. **Degenerative:** Primary osteoarthritis
7. **Others:**
   (a) Chondromalacia patellae
   (b) Osteochondritis dissecans
   (c) Various bursitis: Semimembranosus, prepatellar, infrapatellar
   (d) Osgood Schlatter's disease
   (e) Baker's cyst

HISTORY AND ITS EVALUATION

The patients with knee pathology complain of certain specific complaints:
- Pain
- Swelling
- Instability
- Difficulty in movement
- Locking, pseudolocking
- Clicks
- Malalignment (deformity) or limb-length discrepancy

1. **Pain:** It is the most common complaint, which could be acute or chronic.

   Acute pain is observed in:

   (a) *Acute trauma*: History of trauma

   (b) *Acute infection*: Septic arthritis

   (c) Exacerbation of chronic condition (inflammatory/degenerative/metabolic)

> An important objective of pain assessment is to figure out the nature of pain, i.e. whether it is *mechanical pain* or *rest pain*, as both have different etiologies *(Read Chapter 1)*.
> (a) Mechanical pain is observed in degenerative diseases/mechanical pathologies like meniscal tears/cartilage injury/osteoarthritis.
> (b) Rest pain is observed in inflammation/infection/tumor like rheumatoid arthritis (RA), tuberculosis, etc.

2. **Swelling:** It could arise within the joint or from an extra-articular source (bone, tendon, nerve, vessels, etc.).

   However, the reasons for "swelling arising within the joint" are:

   (a) Effusion (Joint fluid/haemarthrosis/pus)

   (b) Synovial hypertrophy. Alternatively, it could be both.

> ***An important aspect of swelling assessment is the onset of swelling.***
> (A) Swelling which is immediate/within a few hours after the trauma indicates hemarthrosis.
> (B) Swelling after 12–24 hours of the trauma indicates synovial effusion due to the synovial reaction due to injury to the lesser or avascular structures of the joint (meniscus, cartilage).
> (C) Chronic swelling could be due to effusion/synovial hypertrophy or both.

> Hemarthrosis is due to intra-articular # or injury to intra-articular structures which are vascular.

3. **Instability**

   "My knee gives way" or "I cannot trust my knee" while running, jumping, turning, stair climbing, walking on uneven ground, etc. indicates instability of the joint.

   It happens after a twisting injury or a major trauma. Patella dislocation could be atraumatic or can happen even with the minimal trauma.

   An acute significant ligament injury leads to an inability to bear weight, stand and walk for few hours to days. Only a few days later, the patient regains their ability to bear weight. Later, they may experience chronic, intermittent instability.

- A joint is stable due to the integrity of soft tissues (ligaments, capsule), bony, musculotendinous units and other physical factors. Hence, instability indicates the deficiency of one or more structures.
- Common causes of knee instability are: Tear of the ACL, PCL, Collateral ligament or MPFL, trochlear dysplasia, etc.

4. **Difficulty in movement:** Loss of range of movement could be another complaint which could be due to pain, swelling, deformity, mechanical block, or stiffness due to other pathology.

5. **Locking:** It is a pathological condition wherein the knee is locked or stuck in a flexed position. It is a true mechanical block to further movement in any direction, flexion/extension (*Note: pathological locking is different from physiological locking which occurs during terminal extension*).

    It is commonly observed in the *bucket handle tear of the meniscus or loose bodies.*

    *Remember: The knee never gets locked in full extension.

    Pseudo-locking: It is not a true mechanical locking but a mere muscular spasm not allowing further movement. It is *seen in patellofemoral arthritis.*

6. **Clicks:** Audible clicks/thuds are common features of the discoid lateral meniscus. It may also arise out of maltracking patella, meniscal tear or loose bodies.

7. **Malalignment (deformity) or limb-length discrepancy:** Traumatic, metabolic (rickets), infective, degenerative or congenital conditions can cause an alignment disturbance (deformity) or limb-length discrepancy. Various common deformities are:

    (a) *Genu varum*: It is common in childhood but resolves gradually. Also observed in osteoarthritis (OA), rickets and Paget's disease.

    (b) *Genu valgum*: It is also physiological and tends to resolve by the age of 6 years. It is more frequent in females and may be a contributory factor in recurrent dislocation of patella (due to increased Q angle). Also observed in Rickets, Rheumatoid arthritis.

    (c) *Genu recurvatum*: Mostly due to joint laxity. Sometimes observed, after a posterior capsular tear of the knee in combination with PCL and PLC tears.

CLINICAL EXAMINATION

General and Systemic Examination

Meticulous general and systemic examination must be performed if the disease is systemic in nature and has affected the knee, e.g. rheumatoid arthritis, tuberculosis, etc.

Local Examination

The entire lower limb should be properly exposed from pelvis onwards after proper informed consent, privacy and chaperone.

Gait

Gait should be noted and mentioned.

Attitude

Usually knee examinations are performed in supine position. The attitude of the both lower limbs can be described in standard fashion. (Fig. 8.3).

Inspection: From Front, Side and Back

It is done in standing and supine positions.
(A) Standing: It gives an overall assessment of pelvic tilt (if any) and lower limb alignment.
(B) Supine:
  (i) *General findings: Swelling, scar, sinus, ulcer assessment (in standard fashion)*
  (ii) *Specific findings:*
  1. Deformity:
    – *Coronal plane deformities (genu varum/genu valgum)*: Observe from front (Figs. 8.4A and B)
    – *Sagittal plane deformity (flexion deformity/genu recurvatum)*: Observe from side (Figs. 8.5A and B)

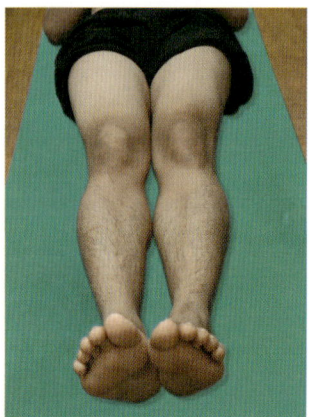

Fig. 8.3: Normal alignment of lower limb.

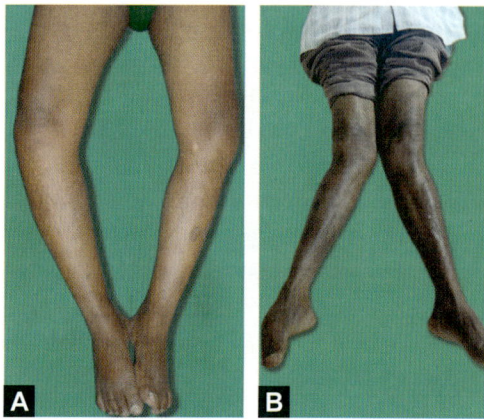

Figs. 8.4A and B: (A) Genu varum. (B) Genu valgum.

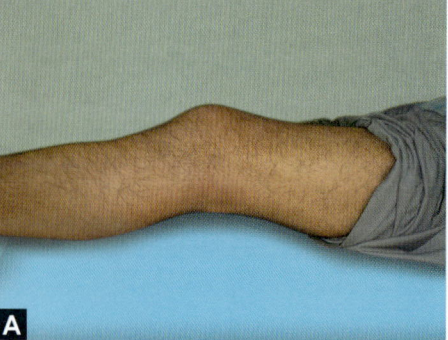

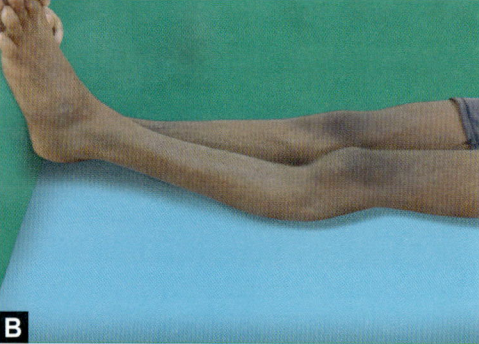

Figs. 8.5A and B: (A) Flexion deformity of the left knee. (B) Genu recurvatum.

Principle of deformity assessment

Always stand in the plane perpendicular to the plane of deformity. For example, varus and valgus of the lower limb are a coronal plane deformity. So, stand in the sagittal plane of the patient (in front of the patient). For recurvatum and flexion deformity (sagittal plane deformity), stand on the side of the patient (coronal plane).

Genu Valgum (knock knee)	Genu Varum (Bow knee)
The severity of G. Valgum is measured by intermalleolar distance.	The severity of G. varum is measured by intercondylar distance.
Mild: 8-10 cm	**Grade 1**: 5-7.5 cm
Moderate: 10-15 cm	**Grade 2**: 7.5-10 cm
Severe: > 15 cm	**Grade 3**: > 10 cm

Genu recurvatum is also known as the hyperextension of the knee. *If bilateral and symmetrical, it is physiological for that person and indicates laxity of ligaments. However, unilateral recurvatum is mostly pathological* indicating a ligament injury, especially PCL, posterior capsule, malunited proximal tibia fracture and weakness in gastrocnemius or biceps femoris.

2. *Muscle wasting*: Thigh and calf
3. *Limb length discrepancy*: Observe level of malleoli and heel with both limbs parallel to each other
4. *Position of the patella*: Normally, the patella is rotated outwards and the lower pole is almost at the level of the joint line.
5. *Swelling*: An intra-articular swelling of the knee joint may give rise to a horseshoe-shaped swelling (Fig. 8.6).

(C) Prone:
   - Examination of *popliteal fossa*: Look for any swelling, pulsation, etc. (Fig. 8.7).

(D) Footwear examination: *A quick* look at the shoe worn by the patient can give an idea of weight-bearing pattern. For example, patients with normal gait get their shoe wear on the lateral border whereas ones with flat feet and genu valgum often have shoe wear on inner border of shoe.

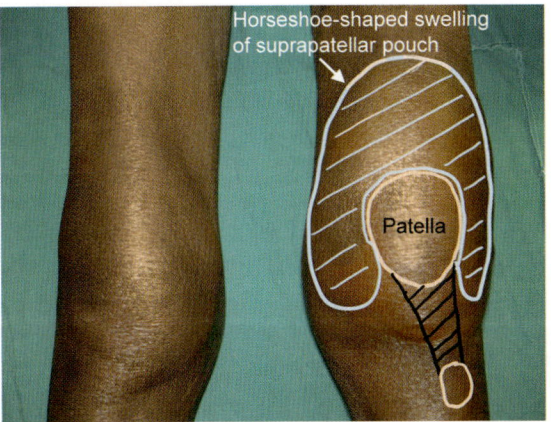

Fig. 8.6: Horseshoe-shaped swelling of the left knee.

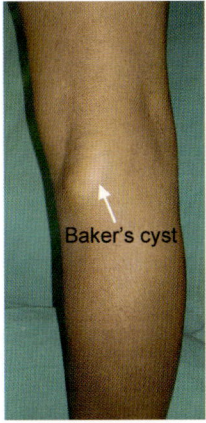

Fig. 8.7: Baker's cyst in the popliteal fossa.

Palpation

(a) *Local rise in temperature.*

(b) *Tenderness:* Always palpate in a sequence to look for tenderness over various bony and soft-tissue points. Some important landmarks are mentioned in the box (Fig. 8.8 and Box 8.1).

> **Box 8.1: Important soft tissue and bony landmarks around the knee joint**
> **Bones:** Femoral condyles (medial, lateral), tibial plateau (medial, lateral), fibular head, patella, tibial tuberosity, epicondyles (medial, lateral)
> **Soft tissue:** Attachments of MCL, LCL, iliotibial band (ITB), patellar tendon, etc.

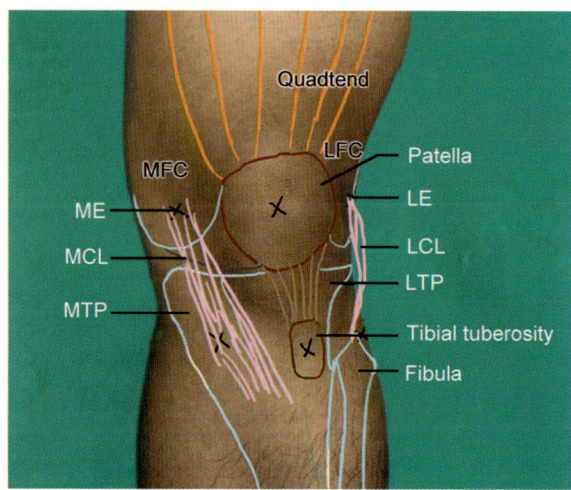

Fig. 8.8: Major soft tissue and bony landmarks for the palpation. (ME: Medial epicondyle; LE: Lateral epicondyle; MCL: Medial collateral ligament; LCL: Lateral collateral ligament; MTP: Medial tibial plateau; LTP: Lateral tibial plateau; LFC: Lateral femoral condyle; MFC: Medial femoral condyle).

(c) *Specific tests during knee palpation:*

I. **Swelling:** It could be intra- or extra-articular.

  i. The extra-articular swelling around the knee should be described as per the standard description of swelling during palpation.

  ii. Intra-articular swelling is usually due to effusion or synovial hypertrophy or both. Effusion usually takes the shape of a horseshoe around the patella (*see* Fig. 8.6). It also makes the "usually empty parapatellar hollows" look full.

II. **Joint line tenderness**

  Method: While patient in supine, the knee is gradually flexed to 90°. The examiner palpates the tibial tuberosity (TT) using their thumb. For the medial joint line, the thumb is advanced proximally just adjacent to the medial side of the patellar tendon until the thumb dips into the soft spot in the joint. Further, the joint line is palpated medially (Figs. 8.9A and B). Similarly, the joint line is palpated on the lateral side.

  Interpretation: A tender joint line indicates arthritis, meniscal tear or mid-substance collateral injury.

> Normally, the knee joint line is located approximately at the level of the lower pole of the patella.

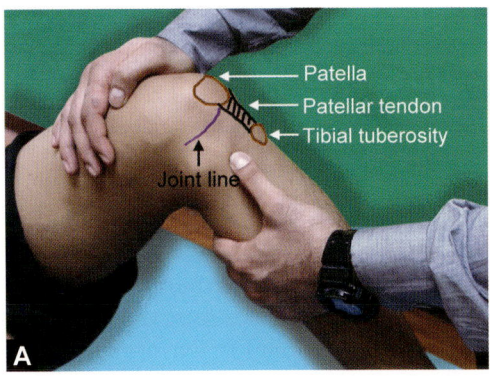
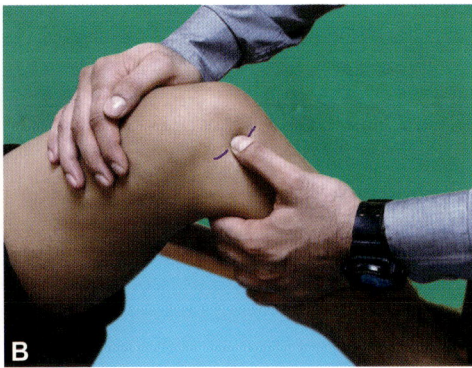

Figs. 8.9A and B: Palpation of the joint line.

III. Patellar tap: To ascertain an excess of fluid in the joint.

Method: Patient lies supine with the *knee in extension*. For the right knee of the patient, the examiner uses his left hand to squeeze the excess fluid in the suprapatellar pouch from proximal to distal direction and then the hand is held in the same position just above the patella (*Note: Suprapatellar pouch extends four finger breadth above the superior border of patella*). Then, tip of all the fingers and the thumb of the right hand are placed together on the anterior aspect of the patella and the patella is pushed towards the femoral trochlea with a "jerk" (Fig. 8.10).

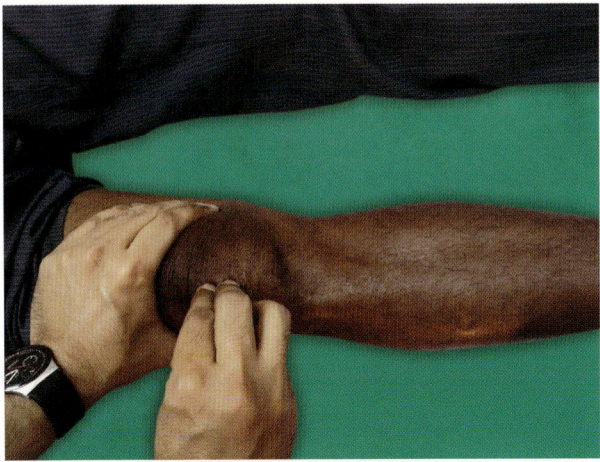

Fig. 8.10: Patellar tap.

In case of an excess of fluid, the patella hits the femoral trochlea and bounces back. Multiple repetitions are performed to confirm the finding.

Interpretation: Positive tap indicates excess fluid in the joint. However, this technique is valid for moderate fluid in the joint. "Tap" is negative in case of minimal or severe effusion.

> In the case of mild effusion, the "tap" is negative due to the minimal fluid, which cannot make the patella float over the trochlea. In addition, "tap" is negative in case of severe effusion as it is hard to displace patella during tap due to excess fluid *(Normal amount of synovial fluid in the knee joint: 5 mL).*

Minimal fluid in the knee joint could be assessed in a standing position where the minimal fluid gravitates to the lower part of the knee joint and then the tap can be performed. However, the quadriceps should be completely relaxed while performing this test.

Stroke/Bulge test for effusion: With patient supine and extended knee; examiner strokes upwards with the edge of the hand on the medial parapatellar side to milk the fluid into the superior and lateral compartment. The test is positive if fluid returns into the medial side of the knee leading to bulge of medial parapatellar gutter.

IV. **Crepitus:** To ascertain the condition of the tibiofemoral or patellofemoral cartilage.
   Method: It is assessed by keeping the hand over the knee while moving the knee though the available range of movement. The crepitus (fixed/mobile) is felt over the palmar aspect of the hand of the crepitus. (*Note: crepitus can also be assessed during movement of the knee*).
   Fixed crepitus: The crepitus felt could be fixed in its location while it is felt. It means that every time the knee is moved through the range of movement (ROM), the crepitus is elicited in the same sector of the ROM. This is observed in OA where there are geographically fixed lesions of the cartilage.
   Mobile crepitus: It implies that the crepitus elicited once might not be felt again or where there is no specific sector in ROM where it is felt. This is observed in case of loose bodies/mobile meniscal flaps wherein a loose body/flap creates crepitus only when it is entrapped between the two articulating surfaces. Once it moves away from the articulating surfaces, the crepitus is not elicited.

V. **Synovial hypertrophy:** Synovial hypertrophy is merely a sign indicating the reaction of the synovium to another existing pathology (infection, arthritis, meniscal tear, loose body etc). But, it does not indicate the etiology.
   Method: With the patient supine and knee extended, the synovial hypertrophy is felt while palpating over MFC (medial femoral condyle) medial to the medial border of the patella (Fig. 8.11).
   Although synovium is present all over the joint, it is easy to palpate it over the MFC because there is no thick tendon over the MFC (as vastus medialis is mostly muscular). However, superiorly thick quadriceps tendon and the laterally taut IT band prevent the palpation of synovium over those areas.

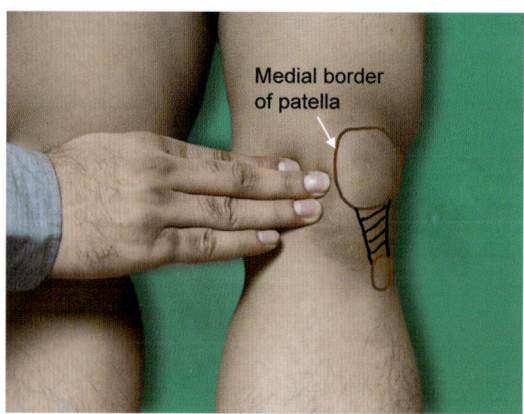

Fig. 8.11: Palpation of synovial hypertrophy.

VI. Retropatellar tenderness: It is performed to ascertain patello-femoral cartilage health. There are two methods to perform this test, patella grinding and the facet tenderness method.

(i) *Patellar grinding test*: This test helps in assessing the lesions of patellofemoral joint (either patella or trochlea). [*Note*: *It should be done at the end of the examination as it is provocative test and could be quite painful*].

Method: With patient supine and knee extended, examiner places his entire hand over the patella , gently presses it against the femoral trochlea and hand is rotated clockwise over the patella (Fig. 8.12).

Interpretation: In case of patellofemoral cartilage lesions, the patient winces with pain.

(ii) *Facet tenderness*: To ascertain the patellar (only) cartilage health.

Method: With patient supine and knee extended; for the left knee, examiner uses the thumb of his left hand and pushes the patella medially uncovering the under surface of the medial facet out of the trochlea. Next, the index finger of the right hand is insinuated onto the under surface of the medial facet of the patella and feel for facet tenderness. Similarly, push the patella laterally with the index finger of the right hand and feel for tenderness under the lateral facet with an index finger of the left hand (Figs. 8.13A and B).

Interpretation: A tender facet, medial or lateral, is suggestive of damage to the patellar cartilage.

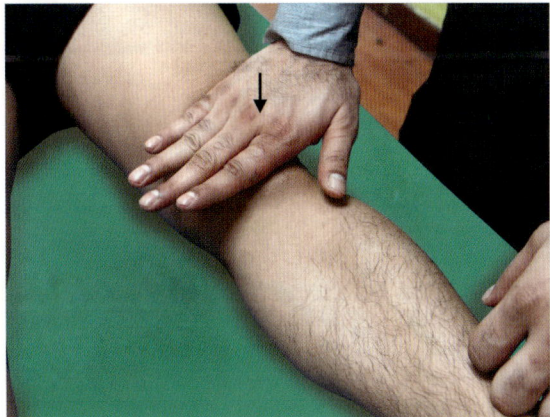

Fig. 8.12: Patellar grinding test.

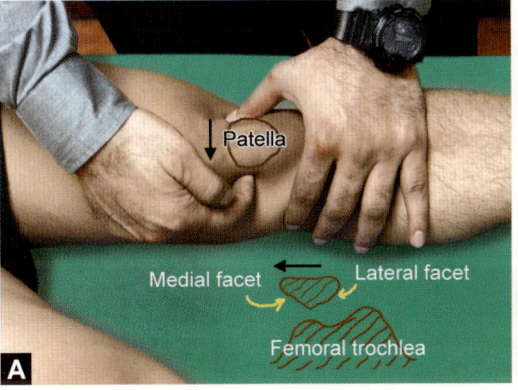
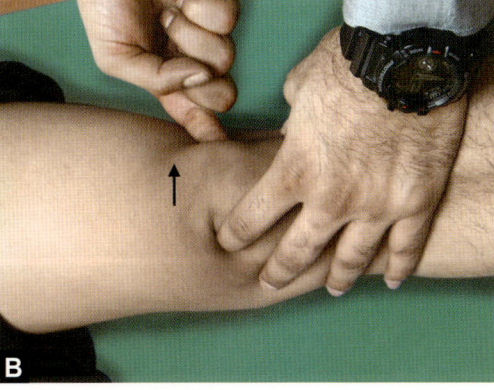

Figs. 8.13A and B: Palpation of medial and lateral facet of patella.

VII. Palpating popliteal fossa: For any swelling, deep tenderness.

VIII. Ligament laxity: Recurrent patellar dislocation (RPD) can have an association with hyperlaxity. One can use the Beighton score to assess the hyperlaxity *(Read chapter 4 for Beighton score)*.

Movements

- Major movements at knee joint are Flexion and Extension, and small degrees of medial and lateral rotations. However, the latter is clinically not recorded.
- **Flexion:** Normal range is 0–140°. It may be a few degree less or more depending upon the bulk of the thigh and calf (Fig. 8.14A).
- **Hyperextension:** Hold the thigh against couch with one hand and try hyperextending the knee while lifting the leg/foot with other hand. This reveals hyperextension, if any. Normally, it is 0° but occasionally it could be up to 10–20° (Fig. 8.14B)
- **Extensor lag:** With the patient sitting, ask him/her to extend the knee against gravity. Note extensor lag, if any. Compare with normal side. (Fig. 8.14C).

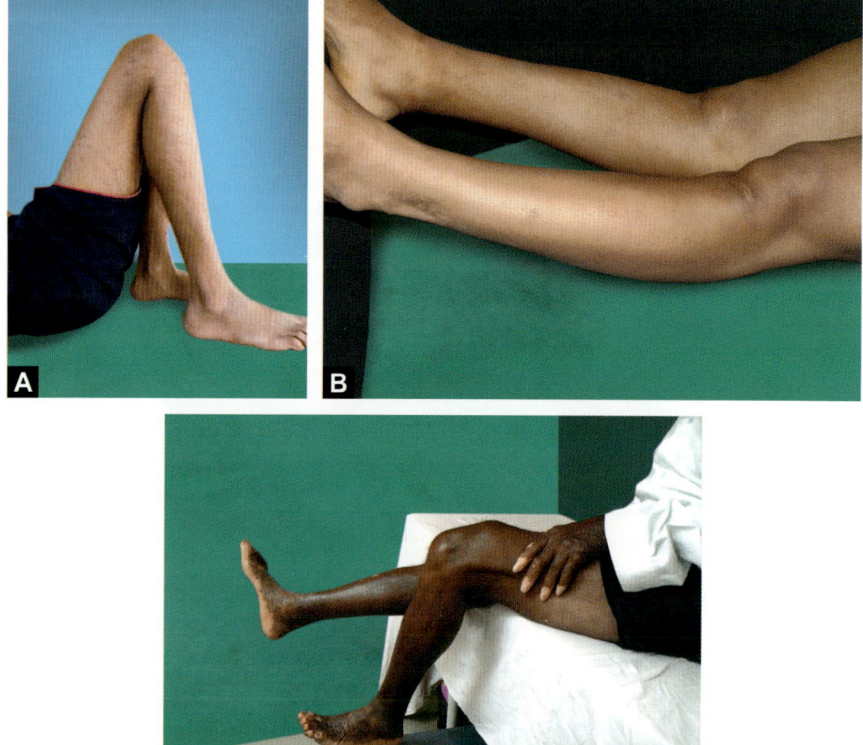

Figs. 8.14A to C: (A) Limited flexion movement of the right knee (see difference in heel levels). (B) Hyperextension of the right knee. (C) Extensor lag in the left knee.

Extensor lag is a condition wherein the knee fails to come back to neutral in full extension or point of starting of flexion (in case of flexion deformity) actively. However, passively the knee can be brought back to the neutral or point of starting of flexion. It is due to a disuse related weakness of quadriceps muscle (not paralyzed).

Measurement

(a) **Length of the limb:** With pelvis squared, the length of the lower limb is measured in the standard fashion [anterior superior iliac spine (ASIS) to medial joint line (relative length of femur); medial joint line to tip of medial malleolus (length of tibia)] (Figs. 8.15A and B).

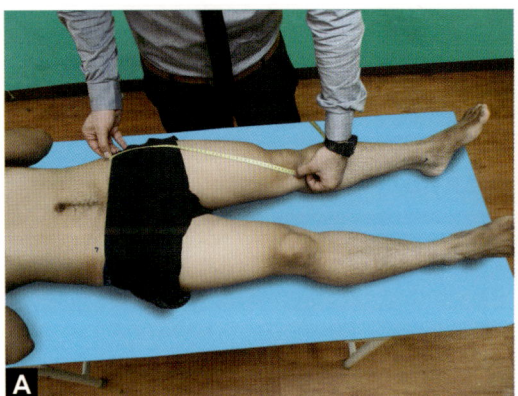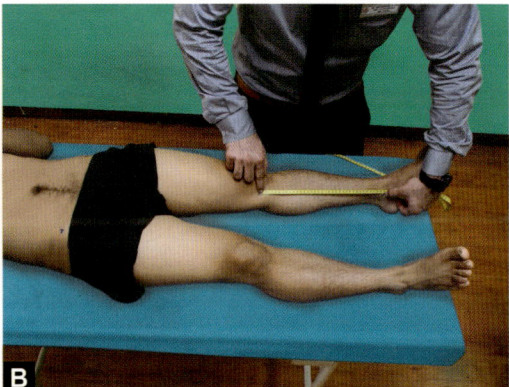

Figs. 8.15A and B: Measurement technique of the lower limb length.

(b) **Wasting of thigh and calf muscles:** Circumferential thigh muscle girth is measured over maximal thigh (15 cm above superior pole of patella) and maximal calf girth from the joint line and compared with the normal side.

(c) **Q angle:** It is the angle between the quadriceps tendon and the patellar tendon. Biomechanically, it is a measure of the lateral pull exerted on the patella by the quadriceps muscle.

Method: Patient lies supine with both lower limbs parallel to each other and quadriceps relaxed. *The most important prerequisite is that the patella should be centered over the knee.* Mark ASIS, the center of the patella and the tibial tuberosity (TT). Join ASIS and the center of the patella with a straight line. Another line is drawn from the center of the patella to the TT. The "inner angle" (α) between the intersection of two lines is the 'Q' angle (Figs. 8.16A and B).

Interpretation: The normal "Q" angle in male and female is 14 and 17° respectively. It is higher in patients with genu valgum.

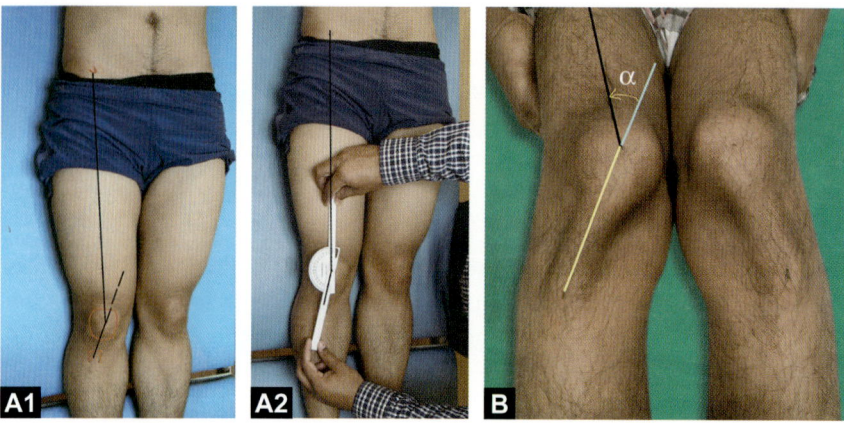

Figs. 8.16A and B: (A) Measurement technique of "Q" angle. (B) High "Q" angle.

Higher the Q angle, the bigger is the risk of lateral patella dislocation due to the larger lateral vector pull over the patella.

Neurovascular Examination of Lower Limbs

As per standard assessment protocol.

Special Tests

(A) Stability test for Anterior cruciate ligament (ACL)
(B) Stability test for Posterior cruciate ligament (PCL)
(C) Medial and lateral collateral ligament stability test
(D) Meniscal tests
(E) Patella stability and other tests
(F) Posterolateral corner of knee stability test

Before we proceed to understand the abnormal opening of the joint due to ligament tear (cruciates and collaterals), we must know the normal opening vs abnormal opening mentioned in the Box 8.2.

> **Box 8.2: Grade of ligament laxity**
> *Grade 0*: <3 mm laxity/opening
> *Grade 1*: 3–5 mm laxity/opening
> *Grade 2*: 5–10 mm laxity/opening
> *Grade 3*: >10 mm laxity/opening

(A) Stability test for ACL

1. **Anterior drawer's test**

   Prerequisite: The knee joint must be flexed up to 90°.

   Method: The patient lies supine on the couch; the knee is flexed to 90° and the hip to 45°. Now, the examiner sits on the forefoot of the patient and stabilizes it. Further, the examiner places both his hands around the upper end of the tibia, palpates the hamstring tendons with the fingers of both hands and feels for its tightness. Ask the patient to relax the hamstrings, if it is found to be taut. Gentle massage over the hamstring too can help in relaxing the hamstrings.

Once the hamstring is relaxed, the examiner places *both the thumbs over the anterior joint line on either side of the patellar tendon.* The purpose of the thumb over the joint line is to feel the normal step off of 1 cm and further relative forward movement of the tibia with respect to the femoral condyle. Now, an anteriorly directed force is given to the upper end of the tibia and then relaxed. This step is repeated a few times to confirm the anterior movement (Fig. 8.17). *One must also feel the end point of 'pull' whether it is hard or soft. A soft end point of 'pull' indicates injury to the ligament whereas hard end point suggests intact ligament.*

Interpretation: In a normal knee with an intact ACL, the tibia cannot be moved more than 1–2 mm forwards beyond the normal step off. The test is considered to be positive if there is soft endfeel, and the tibia moves forwards more than 3 mm. It can be graded as 1, 2 or 3 (Box 8.2).

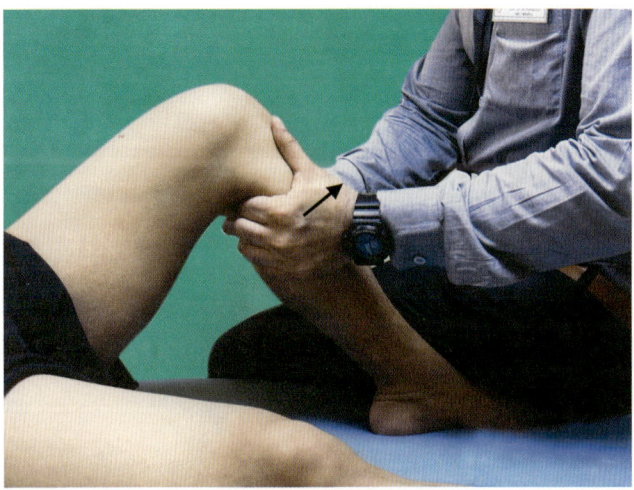

Fig. 8.17: Anterior drawer test.

2. **Lachman test:** It is a *more sensitive* test for ACL tear than the anterior drawer test and is more useful in acute injuries of the knee where the knee cannot be flexed up to 90°.

   Method: The patient lies supine on the couch with knee extended. For the right knee, the examiner holds the lower end of the thigh of the patient with his left hand and the upper end of the leg by the right hand and the knee is gradually brought into 15–20° of flexion. Now, the examiner stabilizes the lower thigh with his left hand while right hand pulls the leg forward and then let loose. The leg is pulled forward couple of times to determine the end point feel (soft/hard) and an estimation of drawer (Fig. 8.18).

   Interpretation: The test is considered positive if the anterior translation >3 mm or the end point feel is soft. If anterior translation <3 mm or the end point is hard, the Lachman is negative.

Modified Lachman test: Performed in obese patients or who have bulky thighs. For right knee with patient supine, examiner flexes the knee upto 15° and places his left thigh under patient's right thigh and places his left hand over patient's thigh to anchor it firmly against his thigh (blue arrow). Now, upper end tibia is pulled forward (orange arrow)to perform Lachman test. (Fig. 8.18B)

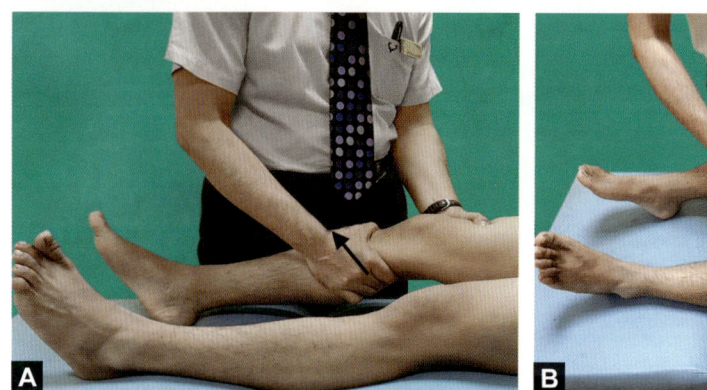
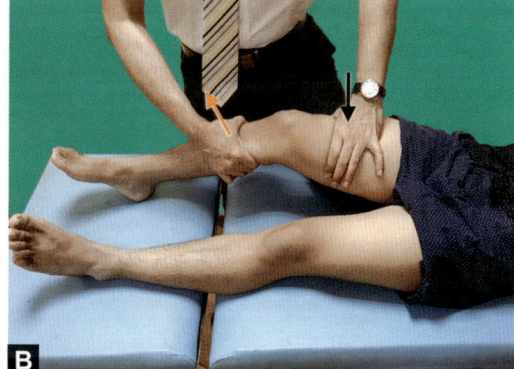

Figs. 8.18A and B: (A) Lachman test. (B) Modified Lachman test.

In case of a complete ACL tear, it is possible to have a positive Lachman but a negative anterior drawer test *due to the **door-stopper effect of the meniscus*** which is effective when the knee is 90° flexed.

In 90° flexion, the intact posterior horn and posterior third of the meniscus blocks the anterior movement of the tibia over the femoral condyle giving a false negative anterior drawer test. However, such a doorstopper effect of meniscus is not seen in 15–30° flexion of the knee while performing the Lachman test.

Another reason why the anterior drawer may be negative despite having an ACL tear is due to either tight hamstrings or pain in the knee leading to hamstring spasm.

3. **Pivot shift test:** *Most specific test for the ACL tear.*

   Basis of the test: In the knee with ACL tear, the knee subluxes in valgus, internal rotation and extended position.

   Method and interpretation: For left side; On an extended knee, the examiner holds patients left ankle with his left hand and holds the upper end of leg with right hand and index finger just below the upper end of fibula. Now, the leg is gently internally rotated with left hand and valgus stress is provided whereas right hand gives counter for valgus. Now the knee is gradually flexed. The knee subluxation (which appeared with knee in valgus, internal rotation and extension) reduces to normal at 20–30° of flexion by a click, jump or a glide which is observed over the anterolateral aspect of knee (Fig. 8.19).

(B) Stability tests for PCL

1. **Posterior drawer's test:**

   Method: The patient lies supine on the couch with index knee flexed to 90° and hip to 45°. The examiner sits on the forefoot of the patient and stabilizes it. Then the examiner places both his hands around the upper end of the tibia, *keeps both his thumbs over the joint line,* and pushes the tibia backwards and again pulls forward. This step is repeated a few times to confirm the posterior movement (Fig. 8.20).

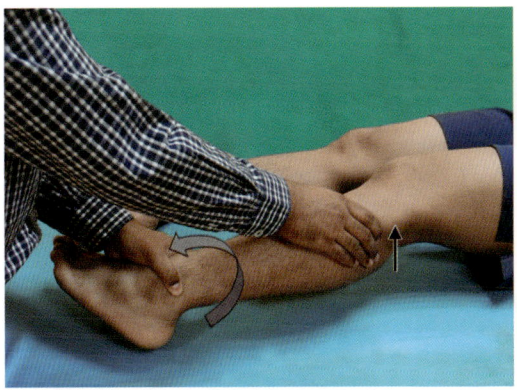

Fig. 8.19: Pivot shift test.

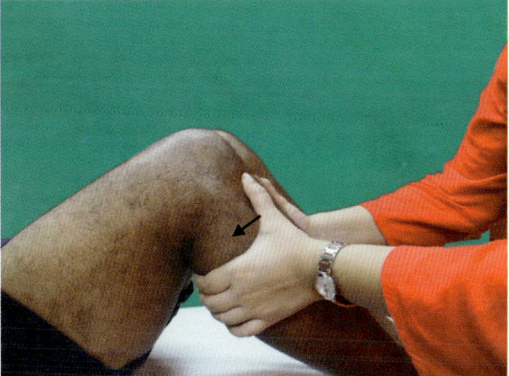

Fig. 8.20: Posterior drawer test.

Interpretation: The thumb over the joint line can simultaneously feel the tibia, femur, and the normal 1 cm anterior step off. In case of a PCL tear, the tibia remains in the "posterior sag position," and the step off between the tibia and femur is not felt. Further, the tibia can be pushed backwards due to lack of posterior support. The amount of posterior shift can vary from 3 mm to 20 mm, rarely more. Also; feel for end point, soft/hard.

2. **Posterior sag sign:**

   Method: The patient lies supine on the couch with both knees flexed to 90° and hips to 45°. Now, the examiner goes on the side of the patient, and tangentially watches the alignment of the tibia to the knee on the index and normal side. Now draw an imaginary line from the shin of tibia towards the patella. In a normal knee, the imaginary line does not touch the patella, and passes few mm anterior to it whereas in case of PCL tear, the imaginary line touches the anterior surface of patella or passes through the patella. (Figs. 8.21A and B).

   One can modify this test by placing a pen over the shin. The pen would touch the patella in case of a PCL tear.

   Interpretation: In case of a PCL tear, the tibia sags posteriorly below the level of the patella, and this leads to an imaginary line or the pen touching the patellar tendon and patella.

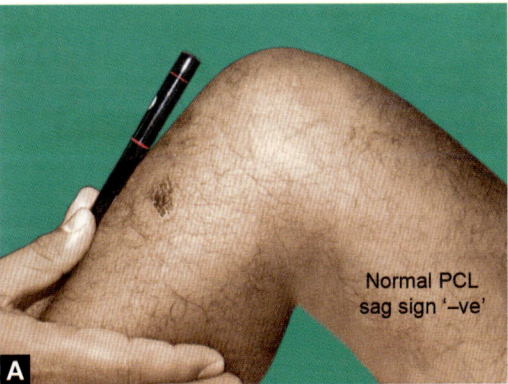

Normal PCL
sag sign '–ve'

A

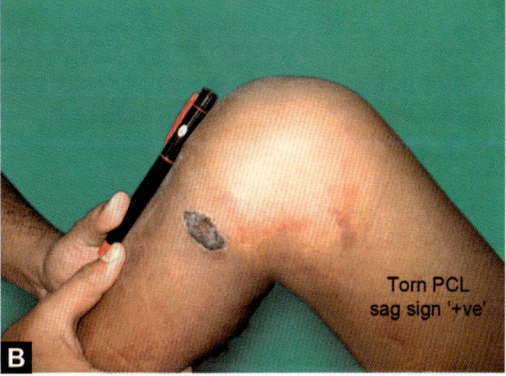

Torn PCL
sag sign '+ve'

B

Figs. 8.21A and B: Sag sign for posterior cruciate ligament.

3. Godfrey's sag sign:

Method: The patient lies supine on the couch, and both knees and the hips are flexed to 90° with both heels at the same level. Now, the examiner goes on the side of the patient and tangentially watches the alignment of the tibia concerning the knee (Fig. 8.22).

Interpretation: Normally, if an imaginary line is drawn from the tibial shin upwards, it does not touch the patella or patellar tendon. However, in case of PCL tear, the tibia sags downwards due to gravity and the imaginary line touches the patellar tendon and patella. Compare with the normal knee.

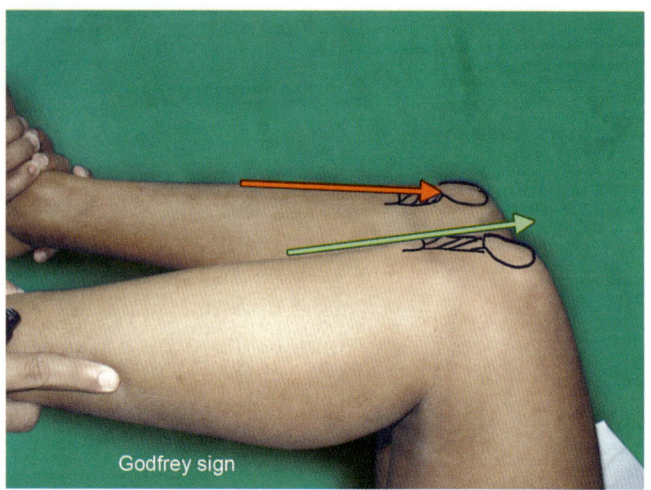

Fig. 8.22: Godfrey sign (Green arrow, normal knee; Red arrow, PCL tear).

4. Quadriceps active test:

Method: The patient lies supine with knee flexed to 90° and hips at 45°. The examiner holds the foot of the patient, anchors it to the examination couch and asks the patient to extend knee while examiners continues to hold foot against the couch. This activates their quadriceps.

Interpretation: In a normal knee, the activation of quadriceps will not lead to any noticeable anterior movement of the tibia (observed at the anterior knee joint line). However, in case of a PCL tear with tibia sagged posteriorly, the quadriceps activation leads to a noticeable anterior movement of the tibia. Repeated quadriceps activation makes it quite obvious.

(C) Medial and lateral collateral ligament (MCL, LCL) stability tests

1. Valgus stress test: For MCL tear

Method: The patient lies supine on the couch with the index knee extended. The examiner stands on the lateral aspect of the leg. For the right knee, the examiner holds the right leg at the level of the ankle while the right hand kept at the level of the lateral aspect of the knee (over the lateral femoral condyle), with a middle finger over the medial joint line. Valgus stress is applied using the hand holding the ankle, whereas the other hand at the level of femoral condyle acts as a fulcrum. The test is performed in 0° extension and 30° flexion.

Another easy method is to hold the right ankle in the axilla between the chest wall and the arm of the examiner while the index, middle and ring fingers of the right hand are kept over the medial joint line. The left hand is kept over the lateral femoral condyle to give valgus support, and the leg is drawn into the valgus (Fig. 8.23).

Interpretation: In the case of an MCL tear, there is abnormal medial opening felt by the fingers placed over the medial joint line.

If there is significant opening in 0° extension, it indicates a tear in the cruciate ligaments as well as the posteromedial structures (posteromedial capsule, posterior oblique ligament, MCL)
If there is significant opening in 30° flexion only, it indicates isloated MCL tear.

2. **Varus stress test:** For LCL tear
   Method: The patient lies supine on the couch with the index knee extended. The examiner stands on the lateral aspect of the leg. For the right knee, the examiner holds the right leg at the level of the ankle. The left hand holds the upper end of leg in such a way that the thumb is kept over the lateral joint line and the remaining fingers are on the medial side to act as a fulcrum. A varus stress is applied using the hand holding the ankle whereas the other hand at the level of the knee acts as a fulcrum. The test is performed in 0° extension and 30° flexion (Fig. 8.24).
   Interpretation: In the case of an LCL tear, there is an abnormal lateral opening felt by the thumb placed over the lateral joint line.

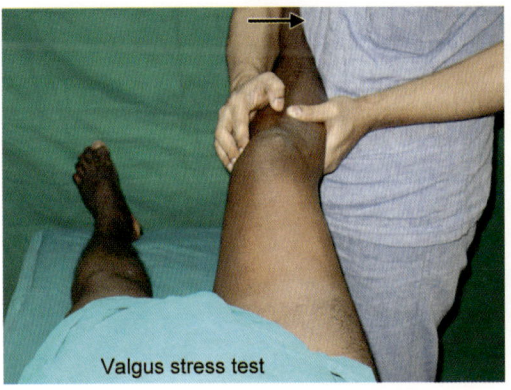

Valgus stress test

Fig. 8.23: Valgus stress test for medial collateral ligament.

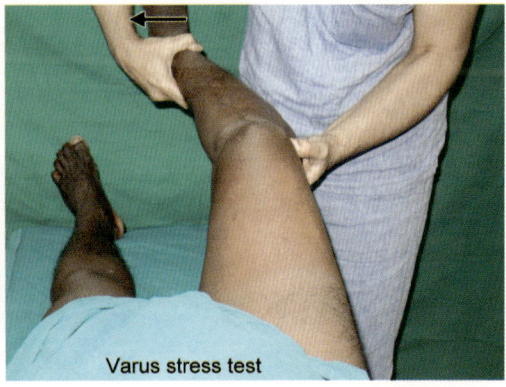

Varus stress test

Fig. 8.24: Varus stress test for lateral collateral ligament.

If there is a significant opening in 0° extension, it indicates a tear of cruciate ligaments as well as the LCL and posterolateral structures.
If there is a significant opening in 30° flexion, only, it indicates LCL tear alone.

(D) Meniscal tests

Joint line tenderness is a more sensitive test whereas McMurray test is a more specific test for meniscus tear

1. **McMurray's test**
   (i) *McMurray for medial meniscus (MM):*
   Method: The patient lies supine on the couch with the knee extended. The *patient is asked to flex their index knee as much as possible* (Note: The examiner must not forcibly flex the knee, as most of the time, the patients have a posterior third tear of the meniscus and they

may experience severe pain if the knee is forcibly flexed). For the left knee, the examiner holds patient's left heel with their left hand while the right hand holds the distal end of the femur. Now, the *leg is externally rotated* and given a valgus stress with left hand, where right hand acts like a fulcrum, and the knee is gently extended (Fig. 8.25).

Interpretation: In case of MM tear, the patient will wince with pain.

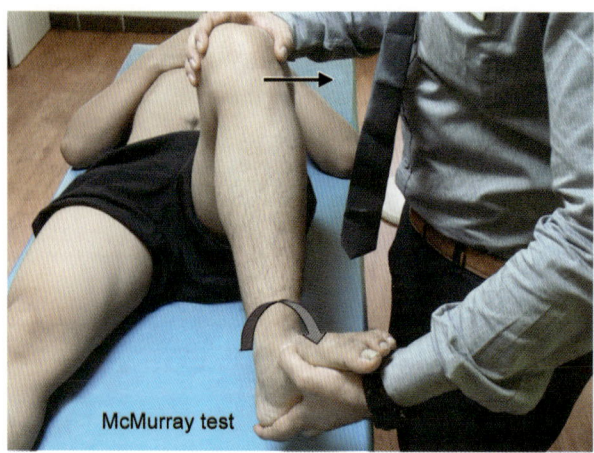

McMurray test

Fig. 8.25: McMurray test for meniscus.

(ii) *McMurray for Lateral meniscus (LM)*:

Method: The patient lies supine on the couch with the knee extended. The *patient is asked to flex their index knee as much as possible.* For the left knee, the examiner holds the patient's left heel with the left hand while the right hand holds the distal end of the femur. Now, the *leg is internally rotated* and given a varus stress with left hand, and the knee is gently extended.

Interpretation: In case of LM tear, the patient will wince with pain.

> *An approximate way to assess the region of the meniscal tear (anterior/middle/posterior third).* From full flexion to extension, the knee moves in an arc of movement. Divide this arc into three-thirds.
> - ***If the pain is felt in the posterior third arc:*** Posterior third tear of meniscus
> - ***If the pain is felt in the middle third arc:*** Middle third tear of meniscus
> - ***If the pain is felt in the anterior third arc:*** Anterior third tear of meniscus

2. **Apley's grinding test:** It is a *useful test to differentiate between meniscal and ligamentous tear.*

   However, this test *is not routinely performed* as there is an element of grinding involved in the test which may "theoretically" damage the meniscus.

   This test *has two parts*: Apley's compression test and Apley's distraction test.

   Method: The patient lies prone on the couch, and the affected knee is flexed to 90°. The patient's thigh is then anchored to the examination couch by the examiner's knee. Then, examiner holds the leg just below the level of the ankle.

Apley's distraction test: The leg is distracted and rotated internally as well as externally. If the patient experiences pain, it is suggestive of ligamentous injury (collateral, cruciate) as the injured ligament is stretched in "distraction" (Fig. 8.26A).

Apley's compression test: The examiner applies downwards force on the foot and the leg is rotated internally as well as externally. This relaxes the ligaments and compresses the menisci. If patient experiences pain, it is suggestive of the meniscal tear and not the ligaments (Fig. 8.26B).

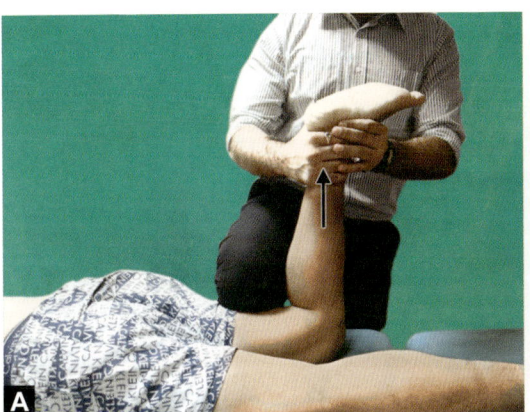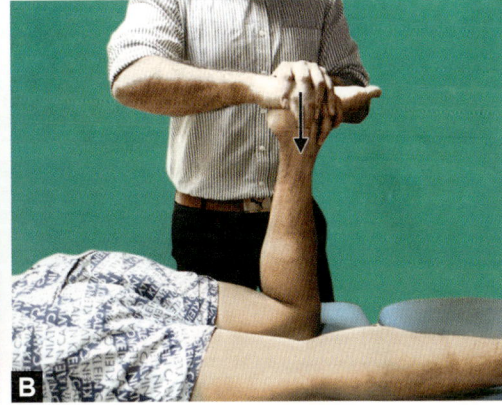

Figs. 8.26A and B: Apley test. (A) Distraction test. (B) Compression test.

3. **Thessaly test:** It is the most sensitive and specific test for a meniscal tear.

    Method: The patient stands on one leg while the examiner supports him/her by holding their palms with his hands. Now the patient flexes his knee to 20° and rotates the thigh and body internally and externally while maintaining the knee flexion. The test is performed first on the normal and then on the index knee (Figs. 8.27A and B).

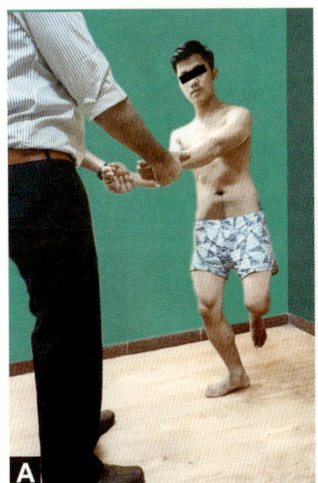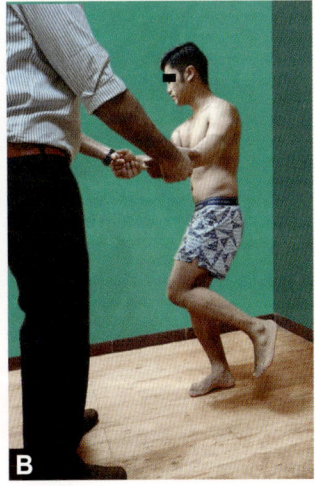

Figs. 8.27A and B: Thessaly test. (A) With internal rotation of body. (B) With external rotation of body.

Interpretation: The patient may experience pain over medial or lateral joint line while rotating their thigh indicating meniscal tear.

(E) Patella stability and other tests

1. Fairbank's apprehension test: The test is performed in *patients with suspected recurrent patellar dislocation (RPD)*

Method: The patient lies supine, and the knee is kept in extension. The examiner holds the patella between their thumb and index finger. Further, the patella is pushed laterally by the thumb of the examiner while the knee is gently flexed from 0° to 30° and extended back to neutral. This step is repeated a few times between full extension and 30° flexion (Fig. 8.28).

Interpretation: In patients with RPD, the patient shows apprehension on their face and stops the examiner from continuing with further flexion or performing this manoever.

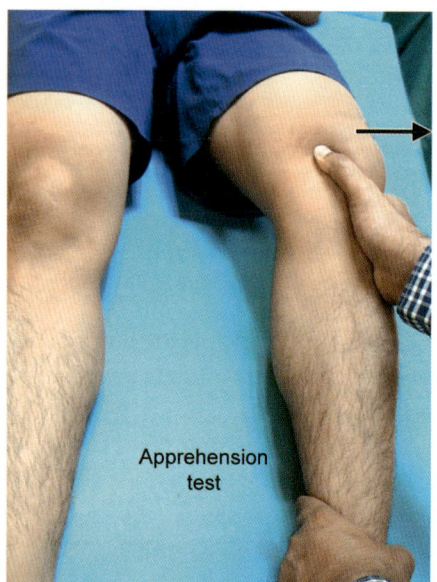

Apprehension test

Fig. 8.28: Apprehension for patellar dislocation.

Rationale of apprehension test

To prevent any lateral subluxation of patella, the major stabilizers are MPFL and trochlear anatomy. Normally, the patella engages into the trochlear groove due to an intact MPFL while it moves from 0° to 30° flexion. A nonengaging patella is due to insufficiency of MPFL which leads to positive apprehension. After 30° flexion, the patella homes in due to normal trochlear anatomy. However, if patella subluxates or dislocates even after 30° of flexion, it may indicate trochlear dysplasia.

---

2. Quadrant test: The test is performed in patients with *suspected patellar dislocation to assess the integrity of the medial or lateral soft tissue structures in extension.*

Method: The knee is kept in extension while the patient is lying supine. Three equally placed vertical lines are drawn over the patella dividing the patella into four vertical quadrants. Then, the patella is pushed medially and laterally with equal force (Fig. 8.29).

Interpretation: Normally, the patella moves a maximum of two quadrants in either direction. Any further movement (three quadrants or more), is indicative of insufficiency of the medial or lateral soft-tissue restraints. Less than a quadrant indicates tight structures. Always compare it with the normal side.

3. **Patella horizontal tilt test:** The test is performed on patients with *suspected tight lateral structures* (lateral retinaculum, IT band).

   Method: The knee is kept in extension while the patient lies supine. Normally, the lateral border of the patella remains at a lower level than the medial, or it remains in external rotation (faces laterally). The patella is held between thumb and index finger of both hands, and lifted and tilted internally to bring lateral border to the same level as the medial border or even a bit higher (Fig. 8.30).

   Interpretation: If one can bring the lateral border of the patella to the same level as the medial or even above, it indicates that the lateral structures are not tight. However, if it cannot be tilted as normal, and remains below horizontal, it indicates tight lateral *structures.* *(Clinical importance: Tight lateral structures tilt patella laterally, and cause lateral excess pressure syndrome or abnormal patella tracking. This may require surgical release!).*

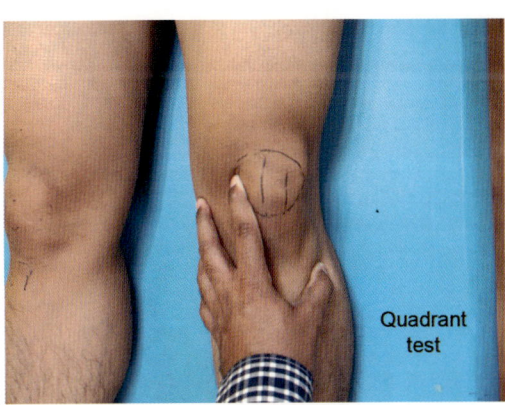
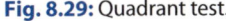

Fig. 8.29: Quadrant test.

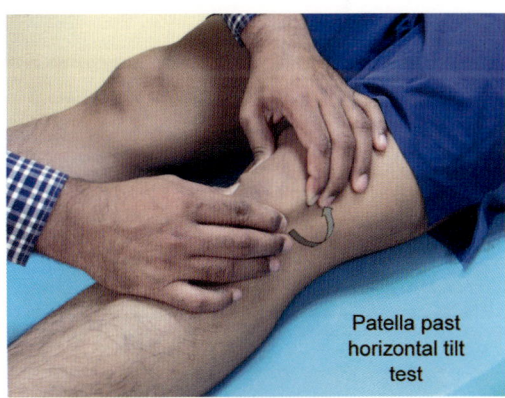

Fig. 8.30: Patella past horizontal tilt test.

4. **Patella maltracking (J-sign):** It is done to assess whether *the patella is tracking or moving in the trochlear groove normally or not, with flexion-extension of the knee.*

   Method: The patient sits on the examination couch with both knees flexed to 90°. Then, the patient is asked to extend both the knees simultaneously and patella movement is observed from 90° flexion until complete extension. This step is repeated several times to observe the tracking pattern (Figs. 8.31A and B).

   Interpretation: Normally, the patella moves upwards in a straight line with a subtle lateral movement at the terminal extension (yellow arrow). However, in cases where the tracking is abnormal, the patella suddenly moves laterally with a jerk (J-sign) [Black arrow].

Positive J-sign is seen in lateral retinacular tightness, VMO deficiency, increased Q-angle, trochlear dysplasia.

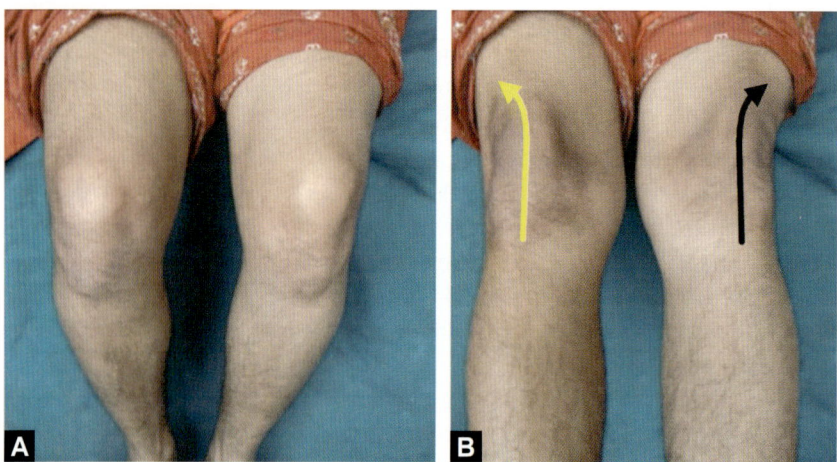

Figs. 8.31A and B: (A) Maltracking assessment of patella. (B) Black arrow is suggestive of sudden jerky outward movement of patella while knee moves in extension from flexion.

Assessment of the Posterolateral Corner (PLC) of the Knee

Isolated PLC injuries are rare, but occur in combination with injuries to cruciate ligaments.

1. **External rotation recurvatum test:** To assess the integrity of the *posterolateral corner (PLC)* structures

   Method: The patient lies supine while the knee is kept in extension. Next, the examiner lifts both the legs off the couch holding both the great toes together with their hands and watches for *"abnormal recurvatum at the knee"* and *"external rotation of the leg"* occurring at the index side in contrast to the normal side (Figs. 8.32A and B).

   Interpretation: Injury to the PLC causes tibia sag in the recurvatum while the leg goes in external rotation.

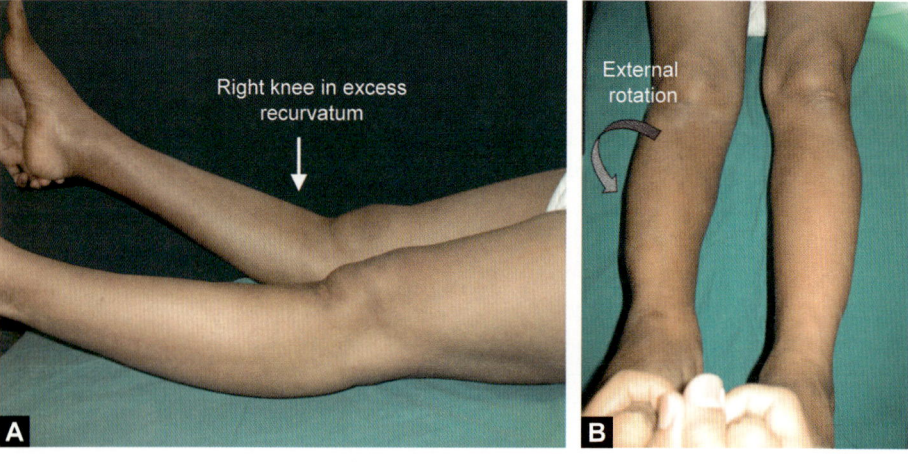

Figs. 8.32A and B: External rotation recurvatum test.

2. **Dial test:** To evaluate the integrity of the PLC structures.

   Method: The patient lies prone on the couch; both knees are flexed to 90° while the plantar aspect of the foot faces upwards. Another assistant can hold both the thighs together to prevent the rotation of the thigh. Now, the examiner holds both the ankles separately and gives an external rotation to the leg while watching for an abnormal external rotation occurring at the level of the knee as compared to the normal side. Watch for the "thigh-foot angle" and compare with the normal side. Then, the knee is flexed to 30°and the same external rotation is repeated and "thigh-foot angle" is observed (Figs. 8.33A). (Note: This test can also be done supine; Fig. 8.33B).

   Interpretation: The index side with damage to the PLC will have excess external rotation (>10°) as compared to the normal side.

   - **If ER is more in 30° only and not in 90°**, it implies injured PLC, and normal PCL.
   - **If ER is more in both 30° and 90°**, then both PCL and PLC are damaged.

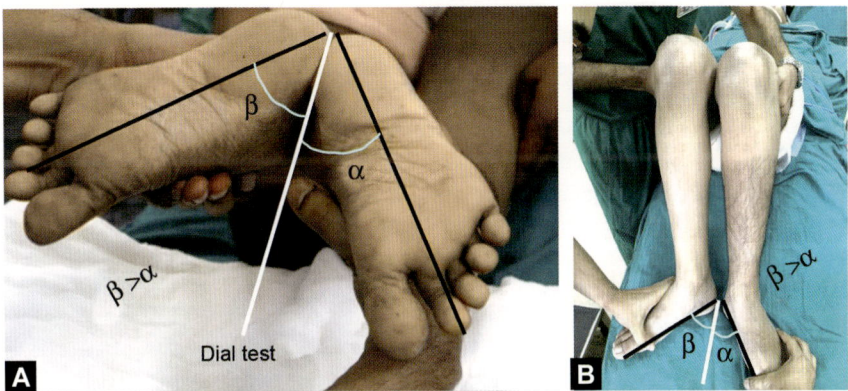

Figs. 8.33A and B: Dial test for posterolateral corner injury.

3. **Reverse pivot shift test:** Performed for diagnosis of PLC injuries (Self reading).

Examination of the Joint Above and Below

- Hip joint and ankle-foot complex

Lymph Node Examination

- Inguinal and popliteal

Knee examination proforma

1. **Gait**
2. **Attitude**
3. **Inspection**
   - **General findings:** *Skin overlying, Swelling, scar, sinus*
   - **Specifics findings of inspection**
     (a) From front
       – Deformity (varus/valgus), muscle wasting (thigh and calf), position of patella, limb length discrepancy, supra/parapatellar swelling
     (b) From side
       – Sagittal plane deformity: flexion/recurvatum deformity
     (c) From back
       – Popliteal fossa, muscle wasting
4. **Palpation**
   - Local rise in temperature
   - Tenderness: soft tissue and bony landmarks
   - Joint line tenderness, patellar tap, crepitus, synovial hypertrophy, Retropatellar tenderness (Patella grinding, Patella facet tenderness), popliteal fossa
   - Hyperlaxity of joints
   - *Confirmation of palpatory characteristics of swelling, scar, sinus, ulcer, deformities*
5. **Movements:** Active and passive
   - Flexion, extension. Look for extensor lag
   - Crepitus, clicks, thud at joint line (in discoid meniscus); if any
6. **Measurements**
   - Limb length, thigh-calf circumference
   - Q angle, extensor lag measurement
7. **Neurovascular examination**
8. **Special tests**
   (a) *Anterior stability tests for ACL*: Anterior drawer, Lachman, Pivot shift test
   (b) *Posterior stability test for PCL*: Posterior drawer, Sag sign, Godfrey test, quadriceps active test
   (c) *Medial collateral stability test*: Valgus stress test in 0° extension and 30° flexion
   (d) *Lateral collateral stability test*: Varus stress test in 0° extension and 30° flexion
   (e) *Meniscus test*: McMurray's, Apley's grinding and Thessaly test
   (f) *Patella stability and other tests*: Apprehension test, quadrant test, patella past-horizontal test, patella maltracking
   (g) *Posterolateral corner test*: External rotation recurvatum test, Dial test, Reverse pivot shift test
9. **Joint above (Hip) and below (ankle)**
10. **Lymph node examination**

**Common conditions affecting the knee joint with
their salient features**

1. **Primary osteoarthrosis of the knee (osteoarthritis)**
   - *Affects*: Adults > 50–55 years of age; obesity is a major risk factor
   - *Presents with*: Mechanical pain, difficulty in walking, squatting, and sitting cross-legged
   - *Pathologically*: Loss of articular cartilage in the joint due to wear and tear
   - *Clinically*:
     – Joint line tenderness
     – Crepitus
     – Painfully restricted ROM
     – Often genu varum and flexion deformity
   - *Diagnosis*: X-ray
   - *Treatment*: Nonsteroidal anti-inflammatory drugs (NSAIDs), physiotherapy, intraarticular steroid or hyaluronic acid injection, arthroscopic debridement, high tibial osteotomy, total knee replacement.

2. *Recurrent instability due to ligament tears (ACL/PCL/MCL/LCL/RDP/combination)*:
   - *Affects*: Mostly young patients
   - *Presents with*: Instability while running/jumping/pivoting sports/climbing stairs, etc. Depending upon the ligament injured, pain and locking, may be associated with ligament laxity
   - H/o twisting injury/road traffic accident (RTA); Usually H/o inability to stand and walk after the injury, immediate swelling
   - *Pathologically*: Complete tear of the ligament
   - *Clinically*: Appropriate tests are positive
   - *Diagnosis*: Magnetic resonance imaging (MRI), X-ray
   - *Treatment*: Rehabilitation, surgical repair/reconstruction: (Arthroscopic/open).

3. *Tubercular arthritis*:
   - *Affects*: Any age
   - *Presents with*: Night pain, deformity, loss of ROM, systemic features (fever/loss of weight, loss of appetite)
   - *Pathologically*: Three stages
     – Stage of synovitis
     – Stage of arthritis
     – *Stage of triple deformity* (stage of triple dislocation: It is a misnomer as there is no dislocation).
   - *Clinically*:
     – Constitutional symptoms ±, synovitis, features of arthritis
     – Triple deformity in late stages: Flexion, posterior subluxation and external rotation at the knee due to "spasm in the biceps femoris tendon," widespread destruction of capsule and supporting structures, arthritis of joint.
   - *Diagnosis*: X-ray, MRI, synovial or bone biopsy
   - *Treatment*: Anti-tubercular therapy (ATT), synovectomy. Biaxial traction to correct triple deformity followed by arthrodesis. Later total knee replacement if required.

4. *Chondromalacia Patella*:
   - *Affects*: Young patients especially females from 2nd decade to 4th decade, often bilateral
   - Usually idiopathic, other etiologies (trauma, infection, inflammation, etc.) are possible

- *Presents with*: Knee pain, especially while keeping the knee bent for long time (in class-room, etc.), climbing stairs, squatting or sitting cross-legged.
- *Pathologically*: Fraying and fibrillation of patellar cartilage
- *Clinically*: Patellar facet tenderness+, Patellar grating+, deep flexion painful
- *Diagnosis*: MRI
- *Treatment*: Activity modification, physiotherapy, analgesics. Usually self-limiting by 6 months to a few years. Rarely, needs arthroscopic debridement of frayed cartilage.

5. *Osgood-Schlatter disease*:
   - *Affects*: Young adolescent kids who are active in sports, often bilateral
   - *Presents with*: Anterior knee pain, especially while running, climbing stairs, squatting
   - *Pathologically*: Avascular necrosis and fragmentation of tibial tuberosity (TT) apophysis
   - *Clinically*: Tenderness + over the tibial tuberosity and TT is prominent (Fig. 8.34)
   - *Diagnosis*: Lateral X-ray of the knee shows fragmented TT
   - *Treatment*: NSAIDs, physiotherapy. Stop/limit sports activity. Usually self-limiting by 6 months to a few years. Rarely needs arthroscopic/open debridement of frayed separated fragments.

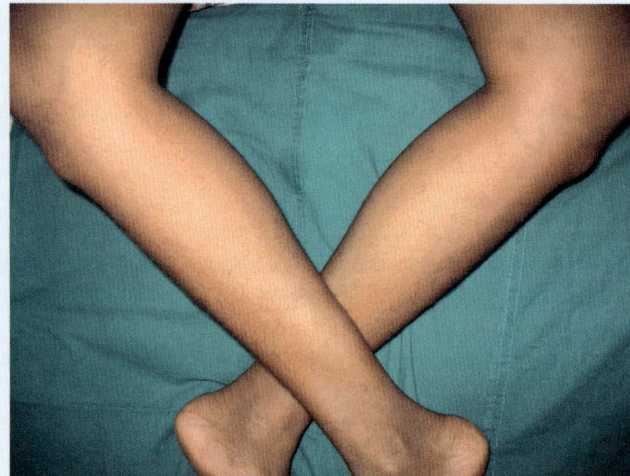

Fig. 8.34: Prominence of bilateral tibial tuberosity seen in Osgood Schlatter disease.

6. *Discoid meniscus (DM).*
   - Congenital disorder; Meniscus is not semilunar, it is like a disc or a coin
   - Usually bilateral, presentation is at any age
   - Lateral discoid meniscus>>>medial DM
   - *Presents with*: Thud and or knee pain with activity
   - *Pathologically*: Large, disk-like meniscus (complete/incomplete)
   - *Clinically*: *Thud/click* present over the joint line. Tenderness over the joint line ±. Meniscal tear test may be positive
   - *Diagnosis*: X-ray, MRI (confirmatory)
   - *Treatment*: Conservative if asymptomatic. For symptomatic cases; Arthroscopic partial meniscectomy (Saucerization).

7. **Bakers cyst**:
   - **Affects**: Mostly in adults or the elderly with coexisting arthritis or intra-articular pathology of the knee
   - **Presents with**: Pain and swelling in the popliteal fossa, coexisting arthritis/synovitis of the knee
   - **Pathologically**: It is *not* a true cyst and is posteriorly located between the medial head of gastrocnemius and capsular reflection of the semimembranosus (oblique popliteal ligament). Whenever there is a chronic synovial irritation due to underlying intra-articular pathology, there is an excess of synovial fluid formation. This leads to the herniation of the knee synovium due to excess fluid pressure through the naturally occurring rent in the posterior capsule of the knee with a unidirectional valve. The excess joint fluid keeps collecting in the cyst due to unidirectional valve.
     (*Note: The fact what we need to remember is that "Baker's cyst is almost always secondary to a primary intra-articular pathology in the knee, like OA or rheumatoid arthritis."*)
   - **Clinically**:
     – Swelling in the popliteal fossa; Firm and prominent on extended knee while soft and less prominent on flexed knee (Foucher's sign)
     – Knee may have features of other pathology like OA/rheumatoid
   - **Investigation**: X-ray, ultrasonography (USG), MRI (confirmatory)
   - **Treatment**: Treat the intra-articular knee pathology, the Baker's cyst may subside. If it remains symptomatic even after primary treatment, it may need excision.
   - **Complication**: Baker's cyst can rupture and mimics deep vein thrombosis of the calf.

Notes

Clinical Evaluation of the Ankle Joint and Foot

▌BRIEF ANATOMY OF THE ANKLE AND FOOT

1. **Basic osteology**
   - The *ankle joint* is formed between the lower end of the tibia, fibula, and talus, whereas the *subtalar joint* is formed between the calcaneum and talus.
   - Twenty-eight bones and fifty-five joints take part in foot-ankle formation
   - The foot can be divided into the hindfoot, midfoot, and forefoot.

Hindfoot	Midfoot	Forefoot
Talus and calcaneum Two joints, ankle and subtalar joint	Midtarsal (3 cuneiforms, navicular, cuboid)	All metatarsals and phalanx

2. **Major ligaments of ankle and foot (Fig. 9.1)**
   - The lower end of the tibia and fibula is bound by the anterior and posterior tibiofibular ligaments
   - *Lateral ligaments of ankle*
     - Anterior Talofibular (ATF), Calcaneofibular (CF) and Posterior Talofibular (PTF) ligament. *[ATF is the weakest of all three, and is most commonly torn in ankle sprain].*
   - *Medial ligament of ankle*
     - Deltoid ligament
   - ***Important ligaments of the foot:*** Spring ligament (plantar calcaneonavicular ligament) and short and long plantar ligaments.

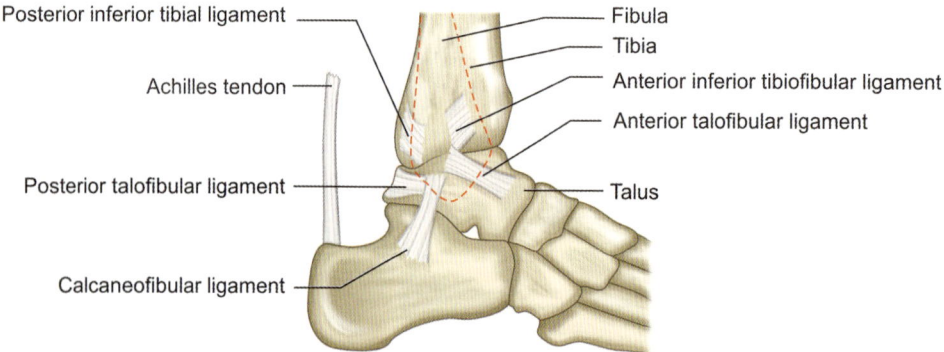

Posterior inferior tibial ligament

Achilles tendon

Posterior talofibular ligament

Calcaneofibular ligament

Fibula

Tibia

Anterior inferior tibiofibular ligament

Anterior talofibular ligament

Talus

Fig. 9.1: Major ligaments of lateral side of the ankle.

3. Arches of the foot (Table 9.1)
- The shape of bones acts as a keystone of the arch short and long plantar ligaments act like staples, Flexor hallucis longus (FHL) acts like tie beam, whereas Tibialis posterior (TP) and Tibialis anterior (TA) are like suspensions of the arch.
- Functions of the arch
  - Divides the weight between various tarsals and metatarsals, makes the foot flexible, easy walking on uneven surfaces, helps in propulsion of body in walking and running and shock absorption.

4. The primary function of ankle and foot is to transmit body weight during locomotion.

5. Structures crossing the ankle under various retinaculum (Table 9.2).

Table 9.1: Types of arches of the foot and their components.

Medial longitudinal arch	Lateral longitudinal arch	Transverse arch
Calcaneum, talus, navicular, cuneiform, and 3 medial metatarsals	Calcaneum, cuboid, and 2 lateral metatarsals	Cuneiform, cuboid, and bases of metatarsals

Table 9.2: Structures crossing the ankle under various retinaculum.

Anteriorly, under extensor retinaculum	Medially, under medial retinaculum	Laterally, under peroneal retinaculum
Tibialis anterior, extensor hallucis longus (EHL), anterior tibial artery, deep peroneal nerve, extensor digitorum longus and peroneus tertius.	Tibialis posterior, flexor digitorum longus (FDL), posterior tibial artery, posterior tibial nerve, flexor hallucis longus (FHL)	Peroneus longus and peroneus brevis

6. Types of joint in ankle-foot
- *Ankle*: Hinge (synovial)
- *Subtalar*: Plane (synovial)
- *Intertarsal, tarsometatarsal*: Gliding
- *Metatarsophalangeal (MTP)*: Condyloid
- *Interphalangeal (IP) joint*: Hinge

7. **Major muscles of foot-ankle, their insertion, nerve supply, and action** mentioned in Table 9.3.

Table 9.3: Major muscles of foot-ankle.			
Muscle	*Insertion*	*Nerve supply*	*Principal action*
Tibialis anterior	Medial cuneiform and first metatarsal bones	Deep peroneal nerve	Dorsiflexion of the ankle, inversion at subtalar joint
EHL	Base of the distal phalanx (dorsal) of the great toe	Deep peroneal nerve	Dorsiflexion of the first interphalangeal joint
EDL	Bases of the distal phalanges (dorsal) of the second, third, fourth, and fifth toes	Deep peroneal nerve	Dorsiflexion of distal interphalangeal (DIP) of lesser toes
Peroneus longus	Plantar side of the medial cuneiform and first metatarsal bone	Superficial peroneal nerve	Eversion, plantar flexion of the first metatarsal
Peroneus brevis	Tuberosity of the fifth metatarsal bone	Superficial peroneal nerve	Eversion
Tendo-Achilles	Calcaneal tuberosity on the calcaneus	Tibial nerve	Plantar flexion of the ankle
Tibialis posterior	Navicular bone (it attaches at all the tarsals except talus)	Tibial nerve	Plantar flexion and inversion
FDL	Bases of the distal phalanges (Plantar) of the second, third, fourth, and fifth toes	Tibial nerve	Plantar flexion at DIP joint of lesser toes
FHL	Base of the distal phalanx (Plantar) of the great toe	Tibial nerve	Plantar flexion of the great toe IP joint

(EHL: Extensor hallucis longus; EDL: Extensor digitorum longus; FDL: Flexor digitorum longus; FHL: Flexor hallucis longus)

Common conditions affecting foot and ankle
1. **Congenital:** CTEV (club foot), flat foot
2. **Traumatic:** Ankle sprain, Fractures, Dislocation
3. **Infections:** Post-traumatic osteomyelitis, Madura foot (rare)
4. **Inflammatory:** Rheumatoid feet with deformities of toes
5. **Metabolic:** Gouty arthritis
6. **Degenerative:** Plantar fasciitis, Retrocalcaneal bursitis, Insertional Achilles tendinopathy, Tibialis posterior tendinitis
7. **Neurological:** Charcot's feet, Morton's neuroma
8. **Neoplastic**
9. **Others:** Sever's disease, hallux valgus, hallux varus

HISTORY AND ITS EVALUATION

The patient may present with chief complaints of:
- Pain and difficulty in walking
- Deformities
- Swelling
- Recurrent instability
- Assessment of disruption in ADL

1. **Pain and difficulty in walking**
   - One must enquire about the onset, duration, site, character, progression, and aggravating-relieving factors of the pain.
   - A constant pain especially at night is a red flag symptom and is suggestive of inflammation, infection, or tumor pathology.
   - The remission and exacerbation of the pain are suggestive of an inflammatory condition.
   - Pain under the heel which begins after placing the foot on the ground and which decreases after walking for few steps is classical of plantar fasciitis.
   - An *acquired deformity in the absence of the pain* gives an idea of Charcot's arthropathy.
   - The history of the trauma should be asked in every case of ankle and foot pain. The ankle sprain or fracture complications must be kept in mind with the history of trauma.

2. **Deformities**
   There are various common deformities of the foot and ankle which may be congenital or acquired. They are hallux valgus/varus, mallet toes, flat foot (plano valgus), congenital talipes equinovarus (CTEV), calcaneovalgus, etc. One must ask about:
   - The **onset** of the deformity is either congenital or acquired. The most common *congenital deformity* of feet is congenital club foot.
     Acquired deformity of the ankle, subtalar and midtarsal joints may be present in underlying neurological, traumatic, infective, or inflammatory disorder.
   - **Progression of deformity:** The deformity due to underlying neurological and inflammatory disorder is usually progressive.
   - **Painless or painful:** Most deformities are associated with pain. However, Charcot's arthropathy and associated deformity are painless.

3. **Swelling** Onset, duration, site of swelling, and progress of the swelling are useful for the clue for the diagnosis.
   - Unilateral or bilateral and localized or generalized swelling should be asked.
   - On and off swelling and redness with pain at first MTP is indicative of gouty arthritis.
   - Isolated proud swelling at the back of heel is suggestive of Haglund's bump/retrocalcaneal bursitis.

4. **Recurrent instability:** It is reported after ligament injury of the ankle. The most common ankle ligament injury is of lateral ligament complex after ankle sprain due to inversion injury.

5. **Assessment of disruption in ADL due to a painful, deformed foot.**

▌ EXAMINATION

General and Systemic Examination

The general and systemic examination is done in standard fashion. It is vital to examine the spine in patients with congenital abnormalities of foot and ankle as the deformities in the foot and ankle could be due to neurological abnormalities of the spine. Hence, it is important to look for deformities of the spine, swelling or any evidence of spina bifida over the spine as Clubfoot or any other deformity of foot and ankle may be secondary to underlying spine pathology.

Generalized ligamentous laxity is commonly responsible for the flexible flat foot. Every child of the flat foot must be examined for hyperflexibility of elbow, wrist, fingers, thumb, knee, and ankle *(refer to Beighton score in shoulder examination)*. The hyperpigmentation of lower leg and ankle may indicate venous insufficiency.

Examination of the Shoe/Footwear

It is quite relevant in the assessment of the foot conditions.
- The shoe of a patient with flat foot would reveal wear on inner side of heel and sole (normally, on outer side).
- Bulging of medial footwear wall indicates an everted foot.
- The normal shoe forefoot area wears in the center.
- Overpronators wear on the medial border, whereas oversupinators wear on the lateral border.

Local Examination

The examination of the foot and ankle should be divided into five parts: *forefoot* (From tip of toes to metatarsals), *midfoot* (cuneiforms, cuboid, and navicular), *hindfoot* (calcaneus and talus), *ankle* and *sole*.

Then, examine the foot-ankle from the side, front, and back, and the patient must be examined in standing and supine positions. One must also examine the leg.

Gait

Check the gait, if the patient is ambulant. It should be observed from the front, the side, and the back. Any asymmetry, limitation, hesitancy, or avoidance of weight bearing should be noted.
- Antalgic gait may be present due to pain in the ankle and foot.
- High-stepping gait in foot drop.
- Check whether the patient is normally walking with the plantigrade foot with equal weight over the heel and forefoot (tripod) or he/she is walking on the heel (calcaneus), forefoot (equinus), or over the lateral border (CTEV).

Attitude

It can be described in sitting or supine positions.

Inspection

It is very important to examine the foot both in standing (if possible) and in sitting positions as dynamic condition like flat foot is best observed in standing position. Ask the patient to stand with both feet a few centimeters apart and to look straight. Now examine the ***forefoot, mid-foot, hindfoot, ankle, sole, size of foot, and skin condition***.

The general finding like swelling, scar, sinus, and ulcers must be noted and described as per standard protocol.

(A) Forefoot

It reveals the *issues related to the toes and nails:*

- Toes (hallux varus/valgus, Mallet toe, hammer or claw toes, hallux rigidus) (Figs. 9.2A and B)
- Splaying of toes (observed in CTEV)
- Nails must be examined for tropic changes.
- *Bunions*: Medial osteophyte and swelling over the first metatarsal (MT).
- Forefoot abduction or adduction should be noted, if any
- All tendons over the dorsum of forefoot.

> **Common toe deformities**
> ***Mallet toe:*** DIP joint flexion deformity
> ***Hammer toe:*** PIP joint flexion deformity
> ***Claw toe:*** PIP and DIP in flexion, whereas MTP in hyperextension
> ***Hallux rigidus:*** Limited dorsiflexion at first MTP joint

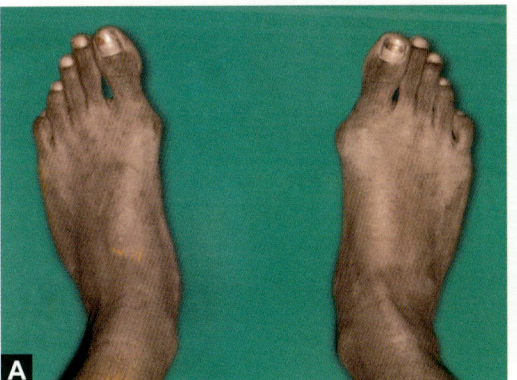 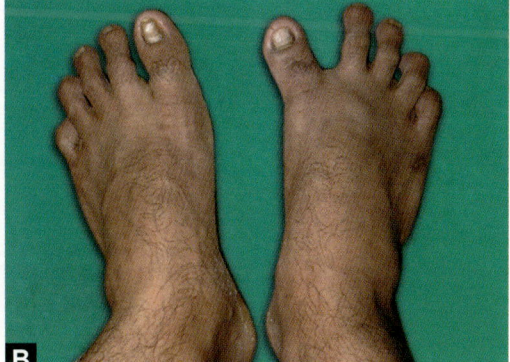

Figs. 9.2A and B: (A) Hallux valgus with bunion over 1st MT. (B) Hallux varus.

(B) Midfoot

The most important aspect to see in midfoot is the assessment of the ***arch of the foot, especially medial longitudinal arch (MLA)***. The height of the MLA apex is about 1 cm. The normal MLA does not touch the ground, and the examiner can insinuate 1–1.5 cm of his index finger under the arch (Figs. 9.3A and B).

- *Exaggerated arch of the foot suggests "pes cavus,"* whereas *attenuated arch of the foot suggests "pes planus" (flat foot)* (Figs. 9.4A and B).
- Further, examiner should differentiate between flexible and rigid flat feet by asking the patient to stand on tiptoe to see whether the medial arch reappears and the heel goes into varus (arch reappears in flexible flat foot). It is known as *heel rise test* (Figs. 9.5A and B).

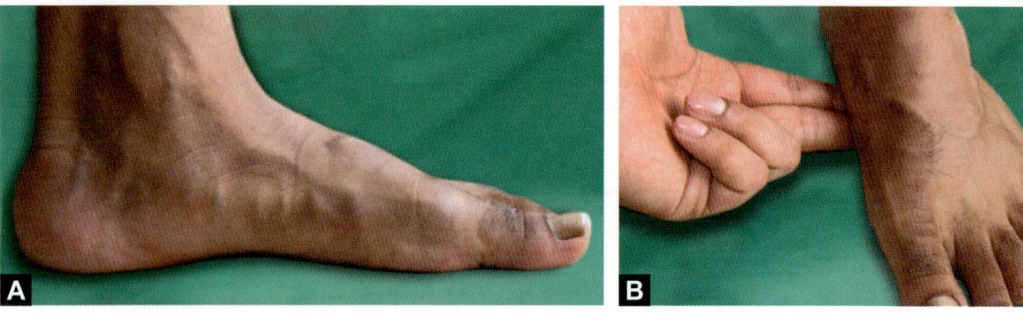

Figs. 9.3A and B: (A) Normal medial longitudinal arch (MLA) of left foot not touching ground. (B) Normal insinuation of finger under the MLA.

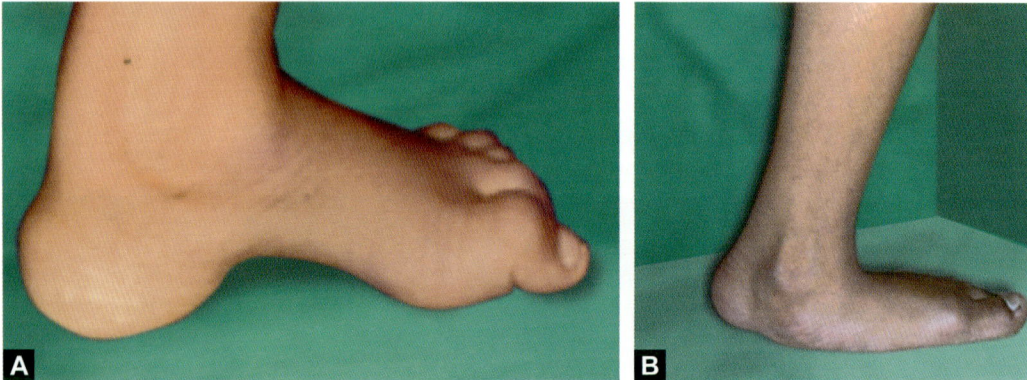

Figs. 9.4A and B: (A) Pes cavus. (B) Pes planus.

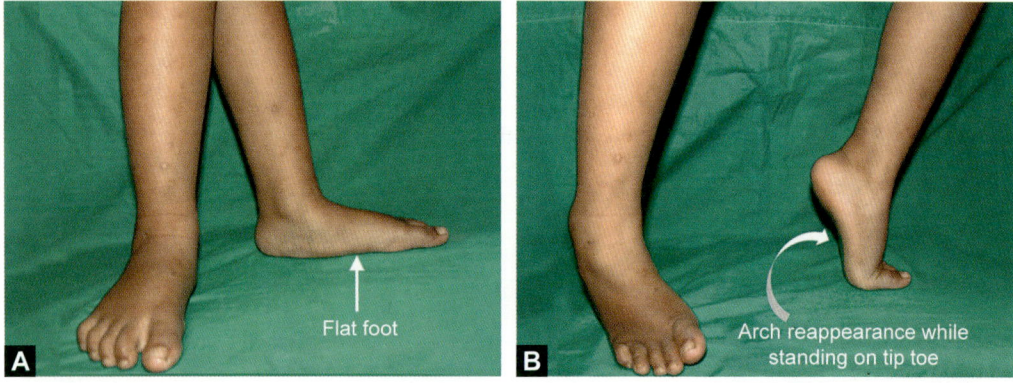

Flat foot

Arch reappearance while standing on tip toe

Figs. 9.5A and B: (A) Pes planus or flat foot. (B) Appearance of arch with heel rise in flexible flat foot.

Common Causes of Flat Foot
1. Congenital
2. Rheumatoid
3. Tibialis posterior tendon dysfunction/tear
4. Neuropathic (Charcot's) foot

(C) Hindfoot and calf

Hindfoot is always examined from "behind and side" especially while standing with feet apart.

- Normal hindfoot alignment is one where the tendo-Achilles (TA) axis and the calcaneum axis fall on the same line (Fig. 9.5C). When observed from behind, only the little toe is seen lateral to the leg.

  The "***too many toes sign***" where too many toes are observed lateral to the leg while standing behind the patient. It is due to forefoot abduction associated with a flat foot (Fig. 9.5D).

- The normal hindfoot alignment can change into hindfoot varus or valgus where the axis of calcaneum is in varus or valgus concerning the axis of TA (Figs. 9.6A and B).

- A ***broadened heel*** may suggest malunited fracture of the calcaneum (Fig. 9.7).

- ***Hindfoot from the side gives an idea of equinus/calcaneus deformity.***

  The hindfoot equinus can be easily detected with the heel off the ground whereas the hindfoot calcaneus reveals heel on the ground with forefoot off the ground.

  - The *small and empty heel* is seen in hindfoot equinus.

- Observe ***silhouette of tendo-Achilles*** (TA) for any swelling (TA tendinitis) or apparent discontinuity (TA rupture)

- Look for any swelling at the ***back of the calcaneum*** (retrocalcaneal bursitis)

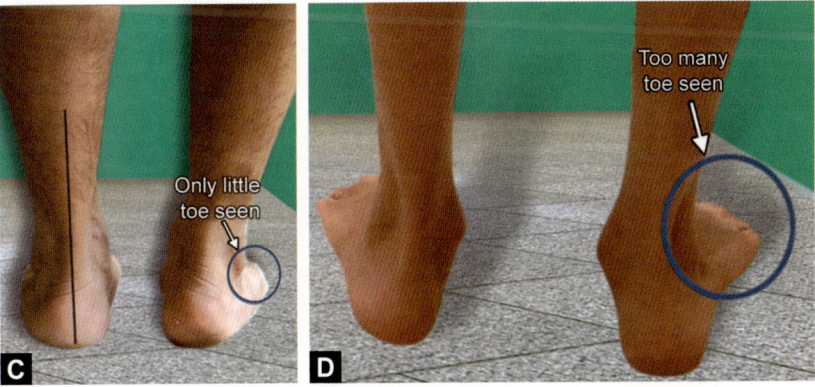

Figs. 9.5C and D: (C) Normal heel alignment and (D) Too many toes sign (white arrow).

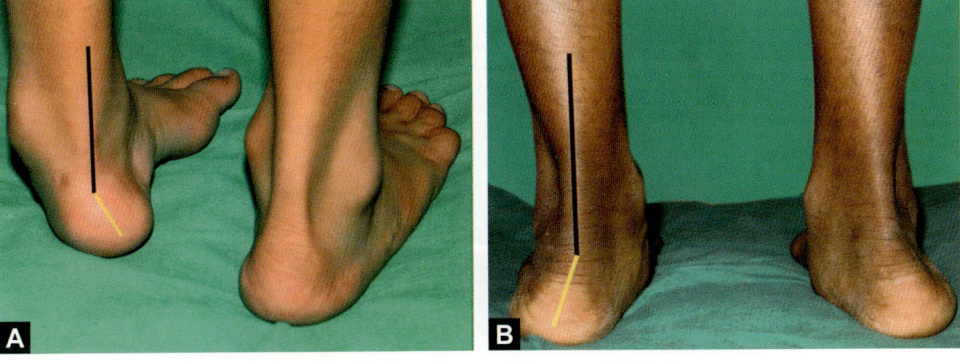

Figs. 9.6A and B: (A) Heel varus (left heel). (B) Heel valgus (left heel).

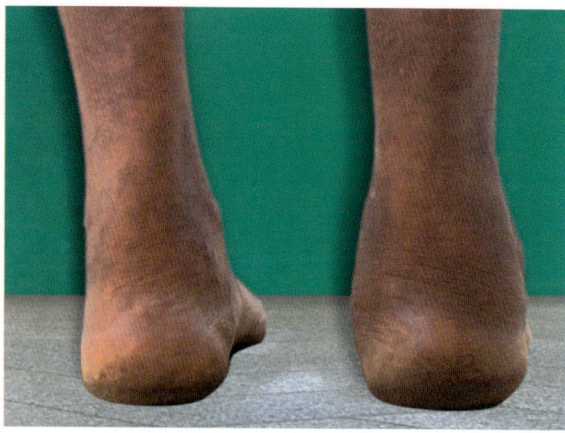

Fig. 9.7: Broad right heel.

- Look for any ***swelling over the posteromedial aspect of the ankle-hindfoot*** over the TP tendon: Tibialis posterior tendinitis
- Look at the ***calf musculature*** for any wasting.

(D) Ankle
- Look for any deformity
- *Observe both malleoli*; their level (lateral is lower than medial), any swelling around
- Prominence of both malleoli (lateral is more in CTEV).

(E) Skin over foot (medial, posterior, lateral, dorsum)
- Look for deep creases, callosities, ulcers, scars, sinus
- ***Skin creases***: Deep medial and posterior creases in CTEV and persistent single deep crease gives an idea of long-standing deformity (as single posterior crease above heel gives a sense of hindfoot equinus) (Fig. 9.8).
- Often, ***callosities*** can be seen on the medial or lateral border when the patient is walking on the medial or lateral border, respectively.
- Swelling, sinus, ulcer, previous scar mark must be noted. It is important to describe these conditions in standard fashion.

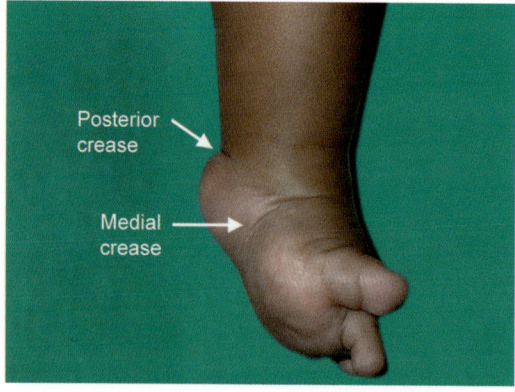

Fig. 9.8: Prominent foot creases in congenital talipes equinovarus.

(F) Sole
- Normally, the sole is mildly concave. However, in rocker bottom foot deformity, it becomes convex (Fig. 9.9).
- The anomalies of the weight-bearing portion of the foot can be assessed during examination of the sole by the presence of abnormal callosities.
- Look for any painful corns or ulcers (painless or painful)
- The excessive load (dirt stain) on the front part with a clean heel suggests equinus contracture.
- Excessive weight on the lateral aspect of the entire foot gives the idea of inversion; excessive weight on the medial aspect of the foot shows eversion/planovalgus foot.

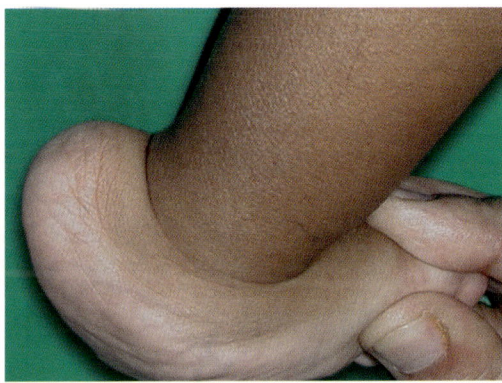

Fig. 9.9: Rocker bottom foot.

(G) Size of the foot
- Normally, the medial border of the foot is longer than the lateral border.
- The lateral column is longer in club foot
- Foot is smaller/bean-shaped in club foot.

Palpation
1. **Local rise in temperature:** Entire foot and ankle
2. **Tenderness:** The tenderness must be felt for specific soft tissue, bony landmarks and joint lines on anterior, lateral, posterior, and medial side of ankle, subtalar, mid- and forefoot, and the sole.

The knowledge of surface anatomy is the key as there are multiple bones, articulations, and structures in the foot.

Tenderness on specific areas may suggest a specific pathology
• **Back of the heel in children**: Severs' disease
• **Back of the heel in adult**: Retrocalcaneal bursitis, TA tendinitis
• **Bottom of the heel in adult**: Plantar fasciitis
• **Anteroinferior to the tip of lateral malleolus**: ATF ligament tear (in ankle sprain)
• **Over sinus tarsi**: Sinus tarsi syndrome
• **First MTP joint**: Gouty arthritis
• **Second/third metatarsal head**: Freiberg disease
• **Over second metatarsal shaft**: Stress fracture/march fracture
• **Between third and fourth metatarsal (with shooting pain)**: Morton metatarsalgia.

(A) Anterior to ankle
  (i) *Ankle joint line*: Normally the ankle joint is situated 1 cm above the tip the medial malleolus (MM). The joint line is felt and confirmed by gentle plantar and dorsiflexion. The joint line tenderness gives an idea of intra-articular ankle pathology.
  Any swelling or bulge along the outline of ankle joint line should be noted. It may indicate synovial hypertrophy/effusion.
 (ii) Just *anteroinferior to the lateral malleolus tip*: Anterior talofibular (ATF) ligament injury.
(iii) *Talar dome*: The anterolateral aspect of talus dome can be palpated just adjacent to anterolateral joint line in complete plantar flexion with inversion. Osteochondritis dissecans of Talus often affects Talar dome.
(iv) Palpate *lower part of the tibia* on posteromedial aspect for any stress # (shin splint)
(B) Lateral: Important landmarks to palpate are (Fig. 9.10):
  (i) *Lateral malleolus*
 (ii) *Peroneal tendons*: Tender in Peroneal tendinitis
(iii) *Calcaneum*
(iv) *Sinus tarsi*: Sinus tarsi is a hollow space an inch anterior and just inferior to the tip of the lateral malleolus. It is tender in sinus tarsi syndrome.
 (v) *Base of fifth metatarsal*: Avulsion fracture.
(C) Posterior: Important landmarks to palpate are (Figs. 9.11 and 9.12A and B):
  (i) *TendoAchilles insertion over back of calcaneum*: Retrocalcaneal bursitis, Insertional TA tendinopathy
 (ii) *Tendoachilles tendon proximal to the insertion over calcaneum*: Tendo-Achilles tendinitis (tender tendon), TA rupture (palpable defect).

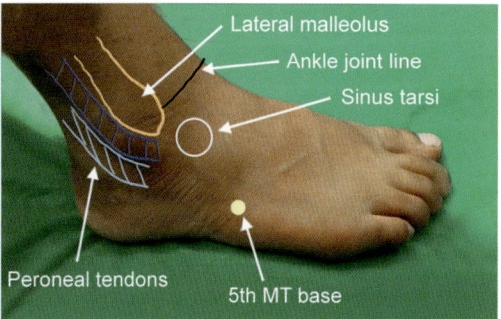

Fig. 9.10: Major landmarks for palpation of anterolateral aspect of ankle and foot.

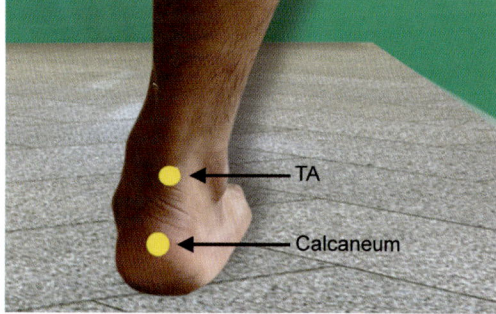

Fig. 9.11: Major landmarks for palpation of posterior aspect of ankle.

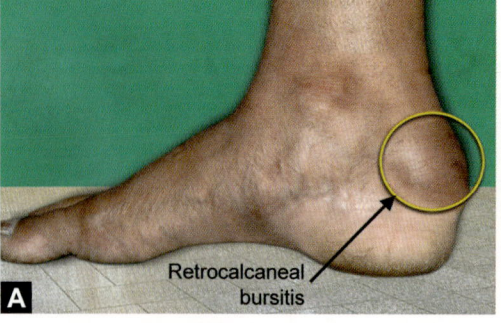

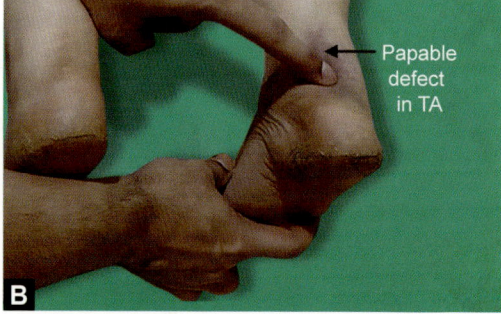

Figs. 9.12A and B: (A) Haglunds bump/Retrocalcaneal bursitis. (B) Palpable gap after TA rupture.

(D) Medial: Important landmarks to palpate are (Fig. 9.13):

 (i) *Medial malleolus*
 (ii) *Tibialis posterior (TP) and other medial tendons*: Just below and behind the MM. TP is often swollen and tender in TP tendinitis. Sometimes, TP is ruptured leading to flat foot.
(iii) *Deltoid ligament*: For sprains/tears
(iv) *Sustentaculum tali*: Fracture
 (v) *Medial tarsals* (Navicular, cuneiforms) and *1st metatarsal*
(vi) *Head of talus*: To palpate the head of talus, palpate the tip of both malleoli. Then move distally in the direction of talus along the foot, till one finds a dip. That is the neck of Talus. Further, one can feel the head which moves with plantar and dorsiflexion.
(vii) *Palpate the tibial nerve* under the medial flexor retinaculum for any nerve entrapment/ neuroma. It can mimic symptoms of plantar fasciitis.

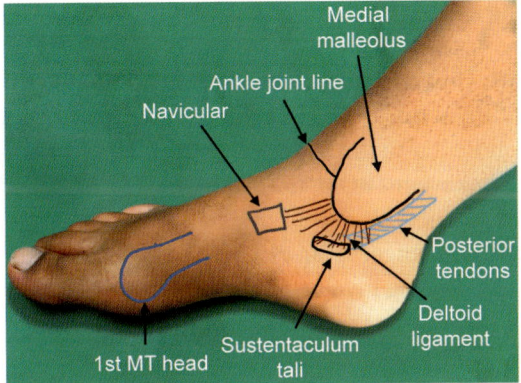

Fig. 9.13: Major landmarks for palpation of medial aspect of ankle and foot.

(E) Subtalar joint palpation: *It cannot be palpated directly. However, can be felt over the height of sinus tarsi.*
(F) Dorsum of foot (midfoot): Palpate all tarsals and dorsal tendons
(G) Forefoot: All metatarsals and toes:
 (i) *Morton's neuroma*: Tenderness between third and fourth metatarsals
 (ii) *Hallux rigidus*: Painful, limited dorsiflexion at the first MTP joint
(iii) *Bunion*: Bony, often painful hump at the base of the big toe.
(iv) *Palpate metatarsals* for stress fracture (second MT shaft in March #).
(H) Sole: Important landmarks to palpate are (Fig. 9.14):

 (i) *Medial calcaneum tuberosity*: Tender in plantar fasciitis
 (ii) *Heel fat pad*
(iii) *Head, shaft, and base of all the metatarsals*
(iv) *Sesamoids of first MT*: Stress #
(I) Medial longitudinal arch: The normal, cavus, or planus must be confirmed. One can perform Jack's test (described in special test) to check flexibility of the arch.

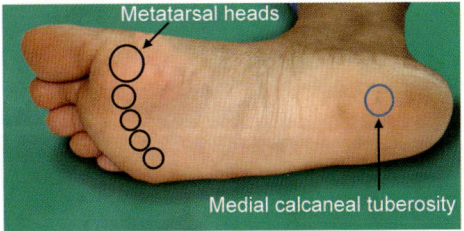

Fig. 9.14: Major points for palpation of sole.

3. Normal intermalleolar relationship

Normally, the tip of the lateral malleolus is situated posterior and 1.25 cm distal to the tip of the MM.

The relationship is altered in the absence of one the malleolus, malunion/nonunion of malleolar or distal tibial-fibula fractures leading to ankle varus and ankle valgus.

4. Deformity correction

One should make an attempt to passively correct the deformity noted on inspection if any. This gives an idea whether the deformity is fixed or correctable (partially/totally/overcorrectable).

5. Ligament laxity

Examine for ligament laxity as patients with ligament laxity may be associated with primary or recurrent ankle sprain.

6. Confirmation of palpatory characteristics of *skin, swelling, scar, sinus and ulcers.*

Movements

1. **Ankle joint: "Dorsiflexion and plantar flexion" (Figs. 9.15A and B):**
   - The neutral position of the ankle is the position of the foot perpendicular to the leg.
   - To assess passive ankle joint ROM, the examiner holds the patient's heel with cup of one hand, and thumb and index finger over the head of

> **Normal ankle and subtalar ROM**
> 1. *Ankle dorsiflexion*: 0–25°
> 2. *Ankle plantar flexion*: 0–50°
> 3. *Subtalar inversion*: 0–40°
> 4. *Subtalar eversion*: 0–20°

   Talus to avoid confounding involvement of the midtarsal movements. The other hand of examiner holds the lower end of leg with knee in flexion to relax Tendoachilles (tight TA would lead to less ankle dorsiflexion estimation). Now the ankle is moved in plantar- and dorsiflexion (Fig. 9.15C).
   - The plantar flexion of the ankle is measured as the angle between the leg and the foot (with maximum plantar flexed position of ankle) minus 90°.
   - The dorsiflexion of the ankle is measured as the angle between the leg and the foot (with maximum dorsiflexed position ankle) minus 90°.
   - The fixed equinus contracture of the ankle is "ankle fixed in plantar flexion". Nevertheless, there is a possibility of further plantar flexion. It can be expressed as "With 20° equinus deformity; the range of motion at ankle is 20–50°".

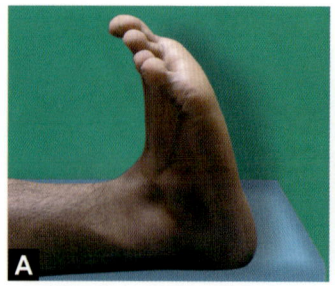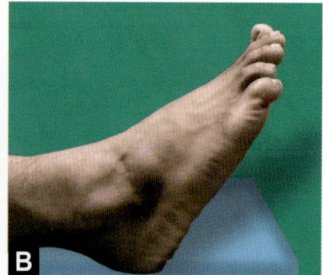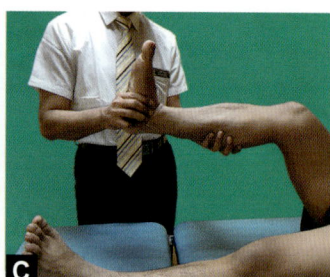

Figs. 9.15A to C: Dorsi- and plantar flexion at ankle.

2. **Subtalar joint: "Inversion-eversion"**

Method to perform inversion-eversion: It is performed by keeping the ankle in full dorsiflexion and holding the back of heel with palm while thumb and index finger holding head of Talus (Fig. 9.16A). The lower end of leg is held by other hand of examiner with knee flexed. By completely dorsiflexing the ankle, the talus is locked into the ankle mortise as broader end of Talus comes inside the mortise (*Talar body is trapezoidal where anterior half is broader and posterior half is narrow*). This precludes any subtle rocking of talus while performing eversion/inversion which may contribute to false eversion/inversion. Then, the heel is inverted and everted to note the range of inversion-eversion (Figs. 9.16A to C).

3. **Midtarsal joint movement:** 10° of adduction and 5° of abduction

Hold the hindfoot with one hand and adduct/abduct the forefoot with the other hand to note the midtarsal movement.

4. **Movement at the toes**
   - *Great toe MTP joint:* Flexion-40°, Extension-65°
   - *Great toe IP joint:* Flexion-60°, neutral in extension
   - *Lesser toes MTP joint:* Flexion-40°, Extension-40°
   - *Lesser toes PIP joint:* Flexion-40°, neutral in extension
   - *Lesser toes distal interphalangeal (DIP) joint:* Flexion-60°, Extension-30°

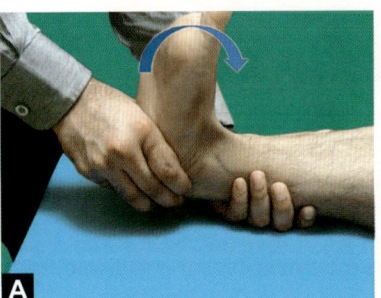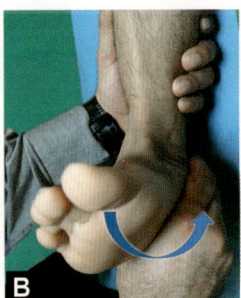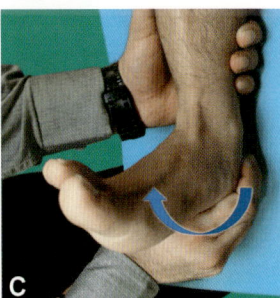

Figs. 9.16A to C: Inversion and eversion at the subtalar joint.

Measurement

1. **The size of the foot** should be measured from the back of the heel to tip of the great toe (medial border) and tip of the fifth toe (lateral border).
   - The practical importance of foot size measurement is to assess the asymmetry of the foot. Also, it helps in the assessment of the sequential correction of the foot. For example, in CTEV, the medial border is smaller than the lateral. With sequential correction, the medial border becomes longer than the lateral.
2. **Calf width** in case of calf wasting.
3. **Heel broadening** (with calipers).

Neurovascular Examination

One must do a complete neurological examination to rule out the involvement of nervous system (sensory, motor, reflexes).

Sensory innervation of foot: The foot is innervated by sural, saphenous, superficial and deep peroneal nerve, and tibial nerve (Fig. 9.17).

Motor innervation: The root value mentioned for specific motor function.
- *Dorsiflexion of the ankle*: L4
- *Dorsiflexion of the great toe*: L5
- *Plantar flexion of ankle*: S1
- *Inversion*: L4, L5
- *Eversion*: L5, S1

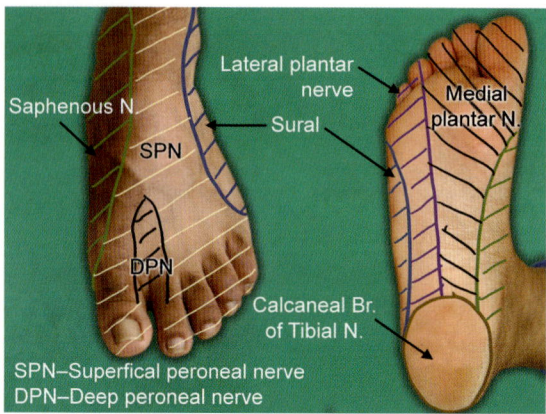

Fig. 9.17: Sensory innervation of the foot.

Special Tests

1. **Tests for ankle stability**
   i. **Anterior drawer test for anterior stability:** To test the integrity of the ATF ligament.
   Method: With the patient sitting on a couch with the knee flexed to 90°, the examiner holds the lower part of the leg from his left hand while the heel is held (cupped) from the right hand and ankle is kept in 10° plantar flexion. Now, an anteriorly directed force is given (anterior drawer) to the heel (Fig. 9.18). Compare with the other side.
   Interpretation: More than 8–10 mm anterior drawer or more than 3 mm compared with the other side indicates insufficiency of ATF ligament.
   ii. **Inversion talar tilt test:** To test the integrity of CF ligament.
   Method: With the patient sitting on a couch with the knee flexed to 90°, the examiner holds the lower part of the leg from his left hand while the heel is held (cupped) from the right hand and ankle is kept in neutral flexion. Now, the ankle is inverted (Fig. 9.19).
   Interpretation: More than 5° tilt compared to the normal side with soft mushy feel and or pain on lateral side may indicate insufficiency of CF ligament.
   iii. **Eversion talar tilt test:** To test the integrity of deltoid ligament.
   Method: With the patient sitting on a couch with the knee flexed to 90°, the examiner holds the lower part of the leg from his left hand while the heel is held (cupped) from the right hand and ankle is kept in neutral flexion. Now, the ankle is everted (Fig. 9.20).
   Interpretation: Increased laxity, soft mushy feel, or pain on injured side compared to the normal side may indicate insufficiency of deltoid ligament.

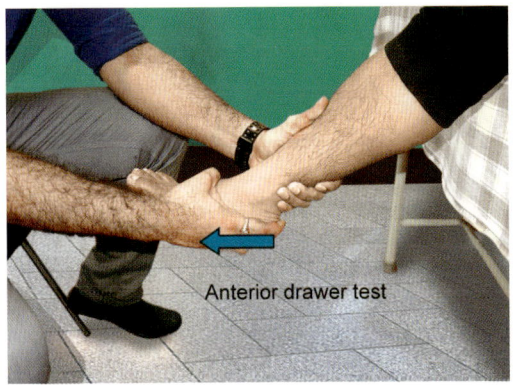

Fig. 9.18: Anterior drawer test.

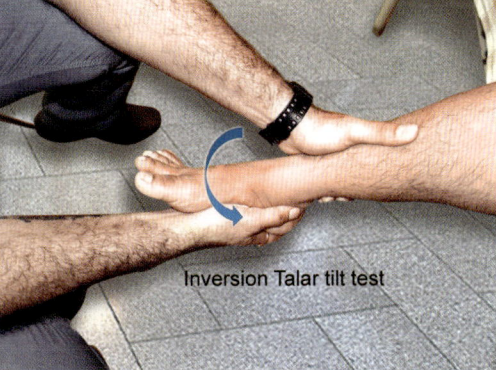

Fig. 9.19: Inversion talar tilt test.

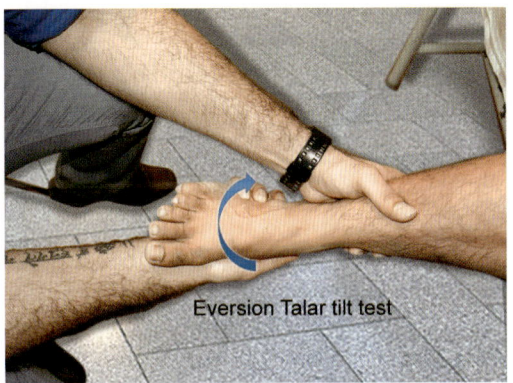

Fig. 9.20: Eversion talar tilt test.

iv. Squeeze test for distal syndesmosis injury

Method and interpretation: With the patient sitting on a couch with the knee flexed to 90°, the examiner holds the lower part of the leg from his hand and squeezes the tibia-fibula together just above the malleolus. Any pain at the distal tibial fibular joint is indicative of syndesmotic ligament injury.

Another method: Hold the lower end of leg with one hand and the foot by the other hand. Now externally rotate the foot. This maneuver can produce pain at the syndesmosis in case of injury.

2. Test for flexibility of MLA for flat foot

i. Jack's test: To check whether the flat foot is rigid/flexible type.

Method: While the patient is sitting; the examiner holds the heel with one hand, and the great toe of the patient is passively dorsiflexed. Observe for MLA exaggeration (Figs. 9.21A and B).

Interpretation: If the MLA exaggerates from its current flat position, it indicates a flexible type of flat foot. If it fails to exaggerate, it indicates rigid type of flat foot (*often due to tarsal coalition*).

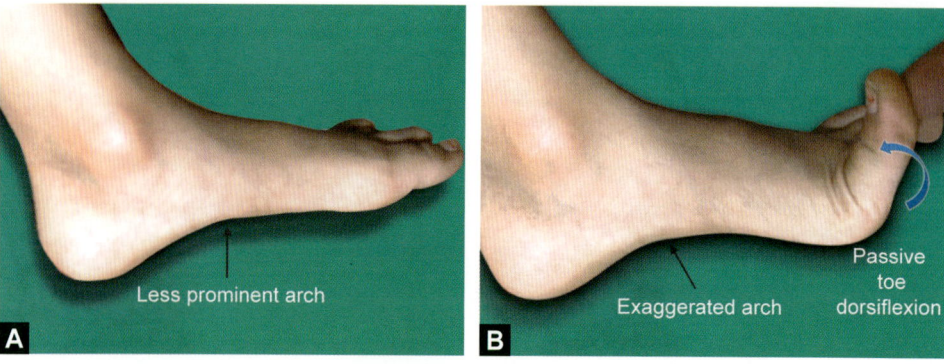

Figs. 9.21A and B: Jack test.

ii. Heel rise test: To check the flexibility of the medial arch/mobile subtalar joint.
   Method: Ask patient to stand on his forefoot and watch for the movement of the heel (*see* Fig. 9.5).
   Interpretation: If the heel moves into the varus (inward) with exaggeration of medial arch, it indicates the flexible type of flat foot. It also indicates that the subtalar joint is still mobile.

3. Coleman block test for hindfoot varus flexibility and forefoot pronation
   Method: While the patient is facing away from the examiner, ask the patient to stand on a wooden block of varying thickness from 2.5 to 4 cm with the heel and the lateral border over the edge of the block while the medial border of the foot and first three toes are allowed to hang freely in plantar flexion and pronation.
   Interpretation: If the heel moves into the neutral (inward), it indicates flexible hindfoot varus and a mobile, supple subtalar joint.

4. Thompson test for integrity of tendo-Achilles tendon
   Method: The patient should lie prone and both the knees should be flexed 90° so that foot faces upward. Now the calf is squeezed gently.
   Interpretation: If the ankle moves in plantar flexion against gravity, this indicates intact Tendoachilles. If it fails to move in plantar flexion, it indicates TA rupture (Figs. 9.22A and B).

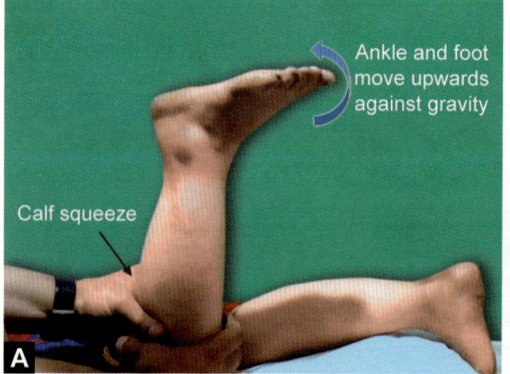
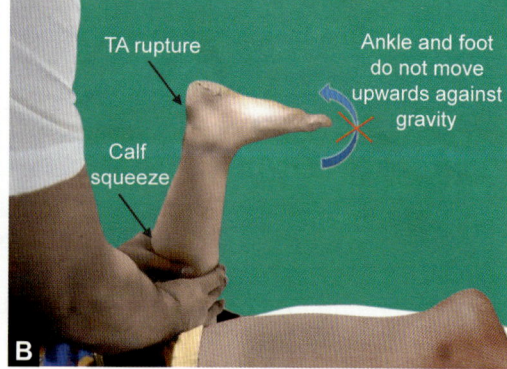

Figs. 9.22A and B: Intact and ruptured tendo-Achilles

5. **Test for calf muscle tightness**
   i. **Silfverskiold test:** To differentiate between gastrocnemius and soleus tightness.
   Method: The patient should lie prone with both knee and hip extended. Now the ankle should be dorsiflexed and the ROM noted. Now flex the knee to 90° to relax the gastrocnemius and again dorsiflex the ankle and note the difference in ROM. Compare with the other side.
   Interpretation:
   • Dorsiflexion improves with knee flexed—gastrocnemius tightness
   • Similar dorsiflexion with knee flexed/extended—soleus tightness

6. **Homan's and Moses' sign for deep vein thrombosis**
   i. *Homan's:* Gentle passive dorsiflexion induces pain in calf.
   ii. *Moses' sign (Bancroft's sign):* Calf muscles are gently compressed forward against the tibia induces pain. (Note: This test is normally not performed due to fear of dislodging the thrombus due to squeezing/compression).

Examination of Other Joints Above

Standard knee, hip joint, and spine examination.

Examination of Lymph Nodes

Inguinal and popliteal fossa lymph node examination.

Ankle examination proforma

1. **Examination of footwear**
2. **Gait**
3. **Attitude**
4. **Inspection:**
   - *General findings*: *All areas for Skin overlying, Swelling, scar, sinus*
   - *Specifics findings of inspection*
     - *Forefoot*: Toes, nails, deformity, abduction/adduction
     - *Midfoot*: Medial longitudinal arch
     - *Hindfoot*: Heel (broadening, deformity), swelling, TA silhouette, Calf musculature
     - *Ankle*: Deformity, level of malleoli
     - *Skin over dorsum and borders*: Skin creases, Callosities
     - *Sole*
     - *Size of foot*
5. **Palpation**
   - Local rise in temperature
   - *Tenderness*: Bony landmark, soft tissues, joint line
   - Anterior, lateral, medial and posterior to ankle
   - Subtalar joint, Midfoot and forefoot, sole, medial longitudinal arch
   - Normal intermalleolar relationship
   - Deformity, ligament laxity
   - Confirmation of palpatory characteristics of swelling, scar, sinus
6. **Movements:** Active and passive
   - *Ankle*: Dorsiflexion and plantarflexion
   - *Subtalar joint*: inversion, Eversion
   - *Midtarsal*: abduction, adduction
   - *Toes*: Flexion, extension
   - **Crepitus, clicks;** if any
7. **Measurements:**
   - Size of foot, calf circumference, heel width
8. **Neurovascular examination**
9. **Special tests**
   - (a) *Test for ankle stability*: Anterior drawer (ATFL), Inversion talar tilt (CFL), Eversion-talar tilt (deltoid ligament), Squeeze test (distal syndesmosis)
   - (b) *Medial longitudinal arch flexibility*: Jack test, Heel raise test
   - (c) *For hind foot varus flexibility and forefoot pronation*: Coleman Block test
   - (d) *Tendoachilles integrity*: Thompson test
   - (e) *Calf muscle tightness Test*: Silfverskiold test
   - (f) *DVT signs*: Moses and Homan's sign
10. **Joint above :** knee, hip and spine
11. **Lymph node examination**

<h3 style="text-align:center;">Common conditions affecting ankle with # their salient features</h3>

1. **Club Foot (CTEV)**
   - *Affects*: Newborn child, common in both sexes
   - *Presents with*: Painless foot deformity, unilateral or bilateral
   - *Pathology*: Congenital deformity of the ankle and foot, soft tissue contracture of the posterior and the medial side of the ankle and the foot
   - *Clinical presentation*: Hindfoot varus, hindfoot equinus, forefoot adduction, forefoot inversion, forefoot adduction
     – Tight tendoachilles, small heel with varus
     – Prominent medial and posterior creases
     – Larger lateral border and smaller medial border of feet
     – Callosities over lateral border of foot in older children
     – Spine, hip, and knee are normal in idiopathic club feet
   - *Diagnosis*: Clinical diagnosis
   - *Treatment*: Serial manipulation and cast application, maintenance with orthosis, surgery in older children.

2. **Congenital Flat Foot/Pes Planus**
   - *Affects*: Children and adults, common in both sexes
   - *Presents with*: Painless deformity
   - *Pathology*: Medial longitudinal arch height is decreased
   - *Clinical presentation*: Present at any age-children/adult
     – Most of the cases are asymptomatic, very few are symptomatic
     – May be unilateral or bilateral, flexible or rigid
     – Hindfoot valgus, low arch, forefoot abduction, forefoot eversion, supination
     – Tight tendoachilles may be present
     – Callosities over medial border of foot in older children/adult
     – *Too many toes sign* (seen from behind) in moderate to severe case
     – Normal neurological examination
     – *Rigid flat foot may be due to tarsal coalition*
     – Spine, hip, and knee are normal in idiopathic flat feet
   - *Diagnosis*: Clinical diagnosis, X-ray may help in tarsal coalition
   - *Treatment*: Usually no treatment is required for the asymptomatic flexible flat foot. Orthosis, surgical intervention for symptomatic/rigid flat foot.

3. **Spina Bifida with Club Foot**
   - *Affects*: Newborn child, common in both sexes
   - *Presents with*: Painless deformity
   - *Pathology*: Failure of fusion of the posterior elements of the spine, which causes the neurological abnormalities (muscle imbalance, sensory loss)
   - *Clinical presentation*: Present at birth, walking age/may present later, tropic ulceration may be the first symptoms:
     – Deformity of the ankle and foot, may be unilateral or bilateral
     – Most of the cases present with neurological involvement (sensorimotor)
     – Trophic ulcer may be present
     – Look for covert or overt signs of spina bifida over spine, surgical scar

- – Bladder and bowel involvement
- – Abnormalities in neurological examination
- **Diagnosis**: Clinical diagnosis, X-ray, MRI, CT, NCV, EMG
- **Treatment**: Serial manipulation and cast application in newborn, maintenance of correction with orthosis, protective footwear, *"correction of underlying muscle imbalance with surgery."*

4. **Plantar Fasciitis**
   - **Affects**: Adult, common in both sexes
   - **Presents with**: Heel pain when patient takes a few steps and walks after a period of rest
   - **Pathology**: Collagen degeneration associated with repetitive microtrauma to the plantar fascia
   - **Clinical presentation**: Very common cause of heel pain in middle age (late 30s–50s):
     - – Heel pain with initial steps which decreases after a few steps
     - – Tenderness present over the medial calcaneal tuberosity over the under surface of calcaneum at the attachment of plantar fascia.
   - **Diagnosis**: Essentially clinical diagnosis; X-ray to rule out other pathologies like infection, tumor, and inflammation
   - **Treatment**: Nonsteroidal anti-inflammatory drug (NSAID), soft heel shoe, rest, steroid injection, rarely surgical release of fascia.

5. **Retrocalcaneal Bursitis (Hump-Bump/Haglund's Deformity)**
   - **Affects**: Adult, common in both sexes
   - **Presents with**: "Back of the heel" pain when the patient takes a few steps and walks after a period of rest with often a swelling
   - **Pathology**: Inflammation of bursa (bursitis) which is located between the Achilles tendon and the calcaneus, may be idiopathic or secondary to inflammatory condition
   - **Clinical presentation**: Posterior heel pain in middle age (late 40s–60s), common in repetitive trauma, sports person:
     - – Back of heel pain which decreases after a few steps, often swelling present at the back of the heel
     - – Tenderness present over the posterior aspect of calcaneum where tendoachilles is attached
   - **Diagnosis**: Clinical diagnosis, X-ray, USG, MRI
   - **Treatment**: NSAID, rest, physical therapy, heel rise, rarely surgery.

6. **Hallux Valgus**
   - **Affects**: Present in adults, common in females, common with narrow shoe habit
   - **Presents with**: Painless or a painful deformity of the great toe
   - **Pathology**: Lateral deviation or subluxation at first MTP joint
   - **Clinical presentation**: Asymptomatic in most cases, pain at MTP in late stage:
     - – Deformity present, later the great toe rides over the second toe
     - – Bunion over the medial aspect of the first metatarsal head is often painful
     - – Normal neurological examination
     - – Rule out rheumatoid arthritis (RA), gout
   - **Diagnosis**: Clinical diagnosis, X-ray
   - **Treatment**: Asymptomatic should be left, orthosis, surgical correction.

7. **Gouty arthritis**
   - *Affects*: Present in adults, common in males
   - *Presents with*: Intermittent acute severe pain
   - *Pathology*: Inflammatory response to the presence of monosodium urate (MSU) crystals in joints common in first MTP joint, causes acute arthritis, chronic arthropathy
   - *Clinical presentation*: Acute-onset pain at first MTP:
     - Most of the cases are symptomatic, intermittent episodes of gouty attack
     - Pain, tenderness, and increased warmth at first MTP Joint. Tophi in soft tissues
     - Normal neurological examination
   - *Diagnosis*: Clinical diagnosis, X-ray, uric acid level, renal function test
   - *Treatment*: NSAIDs, colchicine, allopurinol, febuxostat.

8. **Charcot's Joint/Neuropathic Joint**
   - *Affects*: Diabetes is the most common cause. Other causes are Hansen's disease, multiple sclerosis, syringomyelia, spinal cord injury, spina bifida, tabes dorsalis
   - *Presents with*: Painless deformity and swelling of the foot
   - *Pathology*: Arthropathy of small joints of foot due to sensory loss
   - *Clinical presentation*: Painless, deformed foot. One can observe gross flat foot or acquired rocker bottom deformity
     - Diabetes remains the most common cause of Charcot's joint involving foot
     - Ulcers may be present
     - Exaggerated movement at the ankle and other joints, if involved
   - *Diagnosis*: X-ray is the diagnostic: dense bones, deformity, debris, dislocation of joints, destruction (gross) of the joints
   - *Treatment*: Orthosis, footwear modification. Rarely surgical correction of deformity or exostosis excision is required to prevent/treat non-healing ulcers.

9. **Tibialis Posterior Tendinitis/Insufficiency**
   Most common cause of adult acquired flat foot
   - *Affects*: Mostly women, sixth decade onwards. Other risk factors are inflammatory arthritis (RA), diabetes, obesity, and steroid use
   - *Presents with*: Painless/painful deformity and swelling of the foot
   - *Pathology*: Progression of tendinitis to gradual insufficiency or tear of the tendon. This causes medial arch collapse.
   - *Clinical presentation*
     - Pes planus, hindfoot valgus, forefoot varus
     - Medial side ankle-foot pain and swelling along TP tendon,
     - Tenderness posterior to the tip of medial malleolus along course of Tibialis posterior
     - Unable to perform single limb heel rise
   - *Diagnosis*: MRI
   - *Treatment*: Orthosis, rehabilitation, surgery.

10. **Ankle sprain**
    - *Affects*: Mostly young ones. Lateral ankle sprain with injury to lateral ligaments is quite common as compared to medial side sprain.
    - *Presents with*: History of twisting injury to the ankle (primary/recurrent), pain over lateral aspect of ankle.
    - *Pathology*: Tear of Lateral ankle ligaments (most common- ATF; followed by CF and PTF) due to inversion injury. Medial ankle sprain (eversion injury) with tear of deltoid ligament is quite uncommon.

- **Clinical presentation**
  - H/o primary or recurrent ankle sprain, feeling of instability on uneven surface
  - Tenderness anteroinferior/inferior/posterior to the tip of lateral malleolus depending upon site of ligament injury (ATF/CF/PTF)
  - Painful and limited plantarflexion and inversion
- **Diagnosis**: MRI
- **Treatment**: Orthosis, Below knee cast, rehabilitation, Surgical reconstruction of ligament.

Notes

Clinical Evaluation of the Spine

▌ BASIC FACTS ABOUT SPINE AND SPINAL CORD

1. **Basic osteology of spine**
   - 33 vertebrae: 7 cervical, 12 thoracic, 5 lumbar, and 5 sacral and 4 vertebrae in the coccygeal region, constitute the spinal column.
   - ***Characteristics of the cervical vertebra:*** C1-C7 cervical vertebrae have transverse foramen. Vertebral artery and vein travels through this foramen from C1 to C6.
   - ***Characteristics of the thoracic vertebra:*** It has costal facets for articulation with the ribs.
   - ***Characteristics of the Lumbar vertebra:*** Lumbar vertebral bodies have mamillary process and pars interarticularis (bone between superior and inferior articular process).

2. **Spinal cord, nerve roots, and autonomic nervous system**
   - The 45-cm-long spinal cord starts from the foramen magnum to the lower end of L1 or the upper end of L2 vertebra.
   - The bulbous end of the spinal cord is called as conus medullaris. The lumbar and sacral roots continue to descend down in dural coverings, collectively looks like Horse's tail, known as Cauda equina.
   - 31 pairs of nerve roots and 23 intervertebral discs
   - ***Major ascending tract*** in the spinal cord (with function):
     - *Posterior column tract*: Proprioception (position sense), stereognosis, fine touch, two-point discrimination, vibration, and tactile localization
     - *Lateral spinothalamic tract*: Pain and temperature
     - *Anterior spinothalamic tract*: Crude touch and pressure
   - ***Major descending tract:***
     - *Lateral corticospinal tract*: Main voluntary motor tract (crossed)
     - *Anterior corticospinal tract*: Voluntary motor tract (uncrossed)
   - ***Blood supply to the spinal cord:***
     - *Anterior spinal artery*: Anterior 2/3rd of the spinal cord
     - *Posterior spinal artery*: Posterior 1/3rd of the spinal cord
     - *Artery of Adamkiewicz*: Largest anterior segmental artery from the left posterior intercostal artery and supplies lower 2/3rd of the spinal cord
   - ***Sympathetic nervous system*** originates from lateral horn cells of thoracolumbar outflow (T1-L2)
   - ***Parasympathetic nervous system*** originates from craniosacral outflow (vagus-cranial and S2, 3, 4-sacral outflow)

3. Curvature of spine, mobility and function

- *The normal sagittal curvature of the spine*: Lordosis of the cervical spine, kyphosis of the thoracic spine lordosis of the lumbar spine and kyphosis of the sacrum.
- The spine is straight in the coronal plane.
- The mobility of the spine occurs at the intervertebral disc and facet joint.
- Cervical spine and lumbar spines are most mobile, while thoracic spine is the least mobile due to the rib cage.
- Spine protects the spinal cord, provides attachment to various muscles and ligaments, erect posture and mobility.

4. Movement at the spine

- *Cervical spine*: Flexion–extension (YES movement) at atlanto-occipital junction, rotation (NO movement) at atlantoaxial joint and lateral flexion at lower levels.
- *Dorsal spine*: Upper dorsal spine with predominantly rotation and lateral flexion and lower dorsal spine with predominant flexion-extension and lateral flexion (less rotation). This variation is due to the varying orientation of facet joint in upper and lower dorsal spine. The presence of rib cage and large spinous process limit the flexion and extension.
- *Lumbar spine*: Flexion–extension, lateral flexion.

Common conditions affecting the spine.
Congenital and /deformities: Torticollis, Kyphosis, Scoliosis, and Spina bifida
Infection: Tuberculosis, Brucellosis, Pyogenic
Degenerative: Prolapse intervertebral disc, Spondylosis, Spondylolysis, Spondylolisthesis, Lumbar canal stenosis
Inflammatory: Ankylosing spondylitis
Metabolic: Osteoporosis
Traumatic: Paraplegia/quadriplegia
Tumors: Multiple Myeloma, Secondaries

HISTORY AND ITS EVALUATION

History plays an important role in the diagnosis of the exact etiopathology of the spine disease.

Age: It has a bearing in the etiology of the disease.

- The congenital presentation includes spine abnormalities like torticollis, spina bifida, or scoliosis.
- Infection of the spine can occur at any age. However, the young and middle aged are affected.
- Intervertebral disc prolapse (IVDP) and Ankylosing spondylitis (AS) presents in young and middle-aged.
- Degenerative conditions like Spondylosis (cervical/lumbar), lumbar spondylolysis, spondylolisthesis, and lumbar canal stenosis affect middle to older age population.
- Metastasis involving spine is common in older individuals.

> Pain, deformity, swelling, and neurological deficits are common symptoms in a patient with a spine pathology. The onset, duration, and progression of each symptom are important to differentiate the various pathologies.

A. Pain: It is the most common symptom reported in spine disorders.

1. ***Onset of pain:***

   Acute onset: It occurs in conditions like IVDP *(especially after lifting heavy weight while bending forward, fall on buttock)*, discitis or traumatic conditions. Elderly patient may develop acute pain due to osteoporotic collapse of vertebra.

   Often patients inform that it just started after he/she suddenly extended from flexed position. This may indicate instability of spine or disc pathology.

   Insidious onset: It is suggestive of infection (tuberculosis of the spine), degenerative (spondylosis and osteoporosis), or inflammatory condition like AS.

2. ***Timing of pain:***

   Night pain: It may indicate infection, inflammation, or malignancy.

   Mechanical pain (with activity): Degenerative, osteoporosis

3. ***Site of pain:*** Cervical, thoracic, thoraco-lumbar, and lumbar give an idea of anatomical site of involvement. Local pain can arise from muscular, ligamentous, intervertebral disc, capsule and facet joints etc.

4. ***Nature of pain:***

   Shock-like sensation radiating from spine toward limbs indicates nerve root involvement; burning sensation signifies neurologic origin.

   Mere dull localized pain may arise from any of the spinal structure (bone/soft tissue).

5. ***Radiation:***

   - A backache or neck pain with radiation toward the limbs is suggestive of nerve root involvement.
   - *Area of radiation* should be asked for (scapular region, upper limb, anterior aspect of the thigh, posterior aspect of the thigh, calf, or foot).

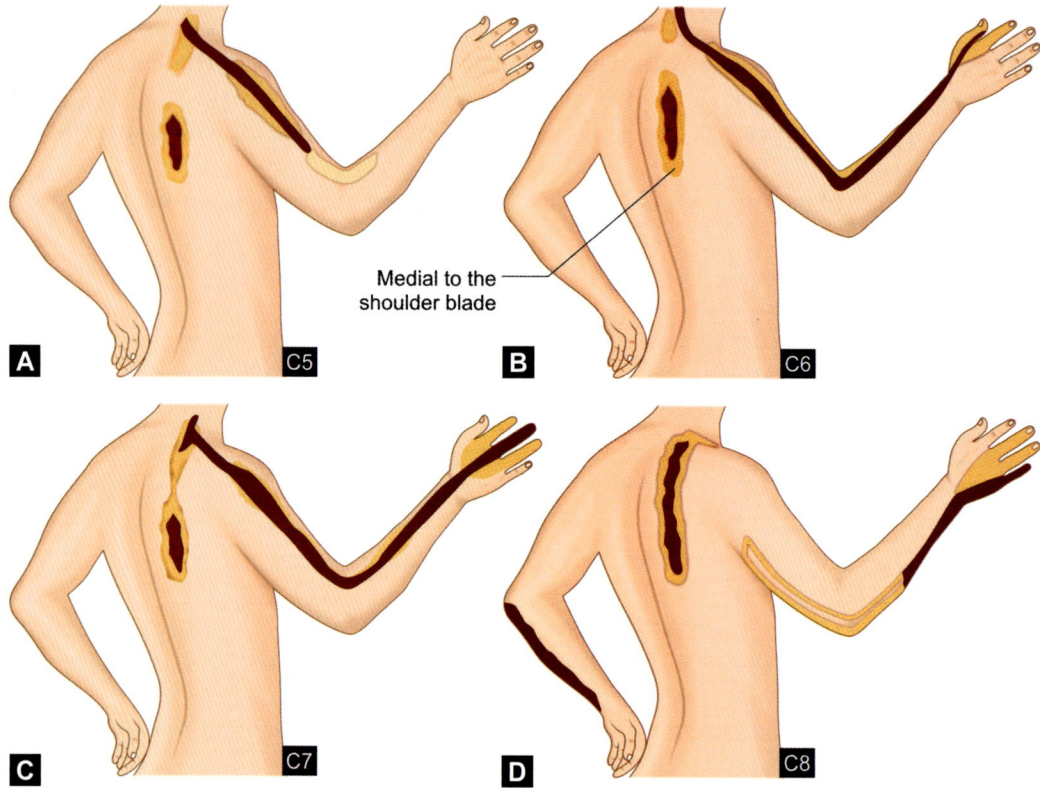

Medial to the
shoulder blade

A C5

B C6

C C7

D C8

Figs. 10.1A to D: Pattern of neck pain radiation towards scapula or upper limb may suggest the root involvement.

In cervical spine, IVDP/cervical spondylosis commonly affects C5,6 and 7 roots, caus-ing radicular pain over the radial (outer) aspect of arm, forearm and hand (thumb and radial two fingers). The pattern of radiation may suggest the root involvement (Figs. 10.1A to D).

- ○ Radiation toward inner aspect of arm and hand is suggestive of thoracic outlet syndrome (TOS) which commonly involves C8, T1, or rarely lower level of cervical IVDP.
- ○ Lumbar spine IVDP/other degenerative conditions commonly lead to L4, L5, and S1 root compression which causes radiating pain toward the back of the thigh, leg, and foot.
- ○ Upper lumbar spine root irritation (L2, 3) is identified with the radiation in front of the thigh.

6. *Aggravating factors*
   - ○ Increase in pain while bending forward, coughing, sneezing or turning in bed is quite typical of acute IVDP of lumbar spine.
   - ○ Pain while bending forward/lifting heavy weight: IVDP of the lumbar spine
   - ○ Pain while bending backward: Lumbar canal stenosis, spondylolysis, spondylolis-thesis, and facet arthropathy

7. *Relieving factors*
   - ○ Pain due to degenerative conditions like spondylosis, canal stenosis, spondylolis-thesis, or osteoporosis, is often relieved at rest.
   - ○ Pain due to inflammatory/infective/tumor pathologies is frequently felt during rest.

8. *Associated stiffness, in morning, and at rest*: Mostly observed in AS and other inflammatory spondyloarthropathies, Rarely in TB of spine.

9. *Walking distance*: In patients with lumbar canal stenosis, the walking distance may decrease due to *neurogenic claudication*. One must make attempts to differentiate neurogenic claudication from vascular claudication (Table 10.1).

Table 10.1: Differences between neurogenic claudication and vascular claudication.

	Neurogenic claudication	*Vascular claudication*
Common cause	Lumbar canal stenosis	Thromboangiitis obliterans, athero-sclerosis of lower limb large vessels
Pain characteristics		
Appears or increases	While standing, walking down-hill, coming down the ramp	After walking for some distance
Ramp/stair climbing	Decreases	Increases
Cycling	No effect	Increases
Pain relieves	Bending forward, climbing up-stairs or ramp	• No effect on bending forward • Increases while going upstairs/ramp
Claudication distance	Variable	Fixed
Associated back pain	Possible	Rare
Distal pulse	Normal	Decreased/absent
Sensory symptoms	Common	Rare
Trophic changes	None	Likely

B. Deformity
- Deformity of neck and trunk is a usual presentation in congenital (torticollis, scoliosis), post-traumatic, infective (TB), inflammatory (AS), or osteoporosis.
- The onset, duration, and progress should be asked to rule out congenital and acquired disorder.

C. Swelling
- Swelling of the neck, back, and the paraspinal region may be the presenting symptoms. It could be congenital (spina bifida) or acquired (cold abscess) in nature.

D. Restriction of motion
- Patient may complain of restricted motion (difficulty in bending forward/backward/rotation) due to pain or stiffness.

E. Neurological symptoms
- Motor weakness or sensory symptoms (tingling, numbness) of the limb indicate involvement of the spinal cord or nerve root.
- Bladder and bowel involvement indicates the involvement of cauda equina/spinal cord.

F. Dizziness
- Sometimes noted in cervical spondylosis due to osteophytes encroaching the vertebral artery foramen leading to vertebrobasilar insufficiency.

G. Systemic symptoms
- Fever, weight loss, loss of appetite, cough, expectoration, and hemoptysis (Infection, tumor of spine).
- Frequent lower respiratory tract infection can happen in AS due to decreased chest expansion.

H. Other conditions
- Pregnancy, Genitourinary or gynecological pathologies (pelvic inflammatory diseases) can lead to back pain.
- Prostate symptoms must be asked for as prostrate malignancy can metastasize to spine and give rise to back pain with/without neurological deficit.

Occupational history
- Desk bound, those involved in heavy manual labor or weightlifting or drivers are more prone for low back pain.

Family history
- Ankylosing spondylitis can have a positive family history.
- Tuberculosis can have history of contact in family or neighborhood.

Past history
- Similar complaint, treatment history should be asked in detail. Any related surgeries done in the past.

Personal history
- Sleep, appetite, Smoking and alcohol intake. Severe pain for weeks, disturbing sleep is a red flag sign.

Menstrual history
- Females with pelvic inflammatory disease can have low back pain.

EXAMINATION OF SPINE

General and Systemic Examination

The general and systemic examination must be performed in the standard fashion.
- Congenital scoliosis could be associated with neurofibromatosis and Café-au-lait spots, which need to be looked for during the general examination.
- Lesions of spine with infective origin (tuberculosis) or tumorous origin (metastasis and multiple myeloma) can have systemic features like pallor and sometimes, cachexia.
- Fever is common in infective and inflammatory conditions.

Local Examination

Gait
- If a person is ambulant, gait is assessed before examining the spine.

> Examination of the patient in standing/sitting position and assessment of gait should be absolutely avoided if there is impending neurological deficit or if loading of spine can lead to deterioration in the neurological status.

Attitude

- The attitude can be commented upon while the patient is examined in standing, sitting, and in supine position.

Inspection

- After appropriate consent, privacy and chaperone; the examination of spine should be performed on a hard bed with the spine completely exposed.
- It should be done in standing, supine, and sitting position.
- The spine examination involves inspection from front, side, and back.

1. **Alignment:** The alignment of the spine should start with inspection of the head, the neck, the shoulder, the pelvis and the natal cleft and should be done from front, side and back.

   From front
   - Normally, head and neck are central. In torticollis, the neck is tilted to one side with the chin rotated to the opposite side (Fig. 10.2).
   - Shape of the chest and abdominal protuberance must be looked for.

   From side
   - Natural *kyphosis of thoracic region and lordosis of the lumbar region* should be noted.
   - Look for abnormality like exaggeration/attenuation of *thoracic kyphosis and lumbar lordosis.*
   - Exaggerated lordosis is mostly compensatory. Often seen in developmental dysplasia of the hip, flexion deformity of the hip, and spondylolisthesis
   - Loss of cervical lordosis is seen in AS
   - Loss of lumbar lordosis is seen in AS, IVDP, spinal infections, or flatback syndrome.

> - *Collapse of single vertebra leads to* knuckle kyphotic deformity
> - *Collapse of two to three vertebrae lead to* angular kyphotic deformity (Fig. 10.3A)
> - *Collapse of four or more vertebrae lead to* roundback kyphotic deformity (*Dowager's hump*) (Fig. 10.3B). It is seen in Scheuermann's disease, Ankylosing spondylitis, multiple osteoporotic vertebral collapse, and Paget's disease.

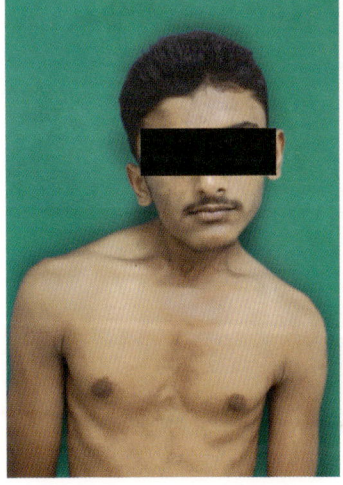

Fig. 10.2: Torticollis of right side.

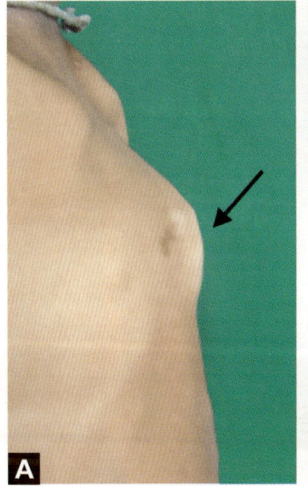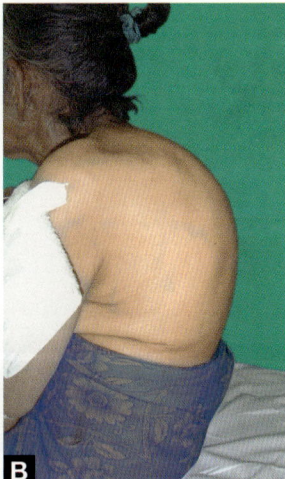

Figs. 10.3A and B: (A) Angular kyphosis. (B) Roundback kyphosis.

From behind

- Normally; *the head, neck, spine, and natal cleft are in one line (**plumb line:** from occiput to natal cleft) and there is no* coronal malalignment (scoliosis) of spine from cervical region to sacrum (Fig. 10.4A).
- *Scoliosis is best noted from behind* (Fig. 10.4B). Scoliosis could be ***functional/structural***.

> Scoliosis is not normal to the spine, and its presence indicate an underlying pathology. It must be examined from behind, in standing and sitting positions.

- ○ *Functional Scoliosis*: While present in standing, it *disappears on* sitting (Figs. 10.4C and D).

  It is often due to limb length discrepancy or acute paraspinal muscle spasm.
- ○ *Structural scoliosis*: It *persists on standing, sitting, or lying down.*

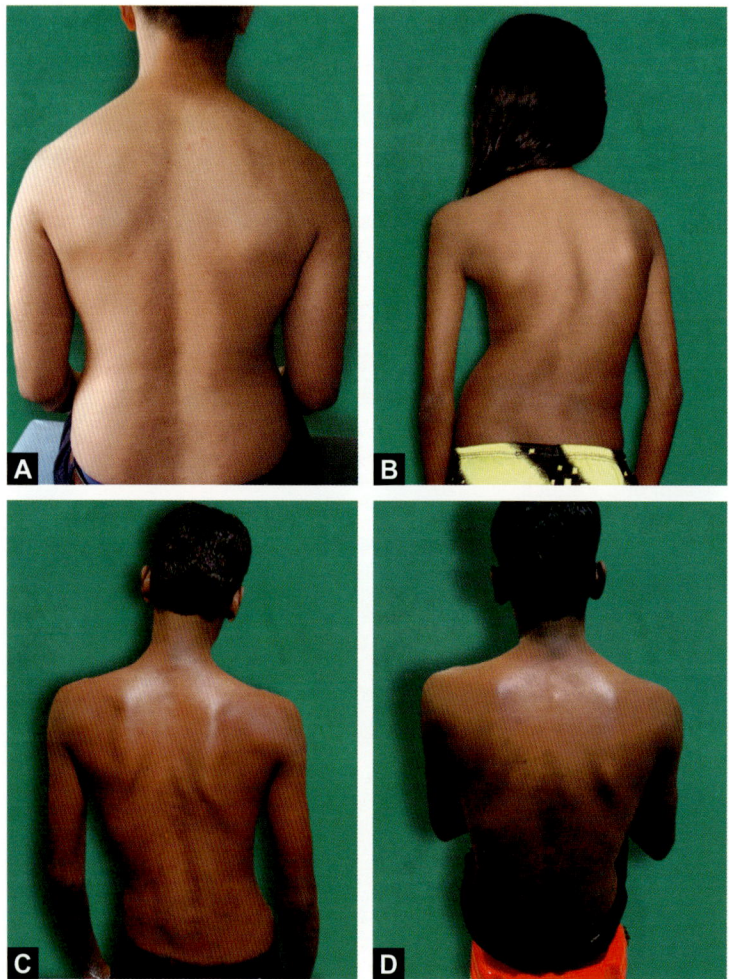

Figs. 10.4A to D: (A) Alignment from back. (B) Scoliosis of dorsolumbar spine. (C and D) Functional scoliosis is noted during standing position whereas it disappears on sitting.

Note the sidedness of the scoliotic curve. Further, patient should be asked to bend forward. If scoliosis disappears on bending forward, it suggests mobile structural scoliosis. If scoliotic deformity does not disappear, it is a rigid structural scoliosis. (Adam's test) (Figs. 10.5A and B).

- *Any list*: Often, acute spasm of the spinal muscles due to pain leads to abrupt lateral shift of the trunk above a certain point (Fig. 10.5C).

  It is also known as *trunk list/lateral shift/acute lumbar sciatic scoliosis/wind swept spine*. It is either ipsilateral or contralateral to the side of the pain. This spasm avoids the irritation of nerve root.

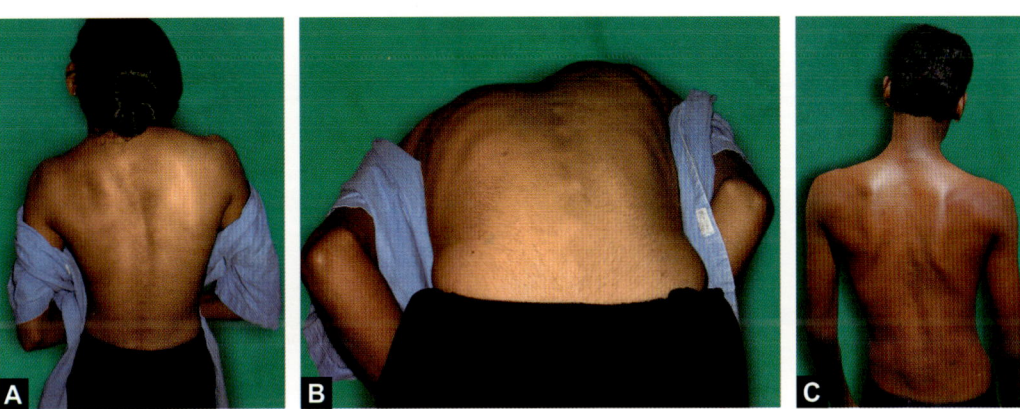

Figs. 10.5A to C: (A and B) Adam's test. (C) List of spine.

2. The level of shoulder and pelvis (from front and back)

- Normally, both shoulders and pelvis (anterior superior iliac spine, ASIS and posterior superior iliac spine, PSIS) are at the same level with head and neck central.
- The tilt of the pelvis, if any, should be noted.

3. Neck and scapula

- Note the hair line: Low hairline is seen in Klippel-Feil syndrome, Turner syndrome
- *Webbing of neck*: Short webbed neck in Klippel–Feil syndrome (Fig. 10.6)
- *Level of scapular spine and inferior angle*: High-riding scapula (Sprengel shoulder)

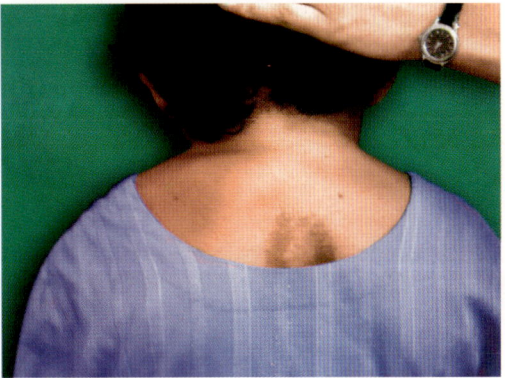

Fig. 10.6: Features of Klippel–Feil syndrome.

4. Skin of the back and elsewhere

- *Presence* of *café-au-lait spots, tuft of hair, dimple* or *hemangioma* should be looked for from cervical to sacral region (Figs. 10.7A to C). café-au-lait spots are seen in Neurofibromatosis which is associated with Scoliosis whereas tuft of hair, dimple or hemangioma are associated with Spina Bifida Occulta.
- The axillary and inguinal region should also be examined for *freckling (Neurofibromatosis, Scoliosis).*

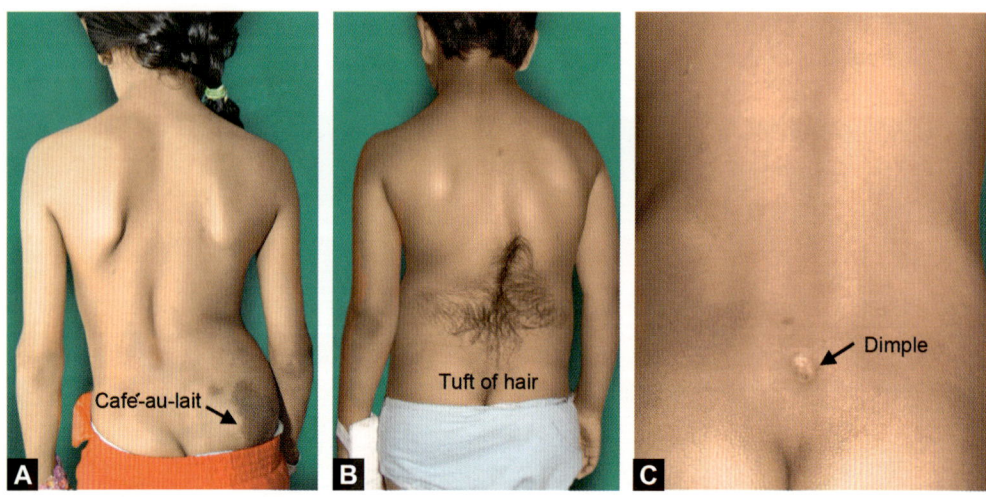

Figs. 10.7A to C: Café-au-lait spots, tuft of hair, and dimple over lumbosacral spine.

5. Swelling

- *Cold abscess*: It should be looked for in the paraspinal region, midaxillary line, intercostal spaces, abdomen, inguinal region as well as Petit triangle (Fig. 10.8A).
- *Rib hump*: Commonly associated with rigid structural scoliosis of the thoracic spine (Fig. 10.8B).
- *Spina bifida aperta*: Swelling on midline over the lumbar spine (meningocele, meningomyelocele).

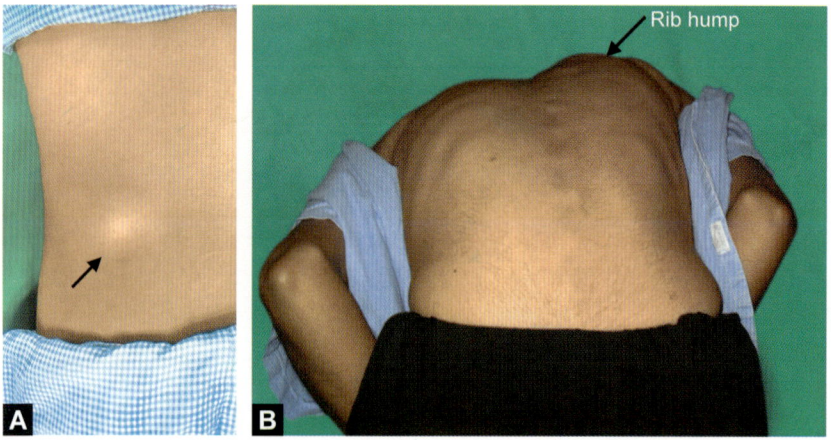

Figs. 10.8A and B: (A) Swelling over the Petit triangle. (B) Rib hump.

Petit triangle (inferior lumbar triangle): It is a triangular space in the lower lateral part of back, bounded medially by latissimus dorsi, laterally by external oblique, and base by iliac crest. The floor is formed by the internal oblique muscle.

6. The attitude and deformity of the upper limb

- Any ipsilateral/bilateral wasting or deformity of upper limbs (claw hand) could be secondary to involvement of cervical spinal cord/roots.

7. The attitude and deformity of the lower limb

- Pes cavus, claw toe, and equinus/calcaneus of one side or both sides may be secondary to involvement of spinal cord/root.

8. Muscle spasm and atrophy of the upper limbs, para-spinal muscle, thigh, and or calf should be noted if any.

Palpation

1. Local rise in temperature: It should be checked over the areas of pain and deformity.

2. Spine tenderness

- It should be elicited over the spine (cervical to sacral region), paraspinal region, along the ribs, and sacroiliac joint. The point tenderness may help in localizing the level of lesion.
- *Method*: *The spinous process could be pressed in*
  (i) Anterior direction (direct tenderness) (Fig. 10.9A)
  (ii) Sideways (twist tenderness)
  Another method to elicit spine tenderness: Gentle thumping (thrust tenderness) along the spinous process of all the vertebrae.
  The level of spinous process involvement must be noted (Fig. 10.9B).
- Absence of spinous process: Noted in the spina bifida.
- Palpable step off between two spinous processes in the lumbar region: Present in lumbar spondylolisthesis.

3. Paraspinal spasm

Method: It is best felt with fingers pressed over the paraspinal muscles. Normally, paraspinal muscles feel soft on palpation, but feel quite firm if in spasm (Figs. 10.9C and D).

4. Normal bony landmarks: Scapula, iliac crest, and PSIS

5. Other soft tissues of the back and neck should be palpated.

6. Deformity of the back, upper and lower limb

- The kyphotic, scoliotic, and lordotic deformities must be palpated and confirmed.
- Always look for any deformities of upper limb, hip, knee, ankle, and foot. Confirm by palpation, if any. Any asymmetry of the lower limb must be noted.

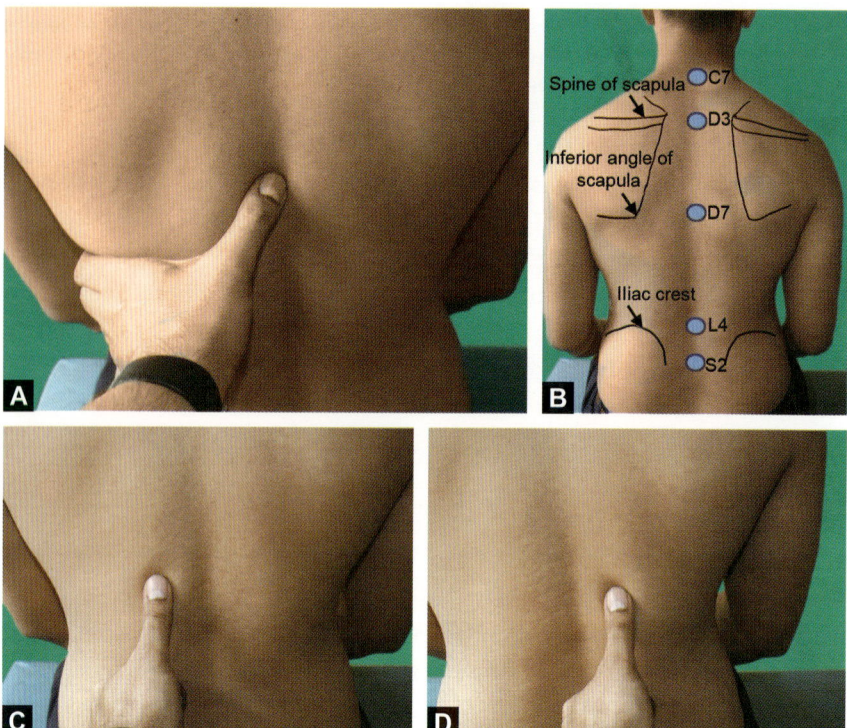

Figs. 10.9A to D: (A and B) Palpation of spinous process and level of vertebra.
(C and D) Assessment of the paraspinal spasm.

Movement of Various Regions of Spine: Cervical, Dorsal, and Lumbar

1. Cervical spine movement: Flexion (0-50°), Extension (0–60°) Lateral rotation (0–80°), and Lateral flexion (0–45°) (Figs. 10.10A to D).

2. Dorsal spine movement: Predominantly lateral rotation (0–50°)

(*Note: Flexion at dorsal spine is limited due to rib cage whereas -extension and lateral flexion is similar to lumbar spine*)

Method: Patient sits on the couch. (Making patient sit on couch fixes the pelvis and hip which can no more contribute to the rotation). Ask patient to keep both the hand over his waist OR cross the arms across the body and keep hands over opposite shoulders, and then to twist the trunk on either sides, one by one (Figs. 10.11A and B).

Interpretation: Lateral rotation must be noted as the angle between the mobile shoulder and static pelvis. Normal lateral rotation is 50° on each side.

3. Lumbar spine movement: *Flexion (0-60°), Extension (0-25°) and Lateral flexion (0-30°)* (Figs. 10.12A to C)

(a) Assessment of lumbar spine flexion: Bending forward, Modified Schober's method

- ***Bending forward method:*** Ask the patient to bend forward and try touching the toes/floor "without bending the knee." If the patient can touch the toes or ground, it includes the movements of the thoracic spine, lumber spine, and hip joint. The patient's movements must be noted as the ability to touch the ground or "how many cm 'away' from the ground"

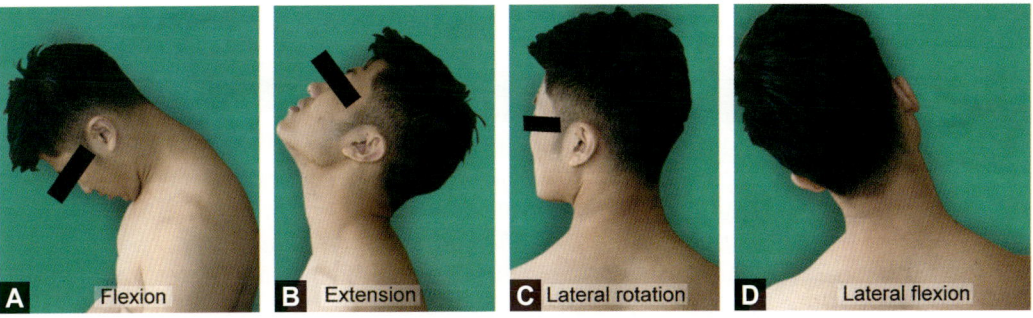

Figs. 10.10A to D: Movements of cervical spine.

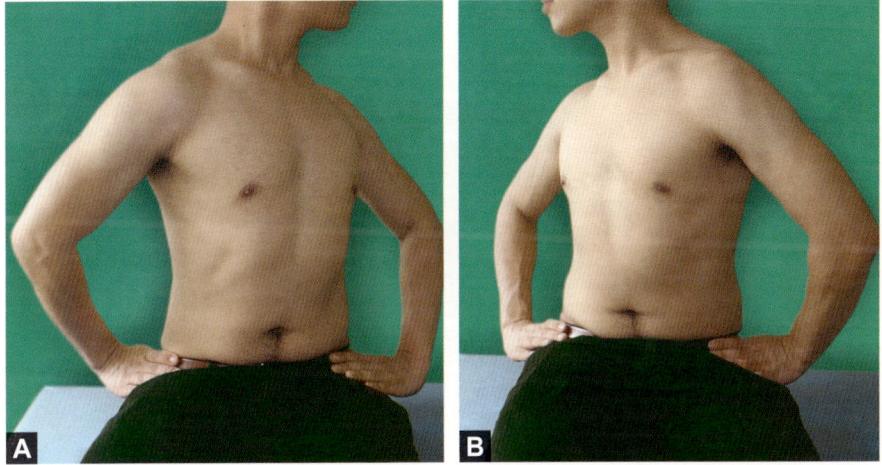

Figs. 10.11A and B: (A and B) Lateral rotation at dorsal spine.

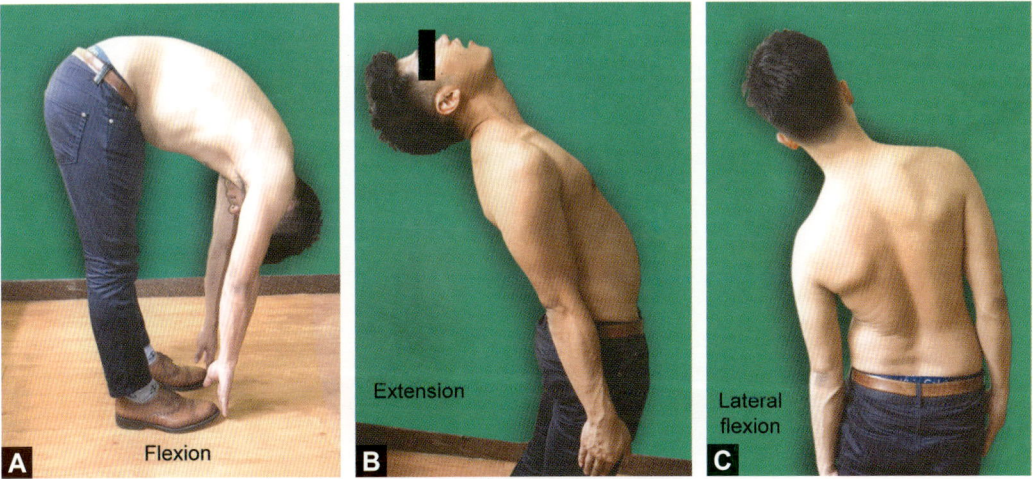

Figs. 10.12A to C: Lumbar spine movements: flexion, extension, and lateral flexion.

- **Modified Schober's method:** Flexion of the lumber spine can also be measured by Schober's method.

  Method: Patient stands erect. Three points are marked over midline of the spine. First mark over the lumbar spine at the level of the dimple of the posterior superior iliac spine, second 10 cm above, and third one 5 cm below the first mark. Ask patient to bend forward as much as possible and measure the distance between highest and lowest mark (Fig. 10.13A). *(In original Schober's method, there are only two points—one at the level of PSIS and other 10 cm above the first one. However, interpretation is the same).*

  Interpretation: The normal distance between the highest and lowest mark during flexion at the lumbar spine increases by 6-9 cm. Less than 5 cm increase in the distance between highest and lowest mark is indicative of decreased lumbar spine flexion. It is decreased in Ankylosing spondylitis.

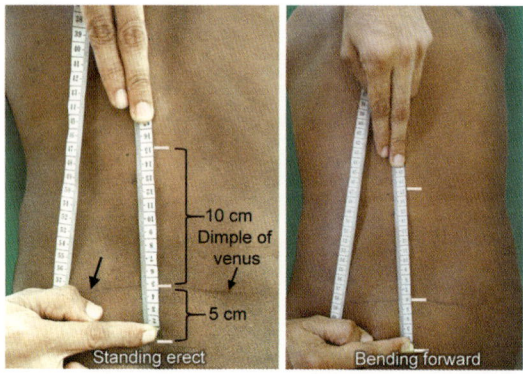

Fig. 10.13A: Modified Schober test.

(b) Extension
Method: Ask the patient to bend backward.

The exact measurement of spine extension is difficult. However, the distance between L1 and S1 should be measured in neutral and backward movement.

- The extension of spine is decreased or not possible in AS.
- Decreased spinal extension in AS is measured by "occiput-wall distance" (Fig. 10.13B). Normally, in completely extended spine, the occiput can touch the wall. However, in the patients with AS, the occiput fails to touch the wall indicating loss of extension in the spine.

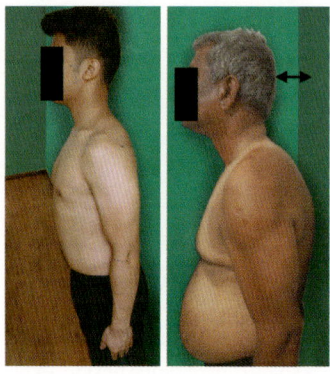

Fig. 10.13B: Normal and increased occiput wall distance.

(c) Lateral flexion

Method: Lateral flexion can be examined by asking the patient to bend on one side. The angle between the imaginary vertical midline axis and the straight line joining T1 and S1 vertebra is measured as lateral flexion of the spine.

> **Note: Painful/painless forward flexion or extension movements of the lumbar spine might provide a clue to the diagnosis.**
> - *Painful forward flexion:* Noted in IVDP
> - *Painful extension:* Noted *in lumbar canal stenosis, spondylolysis, spondylolisthesis, and facet joint arthritis*
> - Both flexion of spine and extension are decreased in ankylosing spondylitis.

Measurement

1. *The linear measurement* of spine has less value in clinical diagnostics.
2. *Chest expansion:* Normal expansion is about 5 cm. It is decreased in AS.
3. *Limb length discrepancy:* if relevant for the case.

Special Tests for Cervical Spine, Thoracic Outlet Syndrome (TOS), Lumbar Spine and Sacroiliac Joint

(A) Special tests for cervical IVDP, spondylosis

1. Spurling test: It is performed in cases where patient complains of radicular pain in the upper limb due to nerve root compression due to cervical IVDP/spondylosis.

Method: Patient is made to sit on a couch. The clinician stands behind the patient and interlocks his fingers of both hands and keeps the volar aspect over the head of the patient. Then, the clinician extends the neck completely, and lateral flexes the neck to 30° and gives mild downward axial pressure over the skull (Fig. 10.14).

Interpretation: With this maneuver, patient experiences radiating pain in the upper limb over the dermatome of the nerve root involved. It indicates nerve root compression and may be seen in cervical IVDP or cervical spondylosis.

> **Basis of Spurling test:** In IVDP/spondylosis, the foraminal area available for nerve root exit near neural foramina is already narrowed due to prolapsed disc and, osteophytes encroaching upon the passage available for the roots. The lateral flexion and axial pressure further narrow the foramina/passage and compresses the nerve root leading to radiating pain in the dermatome of the nerve root involved.

(B) Special test for TOS due to cervical rib or scalenus anterior/medius abnormality

Patient is suspected to have TOS if the cervical radicular pain is toward the medial side of the arm, forearm, and hand as TOS commonly results in pressure over the lower trunk of brachial plexus (C8, T1). *It is in contrast to the IVDP of the cervical spine and cervical spondylosis where the radicular pain in usually over the radial aspect of the arm, forearm, and thumb as latter mostly affects C5, C6 and C7 roots.*

1. Adson's test: Provocative test for vascular component of TOS

Method: Patient sits upright on a couch. The arm on the affected side is extended, abducted, and externally rotated. Then, the neck is extended and rotated *towards the affected* side. Now patient is asked to take a deep breath and instructed to hold. The radial pulse of the affected side is now palpated (Fig. 10.15).

Interpretation: If pulse becomes feeble/disappears, the test is considered to be positive.

2. Wright test: Provocative test for vascular component of TOS

Method: Patient sits upright on a couch. The arm on the affected side is kept extended, abducted, and externally rotated. Then, the neck is extended and rotated *toward normal* side. Now radial pulse is palpated.

Interpretation: If pulse becomes feeble/disappears, the test is considered to be positive.

3. Also in patients with suspected TOS, examine for *sensory and motor disturbance in the region of C8, T1*. There might be intrinsic muscle weakness in hand if there is significant compression of the nerve roots.

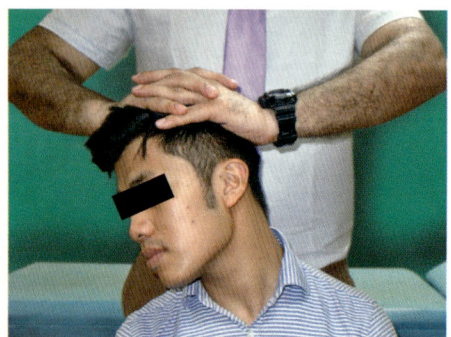

Fig. 10.14: Spurling test.

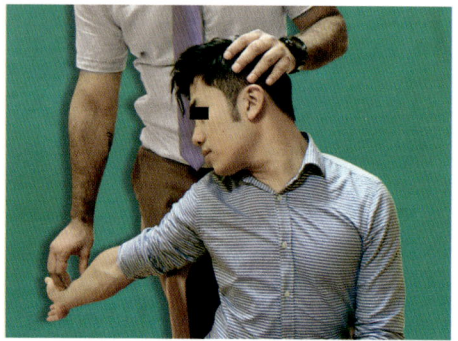

Fig. 10.15: Adson's test.

(C) Special tests for lumbar spine
1. Straight leg raising test (SLRT)
2. Lasegue test
3. Well-leg raising test
4. Femoral nerve stretch test

1. SLRT: Performed to confirm the lumbar nerve root (L4 onwards) irritation/compression.

Prerequisite: No fixed flexion deformity (FFD) at knee and mobile hip

Method: The patient lies supine on the couch. Ask the patient which limb the the pain radiates. At the outset, the normal lower limb is gradually elevated from the couch holding the ankle while keeping the knee in extension (the hand should be kept over the knee to keep it in extension). The angle between the limb and couch is noted. Then, the affected side is gradually elevated and examiner watches the patient's face during the maneuver for any discomfort due to radiating pain in the elevated limb. Ask whether is it pain radiating up to thigh, leg, and foot OR it is mere tightness felt at the back of thigh (Fig. 10.16).

Interpretation: In a normal patient without any root compression, the limb can be raised to 70–90° with ease. However, with nerve root involvement (like in IVDP), the limb cannot be raised more than 60°, and the patient complains of radiating pain to the affected limb way before the normal SLR. Note that in IVDP of lumbar spine with root compression of L4 onwards, the pain always radiates below the level of knee.

In hamstring tightness, patient reports that it is not painful but feels tightness at the back of the thigh.

> **Bowstring test**: After positive SLRT, slightly bent the knee. This reduces or ameliorates the radicular pain. Now, apply pressure to the tibial nerve in popliteal fossa. The test is positive if this reproduces patient's sciatic or radicular pain

2. Lasegue test: Performed to confirm the lumbar nerve root irritation/compression

Method: While performing SLRT, the limb elevation is stopped when patient complains of pain radiating to the lower limb. Then, the lower limb is gradually lowered till the radiating pain reduces completely. Now, the ankle is dorsiflexed which again exacerbates the pain (Fig. 10.17).

Interpretation: Recurrence of pain with dorsiflexion of ankle confirms the root irritation.

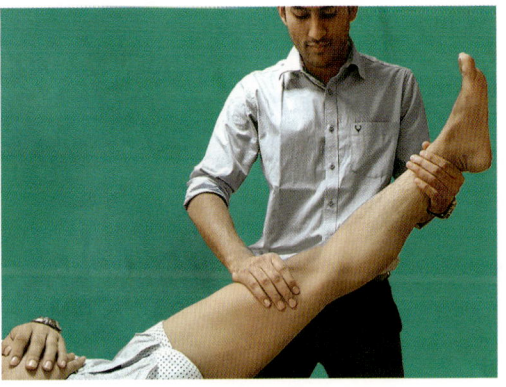

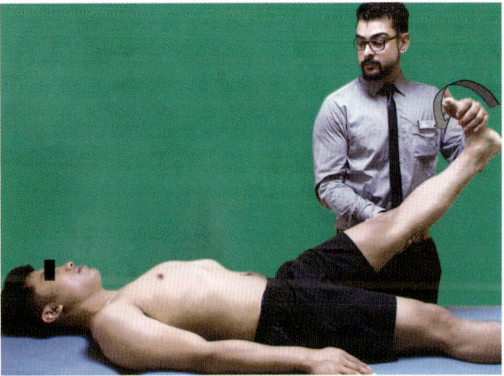

Fig. 10.16: Straight leg raising test.   **Fig. 10.17:** Lasegue test.

3. Well leg raising test/crossed SLRT: It is quite specific for IVDP (axillary type/medial disc prolapse)

Method: It is similar to SLRT but here "only normal limb" is elevated. If the patient complains of radiating pain over the nonelevated/index limb, the test is considered to be positive.

It is *pathognomonic for axillary type of lumbar IVDP.*

4. Femoral nerve stretch test: For L2, 3, 4 root irritation/compression

Method: Patient is made to lie prone on the couch. The affected side knee is flexed followed by gradual extension of the hip (Fig. 10.18).

Interpretation: If this produces tingling/pain in the femoral nerve distribution area, the test is positive.

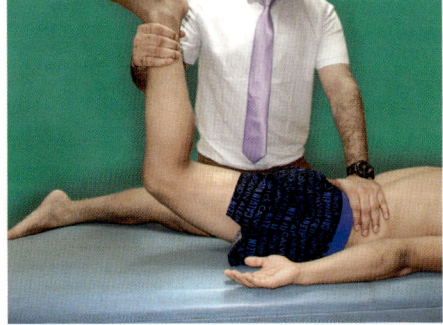

Fig. 10.18: Femoral stretch test.

(D) Special test for sacroiliac joint

1. Figure of four test: To test the involvement of sacroiliac joint (SIJ) especially in inflammatory conditions (Sacroilitis in AS).

Method: Patient lies supine over the couch. The knee is flexed to 90° and the hip is externally rotated. Then, the leg–ankle junction is placed over the lower end of opposite thigh just above the knee. Subsequently, the examiner pushes the knee downward with one hand, and another hand stabilizes the pelvis (Fig. 10.19).

Interpretation: If this maneuver elicits pain over ipsilateral SIJ, it indicates sacroiliitis. The similar maneuver is repeated for the other side.

2. Gaenslen test:

Method: Patient lies supine over the couch. One of the hip and knee are hyper flexed and the other hip is extended over the edge of the couch (Fig. 10.20). If this maneuver causes pain over SIJ (uni- or bilateral), the test is considered to be positive.

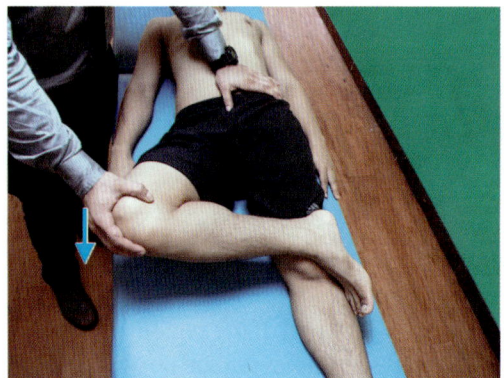
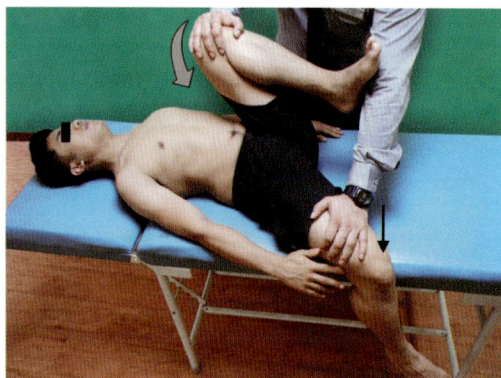

Fig. 10.19: Figure of four test.   **Fig. 10.20:** Gaenslen test.

3. Pelvis compression test:

Method: The patient lies in the lateral position over the couch. Now, the examiner keeps both his hands over the ASIS and exerts a steady downward pressure. This leads to pain over the SIJ (Fig. 10.21A).

The same "pelvic compression" can be applied in supine position too while examiner compresses iliac crest toward each other using his hands placed over both iliac crest.

4. Pelvis distraction test:

Method: Patient lies in supine position over the couch. The examiner exerts a steady downward pressure over the lateral aspect of Ilium causing 'distraction' of SIJ. This leads to pain over the SIJ (Figs. 10.21A and B).

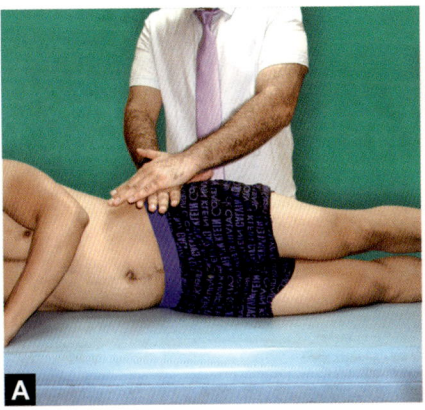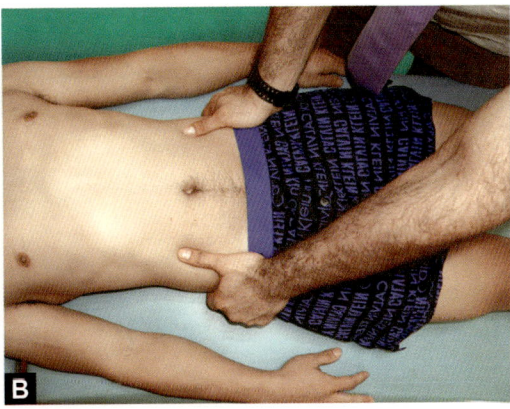

Figs. 10.21A and B: Pelvis compression and distraction test.

Neurological Examination

Though most spinal column/spinal cord pathology may not involve brain and cranial nerves, the neurological examination should be thorough involving a quick assessment of CNS too.

1. *Higher mental function*: Consciousness, alertness, orientation to time-place-person, memory, speech

2. *Cranial nerves*

3. *Sensory examination*: *The principal objective of sensory examination is to ascertain the "level of the lesion".* In case of spinal cord or nerve root involvement, at least one sensation from each tract (posterior column, anterior, and lateral spinothalamic) must be tested The methodology of sensory assessment is outlined in the Box 10.1.

- *Since the pathology of the spine involves spinal cord or the nerve roots, the sensation must be tested as per dermatomal distribution* (Fig. 10.22).

Box 10.1: Method of sensory examination.
- The procedure should be explained to the patient with appropriate consent and privacy.
- With part exposed (never with clothes on), patient must keep his eyes closed during sensory examination.
- The sensation must be tested, dermatome wise.
- Constant stimulus is given over the dermatome bilaterally and simultaneously (to understand the difference between normal and abnormal).
- In between, no stimulus to be given and patient should be asked for sensory perception (to check malingering. It may also indicate that the patient has not understood the procedure)

- *Sensation to be tested*
    - *Touch*: Tested with wisp of cotton
    - *Pain*: Tested with pin
    - *Temperature*: Tested with test tubes containing cold and hot water
    - *Vibration sense*: Tested with 128-Hz tuning fork over bony prominences
    - *Proprioception*: Joint position sense
    - *Stereognosis*: Identify a common object (coin/key) and place in the patient's hand with eyes closed, and ask patient to identify it.
    - *Two point discrimination*: Tested with blunt divider

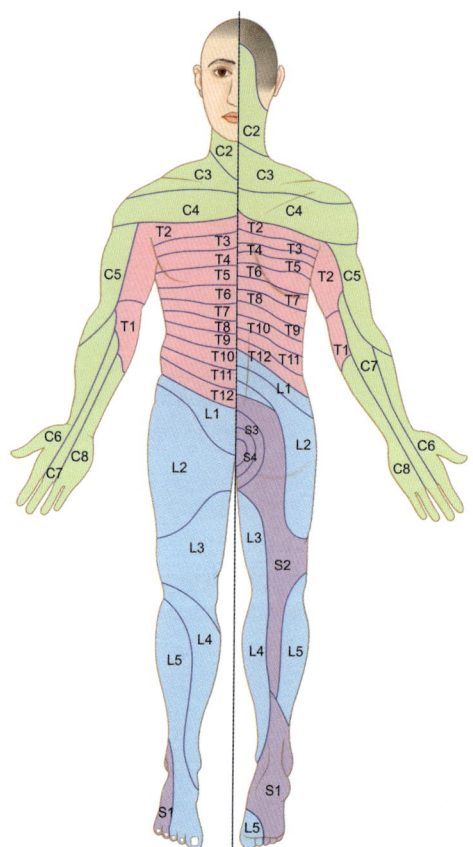

Fig. 10.22: Dermatomes of the body.

4. Motor examination
- *Bulk/nutrition of muscles*: Normal/reduced
- *Tone*: Hypo- or hypertonia. Former is seen in lower motor neurons (LMN) type lesion whereas latter is seen in upper motor neuron (UMN) type lesion (Table 10.2).
- *Power*: Grade the muscle power (0–5) according to MRC grade (Box 10.2)
- *Coordination*: Heel shin test and finger–nose test
- *Involuntary movements.*

5. Reflexes (with root value)
- *Superficial*: Abdominal (T7-T12), Cremasteric (L1, L2), Anal (S3, S4), Bulbocavernous (S3, S4), and Plantar (L5, S1)
- *Deep*: Biceps (C5, 6), Supinator (C6), Triceps (C7), Knee (L2, L3, L4), and Ankle (S1, S2)

6. Abnormal reflexes: Clonus; Patellar and Ankle (observed in UMN lesions)

7. Bladder and bowel status: Normal/automatic/atonic bladder

8. Skin condition: Bed sores grading as per National pressure ulcer advisory panel (NPUAP) (Box. 10.3)

Table 10.2: Differences between upper motor neuron (UMN) and lower motor neuron (LMN) lesion.

	UMN	*LMN*
Wasting of muscle	Less	Pronounced
Tone	Hypertonia	Hypotonia
Superficial reflexes	±	-
Deep reflexes	Exaggerated	Absent
Babinski's	Present	Absent
Clonus	Present	Absent

Box 10.2: MRC grading.

Grade 0: No power
Grade 1: Flicker in muscle
Grade2: Movement + but with gravity eliminated
Grade3: Movement against gravity
Grade 4: Movement against mild-moderate resistance
Grade 5: Movement against full resistance

Box 10.3: NPUAP grading of bed sore.

Grade 1: Erythema of skin, no breakdown
Grade 2: Superficial blisters/peeling
Grade 3: Full thickness skin loss, above deep fascia
Grade 4: Full thickness skin loss deeper than deep fascia, involving deeper structures like bone, muscle, and tendon

Examination of Joints of Upper and Lower Limb

Lymph Nodes Examination

Spine examination proforma

1. **Gait**
2. **Attitude**
3. **Inspection:**
   - **General findings:** *All areas for overlying skin, Swelling, scar, sinus*
   - **Specific findings of inspection**
     (a) Alignment of spine and rest of body
       – *From front:* Head and neck alignment, shoulder level, chest shape and pelvis
       – *From side:* Dorsal Kyphosis and lumbar lordosis (normal/exaggerated/attenuated)
       – *From back:* Alignment of head, neck, spine and natal cleft, scoliosis, List
     (b) Level of shoulder and pelvis
     (c) Neck and Scapula
     (d) Skin of back and elsewhere
     (e) Swelling
     (f) Deformities in upper and lower limb and
     (g) Muscle spasm and atrophy
4. **Palpation**
   - Local rise in temperature
   - Spinous process: Tenderness, step, deformity, any absence of spinous process
   - Paraspinal spasm
   - Other bony (Scapula, PSIS, iliac crest) and soft tissue landmarks, deformities in upper and lower limb
   - *Confirmation of palpatory characteristics of swelling, scar, sinus*
5. **Movements: Active and passive**
   - Cervical spine: Flexion, extension, rotation, lateral flexion
   - Dorsal spine: Rotation
   - Lumbar spine: Flexion (Forward bend, Schober's test), Extension, Wall-occiput distance, lateral flexion
6. **Measurements**
   Chest expansion, limb length (if relevant)
7. **Special tests**
   (a) *Test for Cervical root compression in IVDP/spondylosis:* Spurling test
   (b) *Test for Thoracic outlet syndrome:* Adson's test, Wright test
   (c) *Test for Lumbar spine root compression in IVDP:* Straight leg raising test, Lasegue test, Bowstring test, Well leg raising test, Femoral nerve stretch test
   (d) *Sacroiliac joint test:* Figure of four test, Gaenslen test, Pelvis compression and distraction test
8. **Neurological examination:** Higher mental function, Cranial nerve examination Sensorimotor examination, Bladder and bowel status assessment and skin condition
9. **Joint below:** Hip, knee and ankle-foot
10. **Other areas** like chest, abdomen and lymph nodes of cervical and other areas must be examined in case of suspected spine tuberculosis or malignancy.

Common conditions affecting spine with salient features

1. **Congenital Torticollis**
   - *Affects*: Presents in children. However, may present at any age
   - *Presents with*: Head is tilted to one side, and chin deviates to other side.
   - *Pathology*: Tight sternocleidomastoid muscle due to fibrosis
   - *Clinically*: The head is tilted to tight sternocleidomastoid side, and chin deviates to other side. The lateral rotation of the opposite side is increased while rotation to the same side is decreased. The lateral flexion of the same side is increased while lateral flexion of the opposite side is decreased.
   - *Diagnosis*: Clinical
   - *Treatment*: Bracing, stretching, and bipolar surgical release of the Sternocleidomastoid tendon

2. **Scoliosis**
   - *Affects*: Present in children. However, may present at any age
   - *Presents with*: Deformity in the back; may be thoracic, lumber or both
   - *Pathology*: Idiopathic, vertebral developmental anomaly
   - *Clinically*: Scoliotic deformity, tuft of hair, or neurocutaneous marker present in congenital case. Rigid structural scoliosis does not disappear on flexion of the spine, while functional or compensatory scoliosis disappears on flexion of the spine. Neurological examination is normal in most of the patients.
   - *Diagnosis*: X-ray, computed tomography (CT) scan, and magnetic resonance imaging (MRI)
   - *Treatment*: Bracing/surgery depending upon progression and severity of the curve.

3. **Kyphosis**
   - *Etiology:* Postural, Scheuermann disease, Traumatic, infective (TB), Ankylosing spondylitis, Congenital, Metabolic disorders (osteoporosis).
   - *Presents with:* Kyphotic deformity (normal thoracic kyphosis from T1-T12 is 20-40° of Cobb's angle)
   - *Clinically:* Localized kyphosis indicates infection/trauma affecting spine whereas generalized kyphosis/round back kyphosis indicate Osteoporosis, AS, and Scheuermann disease
   - *Diagnosis:* X-ray, CT scan, and MRI
   - *Treatment:* As per condition

4. **Tuberculosis of the spine**
   - *Affects*: Mostly young adults.
   - *Presents with*: Pain in the back especially in the night, stiffness, fever, weight loss, common in thoracolumbar area especially 'thoracolumbar junction'
   - *Pathology*: Tubercular affection of vertebra; paradiscal is most common. Musculoskeletal TB is always secondary to the primary elsewhere (occult/overt/past history).
   - *Clinically*: Vertebral tenderness and or kyphosis present at site of the vertebral involvement, painful restricted movements of the spine, may have neurological deficit, cold abscess ±
   - *Diagnosis*: X-ray, MRI, and other investigations for TB. *Always investigate for primary focus.*
   - *Treatment*: Anti-tubercular treatment (ATT), bracing, surgical decompression, and stabilization

5. **Intervertebral disc prolapse of cervical region**
   - *Affects*: Mostly young adult
   - *Presents with*: Neck pain with/without radiation to scapular region, suprascapular area, arm, or forearm till the hand

- **Pathology**: Rupture of annulus fibrosis followed protrusion, prolapse, and extrusion of the intervertebral disc.
- **Clinically**: Commonly Intervertebral disc of C4-C5, C5-C6, and C6-C7 regions is affected, vertebral tenderness at affected level, Spurling test, and Upper limb tension test +
- Painful ROM of cervical spine
- Neurological examination is must to correlate the level of disc
- **Diagnosis**: MRI
- **Treatment**: Mostly conservative. Rarely discectomy if worsening neurological deficit or unrelenting pain, which is not responding to conservative treatment.

6. **Cervical rib/TOS**
   - **Presents with**: Pain in the upper limb in C8, T1 dermatome. Occasionally, neck pain
   - **Pathology**: Cervical rib or hypertrophied scalene muscle compresses the lower trunk (C8, T1) of brachial plexus (rarely, upper trunk) causing neurological symptoms or subclavian vein or artery causing vascular features
   - **Clinically**: Neurological features in ulnar nerve or rarely in median nerve distribution area. Typically, the radiation is toward the medial side of the arm and forearm (c.f. IVDP of cervical spine where radiation is over radial aspect as IVDP of cervical spine predominantly occurs in C5-6 and C6-7 regions)
     Sometimes vascular symptoms like swelling (venous congestion), Raynaud's like features in hand, and arterial ischaemia; Adson's and Wright test +.
   - **Diagnosis**: X-ray, CT, MRI, Doppler scan and NCV
   - **Treatment**: Conservative, cervical rib excision

7. **Intervertebral disc prolapse of Lumbar region**
   - **Affects**: Young adults
   - **Presents with**: Low backache with/without radicular pain to one/both lower limbs
   - **Pathology**: Prolapse of the nucleus pulposus via ruptured annulus fibrosus
   - **Clinically**: Vertebral tenderness at affected level, SLRT, Lasegue, or crossed SLR tests are positive, *painful forward flexion*
     Neurological examination is a must to correlate the level of disc. Usually, the root involved is one level below the level of the disc involved in the lumbar spine, e.g. IVDP L4-L5 will affect the L5 nerve root (so will be the sensory and motor features). However, *'far lateral disc prolapse'* can compress the same level root (L4-5 far lateral disc compresses L4 root).
   - **Diagnosis**: X-ray, MRI
   - **Treatment**: Conservative. Rarely discectomy if worsening neurological deficit or unrelenting pain which is not responding to conservative treatment.

8. **Spondylolysis and Spondylolisthesis**
   - **Affects**: Mostly middle age, elderly, and young athletes!
   - **Presents with**: Chronic low back pain ± associated radicular pain; uni or bilateral
   - **Pathology**: Break in pars interarticularis and resultant forward slipping of upper vertebra over lower one
   - **Clinically**: Lumbar spine palpation reveals a *step* between two vertebral spinous process, and *painful extension* of spine
   - **Diagnosis**: X-ray (oblique view) of spine (Scottish Terrier dog sign). Lateral view (in flexion and extension) is helpful.
   - **Treatment**: Conservative, surgical stabilization

9. **Lumbar canal stenosis**
   - ***Affects***: Elderly
   - ***Presents with***: Low back pain with associated radicular pain; unilateral or bilateral, h/o neurogenic claudication
   - ***Pathology***: Stenosed lumbar canal space available for lumbosacral nerve roots due to hypertrophied ligamentum flavum, osteophytes encroachment, facet joint arthritis, and capsule hypertrophy
   - ***Clinically***: Tender lumbar vertebrae, *painful extension* of spine, and neurological signs ±
   - ***Diagnosis***: X-ray and MRI
   - ***Treatment***: Conservative, laminectomy

10. **Ankylosing spondylitis**
    - ***Affects***: Young to middle age males
    - ***Presents with***: Low back pain, morning stiffness, night pain, spinal deformity, hip pain
    - ***Pathology***: Sacroiliitis, and enthesitis
    - ***Clinically***: Kyphotic deformity in dorsal spine, test for sacroiliac joint involvement +, Schober's test +, decreased chest expansion, decreased cervical spine ROM, may not be able to touch occiput against the wall
    - ***Diagnosis***: X-ray and HLA-B27 +
    - ***Treatment***: Conservative, sulphasalazine, physiotherapy, and chest physiotherapy. Rarely surgery

11. **Degenerative lumbar spondylosis (old term: spondylitis)**
    - ***Affects***: Middle age and elderly
    - ***Presents with***: Chronic mechanical low back pain, rarely radicular pain in gluteal region or lower limbs
    - ***Pathology***: Degenerative disorder of lumbar spine
    - ***Clinically***: Tender vertebra, painful ROM, neurological signs are quite rare.
    - ***Diagnosis***: X-ray, MRI
    - ***Treatment***: Conservative

12. **Osteoporosis**
    - ***Affects***: Old age/postmenopausal
    - ***Presents with***: Mechanical low back pain, h/O osteoporotic # in spine, hip, or wrist
    - ***Pathology***: Decreased bone mineral density especially in cancellous bones
    - ***Clinically***: Kyphosis (localized or round back) ±, pathological fractures in hip, spine, and distal radius
    - ***Diagnosis***: X-ray, bone mineral density (BMD) [dual-energy X-ray absorptiometry (DEXA) scan]
    - ***Treatment***: Bisphosphonates, calcitonin, parathormone injection, calcium, vitamin D, braces, and vertebroplasty

13. **Traumatic paraplegia or quadriplegia due to spinal cord injury**
    - ***Affects***: Any age but mostly young adults with h/O trauma
    - ***Presents with***: Traumatic weakness of upper and lower limb with sensory loss
    - ***Pathology***: Injury to the spinal cord
    - ***Clinically***: Sensory loss and motor weakness in limbs, bladder, and bowel involvement, bed sores ±
    - ***Diagnosis***: X-ray, MRI, and CT scan
    - ***Treatment***: Conservative, braces, fracture fixation, and vocational rehabilitation

14. **Spina bifida (aperta/occulta)**
    - *Affects*: *Newborn with a defect, overt/covert*
    - *Presents with*: *Obvious defect in spine, overt/covert*
    - *Pathology*: *Unfused posterior elements of the spine leading to the meningocele, myelocele, meningomyelocele*
    - *Clinically*: *In SB aperta; most patient present with neurological involvement, ankle and foot deformities, trophic ulcer may be present, tuft of hair on the back, and surgical scar present on spine (depends on level)*
      Occulta cases: *Tuft of hair, naevus, dimple, or hemangioma at the site of defect*
    - *Diagnosis*: *X-ray and MRI*
    - **Treatment:** *Surgical closure of the defect (in SB aperta), management of lower limb deformities and ulcers*

15. **Sprengel deformity (Congenital high riding scapula)**
    - Congenital elevation of scapula
    - Usually unilateral, often associated with Klippel–Feil syndrome.
    - More in males (3:1)
    - Often, an omovertebral bar (fibrous, cartilaginous, or bony) connects superomedial angle of scapula to cervical spine (spinous process/lamina/transverse process)
    - Limited shoulder movements

16. **Klippel–Feil deformity**
    - Characterized by abnormal fusion of two or more vertebrae of the cervical spine
    - Often associated with elevated scapula
    - Low hair line, restricted neck movements and shoulder abduction
    - Fused ribs
    - Other malformations in craniofacial region (cleft palate), urinary tract (horse shoe kidney), cardiac anomaly, etc.

17. **Fibromyalgia**
    - Widespread musculoskeletal pain accompanied by fatigue, sleep, memory, and mood issues
    - Pain must be on both sides of body, below, and above the waist.
    - Women are more affected than men
    - Often associated with irritable bowel syndrome, migraine, interstitial cystitis, and jaw pain
    - Bilateral multiple tender spots over the base of the skull, cervical paraspinal muscle and sternocleidomastoid muscle, trapezius, supraspinatus, rhomboids, lateral edge of upper part of breast, lateral epicondyle, upper outer buttocks, greater trochanter, and just above the medial side of the knee

18. **Scheuermann's kyphosis (juvenile kyphosis)**
    - Progressive kyphosis in thoracic region in adolescence
    - Due to osteochondrosis of secondary ossification center of vertebral bodies and aseptic necrosis of "ring vertebral apophyses." Often 7–10th thoracic vertebra is affected.
    - Excess weight lifting may be a predisposing factor
    - **Presents with** back pain and round back kyphosis. The kyphosis is not correctable by changing posture.
    - *Radiographic abnormality*: Thoracic kyphosis > 40° (normal: 25°–40°), at least three adjacent vertebra demonstrating more than 5° of wedging, more anterior disc space narrowing and Schmorl's nodes.
    - *Treatment*: Conservative (<50° kyphosis), bracing (50–75°), and surgery (>75° kyphosis)

Notes

Clinical Evaluation of the Peripheral Nerves

▌ BRIEF ANATOMY AND FUNCTION OF A PERIPHERAL NERVE

Each segment of the spinal cord gives rise to a spinal nerve (A total of 31 pairs). Each spinal nerve is a mixture of motor and sensory components.

- The union of ventral and dorsal roots forms a 'spinal nerve' which is further divided into ventral and dorsal ramus.
- A peripheral nerve is formed distal to the spinal nerve roots (Fig. 11.1).

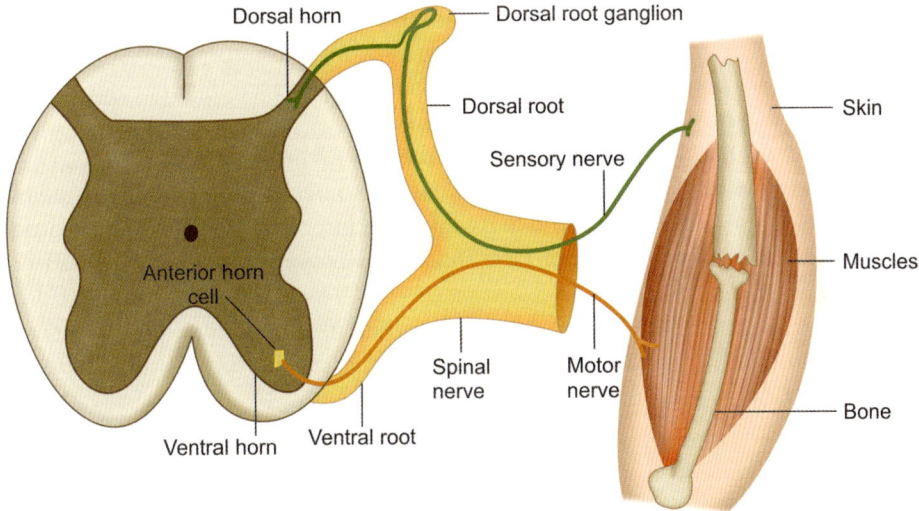

Fig. 11.1: Basic formation of peripheral nervous system.

- The basic unit of a peripheral nerve is an axon (Fig. 11.2). An axon has a cell body (lies in the anterior horn of the spinal cord), an axonal cylinder which is covered by a myelin sheath. The neurilemmal sheath covers the axon and myelin sheath. The axonal cylinder terminates in the neuromuscular junction in case of a motor fiber or a sensory organ in case of a sensory nerve.
- The axonal cylinder is responsible for ante- and retrograde conduction from the cell body to axon terminal and reverse.
- Any affection of the peripheral nerve can affect the sensory, motor and autonomic function of the extremity.

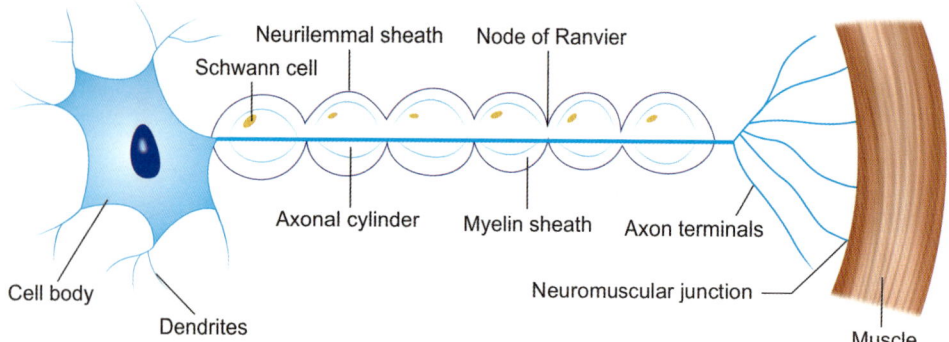

Fig. 11.2: Detailed structure of a neuron.

- **Nerve injury could be neuropraxia/axonotmesis/neurotmesis type (Seddon classification)**
- Nerve affection could be mononeuropathy/polyneuropathy:
  - *Mononeuropathy:* Mostly traumatic, compressive (carpal tunnel syndrome, tumor compression, etc.) or infective (Hansen's disease)
  - *Polyneuropathy:* Generalized causes like metabolic and endocrinal (DM, vitamin B complex deficiency), exposure to chemicals, inflammatory diseases [rheumatoid arthritis (RA), systemic lupus erythematosus (SLE), vasculitis], chronic alcoholism, and medications (INH, Dapsone, Phenytoin etc).
- *Structural nerve injury (Axontmesis, Neurotmesis) leads to Wallerian degeneration followed by regeneration.* Wallerian degeneration is oberved in Axontmesis and Neurotmesis while regeneration is observed in Axontmesis and 'surgically repaired' neurotmesis. *No Wallerian changes (degeneration) are observed in Neuropraxia as there is no anatomical/structural damage to the nerve.*
- While taking the history and examination, one has to differentiate between peripheral nerve affection (LMN, lower motor neuron) and brain-spinal cord affection (upper motor neuron, UMN).

Common conditions affecting nerves (mono/polyneuropathy) are shown in Table 11.1. Common site or condition affecting specific nerve injury are shown in Table 11.2.

Table 11.1: Common conditions affecting nerves (mono/polyneuropathy).
1. *Traumatic:* Mechanical, thermal, chemical, surgical (iatrogenic)
2. *Metabolic and endocrinal:* Diabetes, vitamin deficiency: B_1, B_6, B_{12} deficiency
3. *Infection:* Hansen's disease, Lyme's disease, HIV, Herpes simplex
4. *Compressive neuropathy:* Malunited or displaced fracture, tumor compressing nerves
5. *Autoimmune diseases:* RA, SLE, Sarcoidosis, Guillain–Barre' syndrome
6. *Alcohol, chemicals:* Chronic alcoholism, Lead toxicity, exposure to glue, solvents, insecticides
7. *Genetic:* Friedreich's ataxia, Charcot–Marie–Tooth disease, Fabry's disease
8. *Others:* Medication (anticonvulsant, anti-HIV), radiation

Table 11.2: Common site or condition affecting specific nerve injury.	
Nerve	*Common site/etiology of injury*
Spinal accessory	Surgeries in posterior triangle of the neck (lymph node biopsy, etc.)
Suprascapular	Entrapment under transverse scapular ligament and spinoglenoid notch cyst
Long thoracic	Radical mastectomy, injury to the ribs, and axillary lymph node dissection
Axillary	Dislocation of shoulder and surgical neck humerus fracture
Radial	Fracture shaft humerus, Holstein-Lewis fracture, and fracture supracondylar humerus (extension type)
Posterior interosseous	Monteggia fracture dislocation
Median	Elbow dislocation, fracture supracondylar humerus, entrapment near ligament of struthers, under biceps tendon (lacertus fibrosus) or pronator teres, carpal tunnel syndrome, and lunate dislocation
Ulnar	Fracture supracondylar humerus (flexion type), medial epicondyle fracture, cubitus valgus leading to tardy ulnar nerve palsy, cubital tunnel syndrome, tight flexor carpi ulnaris (FCU) aponeurosis, and entrapment in Guyon's canal
Sciatic	Posterior dislocation of the hip, posterior surgical approach of the hip during hip replacement or acetabular surgeries, and injection to the gluteal region
Common peroneal	Fracture neck fibula, posterolateral dislocation of the knee, tight plasters or splints compressing nerve around the neck of fibula, and upper tibial skeletal traction
Tibial	Posterior dislocation of the knee and entrapment under the flexor retinaculum behind the medial malleolus (tarsal tunnel syndrome)

▌HISTORY AND ITS EVALUATION

The patients with nerve injury mostly come up with two specific categories of complaints, cause (etiology) and effect. First (etiology), which has led to the affection of nerve (trauma, infection, etc.), and second (effect) arising out of the nerve involvement (motor, sensory and autonomic features). So, the history taking in nerve affection is bifacetal which involves finding the etiology of nerve injury and its effect on the nerve. *Further, clinician must always probe into how the nerve involvement has affected patient's activities of daily living (ADL).*

The effect of injury or disease on nerve leads to motor, sensory, and autonomic symptoms.

1. **Motor symptoms:** Inability or weakness to use a specific part or move a joint due to muscle involvement.
2. **Sensory symptoms:**
   - Loss or blunting of sensation in a specific area
   - Tingling, numbness, or radiation of pain
   - Shock like sensation in the limb
3. **Autonomic symptoms:**
   - Altered sweating pattern in the extremity
   - Altered sensitivity to pain and temperature.

While asking these symptoms, one must ask about onset, duration, and progression of complaints. It is important to understand that whether nerve affection is static, improving or deteriorating.

As far as etiology of the nerve injury is concerned, the following could be reasons for nerve injury/affection and details about the etiology must be probed.

1. **Trauma:** Traumatic injuries are one of the common causes of the nerve injury. The injury may be closed or open type.

   Blunt or a closed injury (fracture or dislocation) commonly causes neuropraxia or axonotmesis, and rarely neurotmesis. A major traction injury to the limb can cause extensive injury to a single or group of nerves, e.g. upper limb caught in a moving/rotating object can twist and pull the entire extremity causing extensive injury to the brachial plexus resulting in combination type (axonotmesis and neurotmesis) of nerve injury..

   An open injury (laceration, crush injury, and gunshot) can cause neurotmesis.

   The site of injury may give a clue to the type and level of nerve injury, e.g. a sutured wound over palmar aspect of the wrist may indicate injury to the median nerve or a wound over the fibular neck indicates injury to the common peroneal nerve.

   A tight plaster cast can cause compartment syndrome and resultant Volkmann's ischemic contracture (VIC). Compartment syndrome can cause damage to the nerves leading to variable motor and sensory disturbance in the limb.

   A temporary pressure over the nerve (Saturday night palsy) can cause temporary palsy of the nerve (usually neuropraxia).

   Delayed onset paralysis after a fracture may indicate nerve entrapment in the callus or fibrous tissue. It may also be affected due to the friction over a deformed fragment like tardy ulnar nerve palsy due to cubitus valgus.

   Iatrogenic injury wherein patient complains that his movements and sensations were normal before the surgery to the index limb. An incision around the peripheral nerve location may hint unintentional injury to the nerve during the surgery caused by prolonged traction or transection of the nerve.

   History of an injection given near a major nerve. An injection injury could damage a nerve in two ways: first, by *chemical injury to the nerve* (due to preservatives in the injected medicine) and second, by *direct trauma to the nerve.* Such injury could lead to extensive inflammation and fibrosis to the substance of nerve, and hence, recovery is far delayed, or nerve may not recover at all.

2. ***Infective cause (Hansen's):*** Such patients give a history of hypopigmented or erythematous numb skin patches in other parts of the body along with single or multiple nerve palsy.

   History suggestive of poliomyelitis: A sudden onset patchy paralysis in a limb without sensory loss could be an indication of postpolio paralysis. Such patients may give a history of fever with diarrhea before the onset of paralysis.

3. ***A tumor*** near a nerve can compress, stretch, or infiltrate into the substance of a nerve, which could affect the functioning of the nerve.

4. ***Metabolic conditions like diabetes*** usually cause sensory affection, but motor palsy could be a rare possibility. Chronic diabetic neuropathy can lead to Charcot's arthropathy.

5. **Guillain–Barré syndrome** can cause sudden onset of ascending type of bilateral lower limb paralysis.
6. **Certain drugs** used in chemotherapy and HIV treatment can cause peripheral neuropathy (PN).
7. **Toxins** like lead or arsenic poisoning can cause PN.
8. **Vitamin B12 or folate deficiency**
9. **Connective tissue disorders** like RA, SLE, and Sjogren's syndrome
10. **Hereditary diseases** like Charcot–Mary–Tooth disease and Friedreich ataxia
11. **Chronic alcohol intake, chronic kidney, or liver disease** can cause PN.

This list is exhaustive but the student must probe into the etiology of the nerve affection as the management involves the treatment of the cause too.

▌ EXAMINATION

General and Systemic Examination

The etiology of the nerve affection could be systemic. Hence, a thorough general and systemic examination is recommended.

Local Examination

The entire limb should be properly exposed, including normal side for comparison. If patient is ambulatory, **Gait must be examined in patients with involvement of nerves of the lower limb.**

1. Attitude

The attitude of the affected limb should be described in standard fashion.

2. Inspection

(a) **Deformity:** One must look for deformity in the affected part (Figs. 11.3A to C).

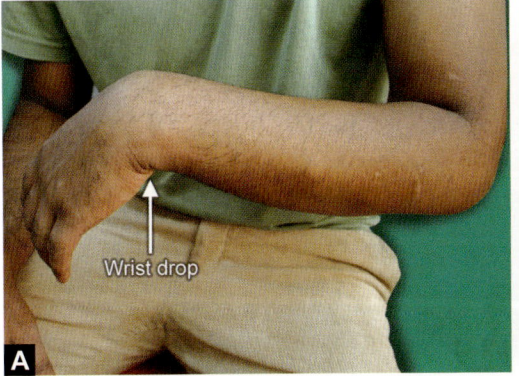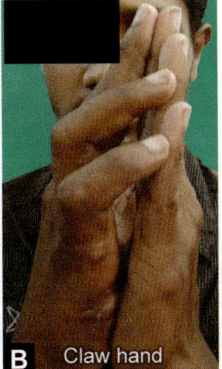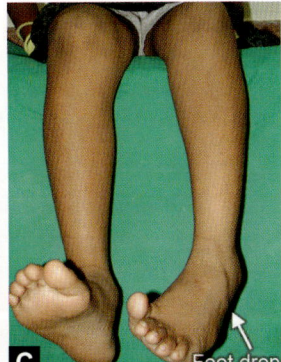

Figs. 11.3A to C: (A) Wrist drop (arrow). (B) Claw hand. (C) Foot drop (arrow).

Classic deformities in nerve palsy
• *Wrist and finger drop*: Radial nerve palsy
• *Claw hand*: Ulnar/median-ulnar nerve palsy
• *Scapula winging*: Long thoracic (serratus anterior)/spinal accessory nerve (trapezius) palsy
• *Policeman's tip hand*: Erb's paralysis
• *Foot drop*: Sciatic/common peroneal nerve palsy

(b) Wasting of muscles

Due to nerve palsy-related muscle disuse and less function of extremity.

(c) Scars

Due to previous injury/surgery. A scar overlying the anatomical location of the nerve may explain the cause of nerve injury (Figs. 11.4A and B), e.g. scar due to a lymph node biopsy in the posterior triangle of the neck may suggest injury to the spinal accessory nerve causing trapezius palsy and consequent scapular winging.

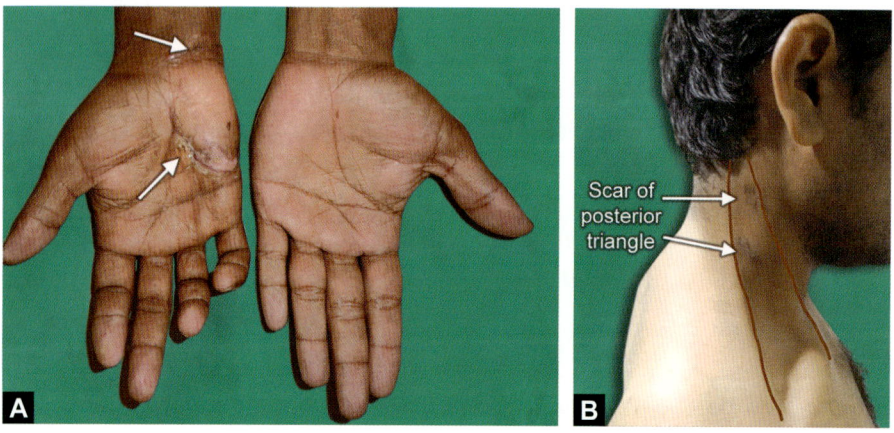

Scar of posterior triangle

Figs. 11.4A and B: (A) Scars over the wrist (ulnar nerve site). (B) Posterior triangle (spinal accessory nerve site).

(d) Skin

Skin shows variable changes due to the dysfunctional sympathetic nervous system.

In early stages: Erythematous and glossy

In late stages: Dry and scaly.

It may have trophic ulcers due to loss of sensation.

(e) Nail changes

Brittle and ridged.

3. Palpation

(a) **Temperature difference** compared to normal side

Early stage: Increased (Warmer)

Late stage: Decreased (Colder)

(b) **Scar tenderness**

(c) **Point tenderness along the course of nerve:** May indicate the neuroma formation or peripheral neuritis.

(d) Palpation of any swelling, scar, bony irregularity, deformity or any other *characteristics of the local etiology* responsible for nerve palsy must be performed.

4. Movements

(a) **Passive movement of the affected joints:** It gives an estimate of the stiffness at the joint.
(b) **Active movement of the affected and uninvolved joints:** It helps in assessing the grade of the power of involved muscles.

5. Measurement

(a) The **length of the limb** should be measured in standard fashion.
(b) **Wasting of muscles**: It indicates chronicity of disease and motor involvement.

6. Neurological Examination

It is important to understand that examination of the central nervous system (CNS) disorder is different and more elaborate from the peripheral nervous system (PNS). Sometimes, what appears to be a PNS disorder could have a CNS component too, e.g. preganglionic type of brachial plexus injury due to root avulsion may have associated spinal cord involvement. So, it is prudent to perform a quick survey of CNS which involves assessment of higher mental function, cranial nerves, and any evidence for UMN type of lesion. Once it is clear from history and a quick CNS survey that the patient has only isolated PNS disorder, the examination of the involved part can be focused onto:

(i) Sensory examination
(ii) Motor examination
(iii) Autonomic examination
(iv) Nerve recovery pattern: Tinel's sign and motor march

(a) **Sensory examination:** The main objective of the sensory examination is that it establishes the level or site of the lesion. The fundamental difference between the sensory examinations of CNS vs PNS is mentioned below.

- *CNS/UMN disorder:* "As per dermatomal distribution" of nerve roots.
- *PNS/LMN disorder:* "As per nerve' distribution."

However, sometimes even in PNS, a dermatomal assessment of sensation would be required especially in brachial or lumbar plexus injuries where the injury is beyond spinal cord but before the formation of spinal nerve. Further in PNS, one has to carefully look for "adequateness" of sensation in the autonomous zone of individual nerve.

Method of performing sensory examination
- Explain the patient about the examination, obtain the consent, ensure privacy and chaperone.
- Expose the part completely. The sensory examination should not be attempted over a part covered with clothing.
- The patient must keep his eyes closed during the sensory examination.
- Perform the sensory test (especially comparative sensations like touch and temperature) on normal and index side simultaneously and ask the patient for "if any difference" in sensory perception between the sides.
- It is also important to do "negative test" to ensure that patient has well understood the test and he/she is not malingering.

Which sensation to test in PNS and CNS?
- **In PNS:** Since the entire nerve is affected which carries all type of sensations; *mostly touch (light/crude) is commonly tested.* It can give a fair assessment about sensory capability of a nerve.
- **In CNS:** All sensations from a peripheral nerve finally are distributed to three major sensory tracts of the spinal cord (posterior column, anterior, and lateral spinothalamic tract). Hence, *at least one sensation from each tract* must be checked to confirm the integrity of all three sensory tracts.

Autonomous zone of major peripheral nerves
- **Axillary nerve:** Upper lateral aspect of arm (also known as regimental badge sign)
- **Radial nerve:** Dorsum of first web space of the hand
- **Median nerve:** Volar tip of the index finger
- **Ulnar nerve:** Ulnar border of the little finger
- **Superficial peroneal nerve:** Dorsum of foot
- **Deep peroneal nerve:** First interdigital space of dorsum of foot

---

(b) **Motor examination:** The motor exam should be done under the following heads:
  (i) ***Bulk and nutrition*** of the muscles
  (ii) ***Tone of muscles:*** LMN lesion cause hypotonia/flaccidity in muscles while UMN lesion cause rigidity.
  (iii) ***Power of muscles:*** It should be graded according to the MRC (medical research council) from 0 to 5.
  Individual peripheral nerve should be examined as per standard test described *(Read description in later part of chapter).*
  (iv) ***Reflexes*** *(Superficial and deep tendon):* Both superficial and deep tendon reflexes (DTR) must be assessed in a case of UMN lesion whereas only DTR assessment in a case of LMN lesion.
  (v) ***Coordination and abnormal movements:*** In UMN lesion

---

Principles/method of motor power examination
- Always start power assessment from the "normal" side.
- Check passive ROM at the affected joint on the index side.
- Always palpate the muscle being tested to avoid trick movement.
- Start with grade III power assessment on index side. If grade III is present, check grade IV/V.
- If grade III is absent, check grade II power.

(c) **Autonomic system examination:**
  - *Vasodilatation:* Warm and pink limb
  - *For anhydrosis:* Starch-iodine test
  - *Sudomotor:* Axon reflex test
  - *Trophic changes in nail and skin:* Brittle, ridged nails; scaly skin

(d) **Nerve recovery pattern:**
  (i) **Tinel's sign:** It is a sign of nerve recovery.
  Method: The part is exposed, and the procedure is well explained to the patient that while tapping the nerve, he/she may experience a tingling or shock-like sensation along the course of the nerve.
  Now, gentle tapping is performed with index finger *along the course of nerve from distal to proximal,* and the patient may report a sudden shock/current like sensation along the course of the nerve in case of positive Tinel sign.

Interpretation: A Tinel's sign is considered to be positive only if it is progressing distally with every follow-up. It implies that at every follow-up, it should be elicited at a level, distal than the previous one. If it remains static (i.e. at every follow-up, the shock like sensations are elicited at the same level), it indicates a neuroma formation (tapping a neuroma too elicits a shock like sensation). A static Tinel sign is a poor sign and indicates no recovery. Remember that nerve recovers at the rate of 1 mm/day. Hence, if Tinel's sign is elicited after 3 months (90 days) of injury, perhaps it should be elicited approximately 90 mm (9 cm) distally from the site of affection.

(ii) ***Motor march phenomena:*** It is another sign of nerve recovery where the nerve supply to the various muscles is restored from proximal to distal.

> Tinel's sign and motor march phenomena happen during Wallerian regeneration, which is observed after axonotmesis or surgically repaired neurotmesis, or in partial neurotmesis where some fibers are in continuity. It is not seen in neuropraxia, as there is no Wallerian degeneration or regeneration.

Individual Peripheral Nerve Examination

1. Spinal Accessory Nerve

It supplies sternocleidomastoid and trapezius muscle (Table 11.3).

Table 11.3: Spinal accessory nerve.		
Muscle	**Action**	**How to test function**
Sternocleidomastoid	Rotate the head to opposite side and flexion of the neck. "Turn-Tilt-Flex"	Ask patient to • Turn his head to opposite side (Fig. 11.5) • Tilt the neck to the same side • Flex the neck
Trapezius	Elevates scapula and rotates it outward	• Shoulder shrugging (Fig. 11.6A) • Shoulder retraction (Fig. 11.6B) • Forward flexion of the shoulder in the prone position

Spinal accessory nerve paralysis leads to mild winging of scapula *(lateral winging)* and inability/difficulty to sustain abduction in midrange of abduction in scapular plane (Figs. 11.6C and D). *[Also read triangle sign at the end of the chapter]*

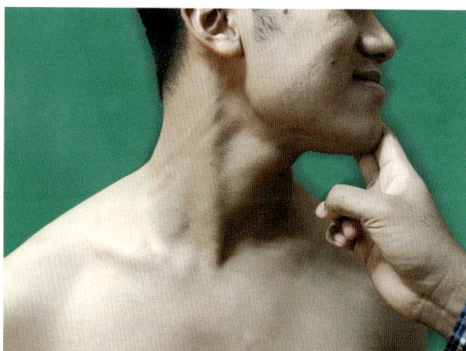

Fig. 11.5: Test for sternocleidomastoid.

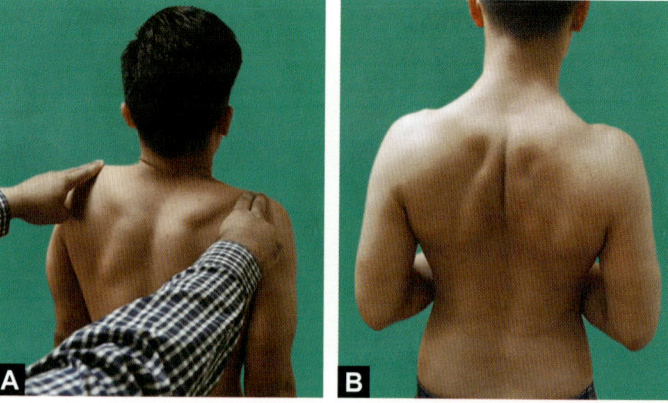

Figs. 11.6A and B: Shoulder shrugging and retraction to test trapezius.

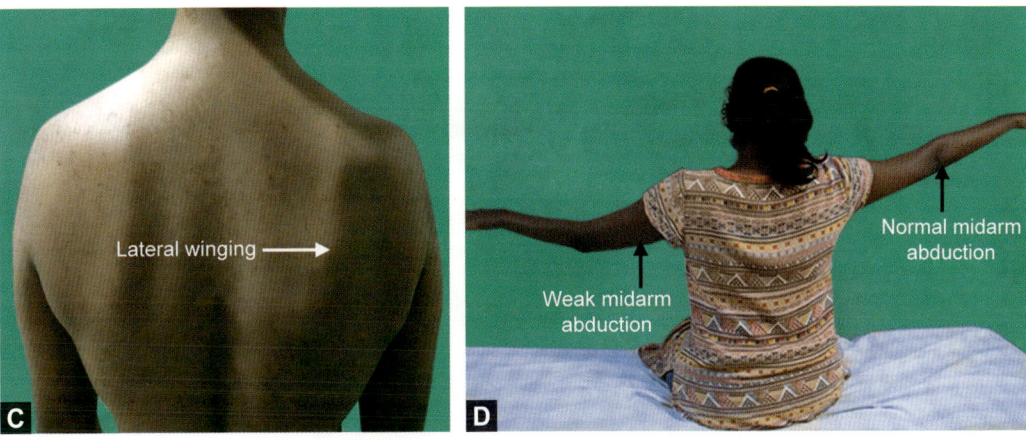

Figs. 11.6C and D: (C) Lateral scapular winging and (D) Weak midarm abduction in spinal accessory nerve palsy.

2. Long Thoracic Nerve (LTN, Nerve of Bell)

It supplies serratus anterior muscle (boxer's muscle) (Table 11.4).

Table 11.4: Function of supplies serratus anterior muscle.	
Function of serratus anterior	*How to test function*
Protraction and elevation of scapula	Patient is asked to push against the wall (Fig.11.7A)

Long thoracic nerve paralysis leads to winging of scapula *(medial winging)* and inability to push against wall wherein winging of scapula becomes prominent (Fig. 11.7B).

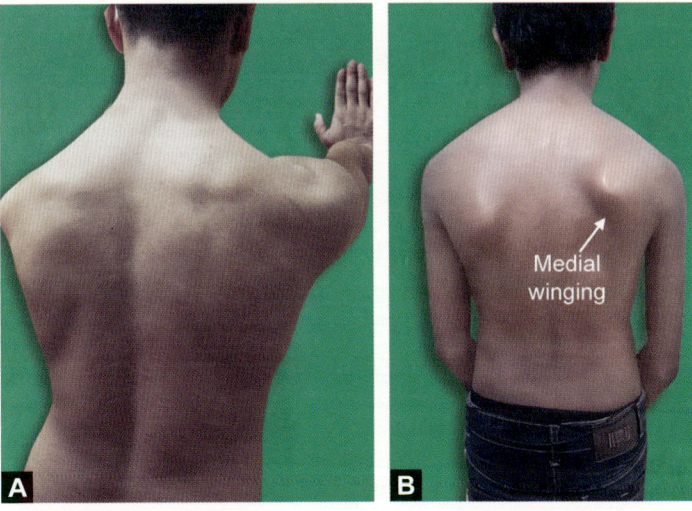

Figs. 11.7A and B: Wall push'test for serratus anterior (A) and medial winging in long thoracic nerve palsy (B).

3. Thoracodorsal Nerve

It supplies latissimus dorsi muscle (Rower's muscle) (Table 11.5).

Table 11.5: Function of latissimus dorsi and its evaluation.

Function of latissimus dorsi	*How to test function*
Extension, adduction, and internal rotation at shoulder (pulls humerus toward trunk and extension)	Ask the patient to abduct arm to 90° in the scapular plane. Now palpate the muscle and ask patient to extend and medially rotate the arm (like an effort to row a boat) while examiner applies resistance (Fig. 11.7C)

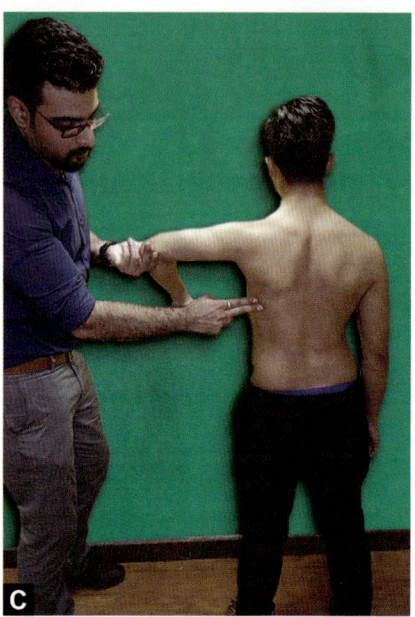

Fig. 11.7C: Test for latissimus dorsi.

4. Medial and Lateral Pectoral Nerve

It supplies pectoralis major muscle (Table 11.6).

Table 11.6: Function of pectoralis major and its evaluation.

Function of pectoralis major	*How to test function*
Flexion (throwing a ball underhand and in lifting a child), adduction (flapping arms), and internal rotation of humerus (arm wrestling)	***Sternal head***: Abduct the arm till 120° and ask patient to pull arm close to chest while the examiner offers resistance ***Clavicular head***: Abduct the arm till 60° and ask patient to pull arm close to chest while the examiner offers resistance (Figs. 11.7D and E)

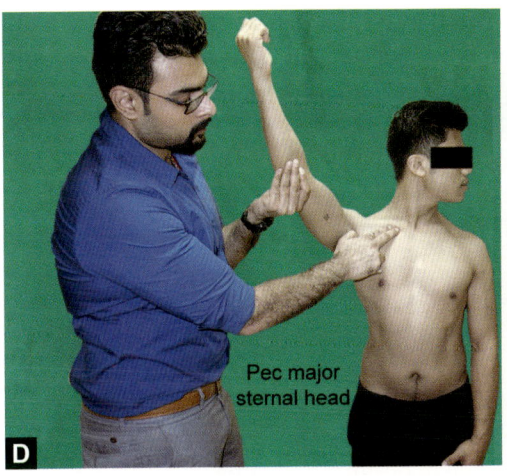
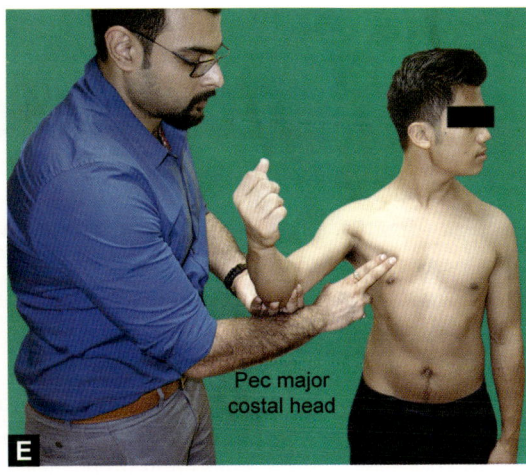

Pec major
sternal head

D

Pec major
costal head

E

Figs. 11.7D and E: Test for pectoralis major: sternal head (D) and costal head (E). (Pec: Pectoralis)

5. Axillary Nerve

It supplies the skin over lower part of the Deltoid for sensation (upper deltoid skin by supraclavicular nerves) and motor supply goes to Deltoid and Teres minor.

- **(a)** *Sensory:* Check sensation over the *lower lateral aspect of the deltoid.* Loss of sensation over this area known as "Regimental batch sign" (Fig. 11.8A).
- **(b)** *Motor:* The motor testing of axillary nerve is discussed in Table 11.7.

> Axillary nerve paralysis leads to loss of shoulder contour due to Deltoid palsy (Fig. 11.8C), regimental badge sign+, loss in power of abduction, and Hornblower sign + for Teres minor palsy.

Table 11.7: Motor testing of axillary nerve.

Muscle	Action	How to test function
Deltoid	**Anterior penna:** Flexion and IR of arm **Middle penna:** Abduction of arm **Posterior Penna:** Extension and ER of arm	**Overall function of Deltoid, and middle penna:** With elbow in 90° flexion, patient is asked to abduct the shoulder. With another hand, the clinician palpates the contraction of the deltoid. (Fig. 11.8B) **Anterior penna:** With elbow extended and shoulder 90° abducted, the patient is asked to perform horizontal adduction and examiner palpates the anterior deltoid fibers. **Posterior penna:** With elbow extended and shoulder 90° abducted, the patient is asked to perform horizontal extension and the examiner palpates the posterior deltoid fibers. *Other tests for deltoid:* Swallow tail sign and Akimbo test
Teres minor	External rotation of arm	Ask the patient to hold the shoulder in 90° abduction and 90° external rotation. The examiner gives resistance against external rotation. If the Teres Minor is paralyzed, the arm falls in internal rotation (Hornblower's sign) (Figs. 11.8D and E)

Other tests of Deltoid function: Swallow tail sign and Akimbo test are required as it is difficult to assess deltoid abduction power in patients with massive rotator cuff tear with pseudopalsy, isolated suprascapular nerve palsy with inability or difficulty to abduct the shoulder or in upper trunk brachial plexus injury where both deltoid and rotator cuff is involved.

- **Swallow tail sign:** In shoulder extension, there is a role of latissimus dorsi, triceps, and infraspinatus. However, in the presence of palsy of posterior deltoid fibers, complete extension cannot be achieved.

  Method: In standing position, the patient is asked to extend both his shoulder simultaneously and examiner watches from side. The affected side fails to extend completely (Fig. 11.8F).

- **Akimbo test:** It is another test to detect deltoid function.

  Method: The patient is asked to keep his hand over iliac crest, flex the elbow, and pronate the forearm. A patient with deltoid palsy is unable to perform the same.

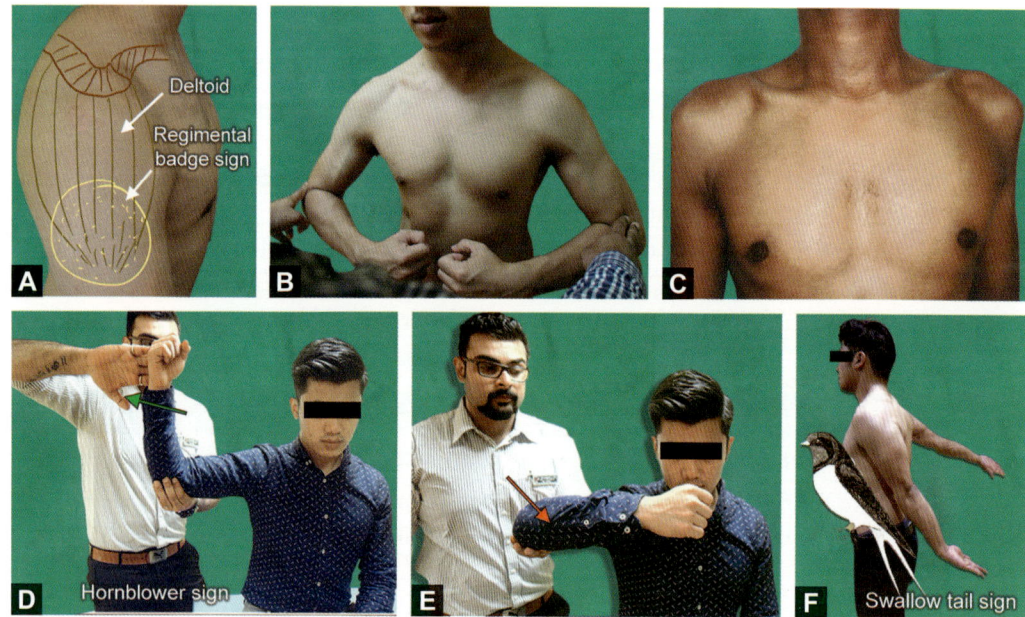

Figs. 11.8A to F: (A) Regimental badge sign. (B) Test for Deltoid. (C) Wasting of left Deltoid. (D and E) Hornblower sign. (F) Swallow tail sign.

6. Musculocutaneous Nerve

It innervates lateral aspect of the forearm (via lateral cutaneous nerve of forearm) for sensation and motor supply goes to biceps, brachialis, and coracobrachialis.

- **(a)** **Sensory:** Lateral aspect of forearm
- **(b)** **Motor:** The motor testing of musculocutaneous nerve is discussed in Table 11.8.

> Musculocutaneous nerve paralysis leads to loss of elbow flexion, mild loss of supination strength of forearm (as biceps is also a supinator) and loss of sensation over lateral aspect of forearm.

Table 11.8: Motor testing of musculocutaneous nerve.		
Muscle	**Action**	**How to test function**
Biceps	Elbow flexion	Ask patient to flex the elbow with forearm supinated (Fig. 11.9A)
Brachialis	Elbow flexion	Ask patient to flex the elbow with forearm pronated (Fig. 11.9B)

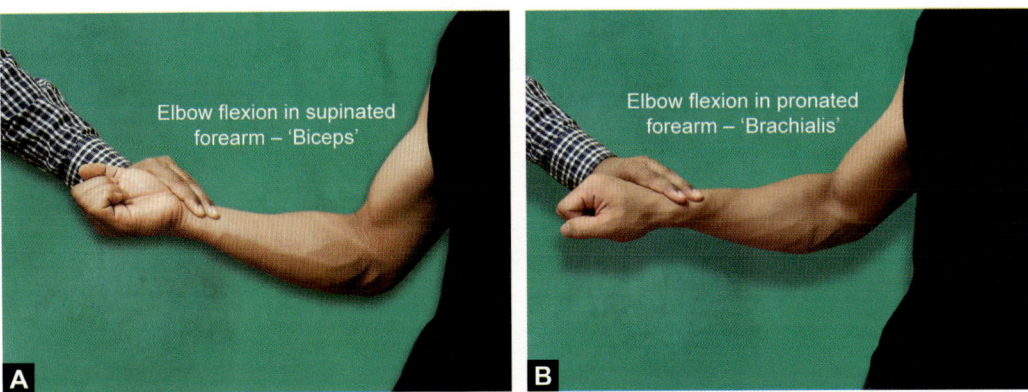

Figs. 11.9A and B: (A) Test for biceps muscle. (B) Test for brachialis muscle.

7. Radial Nerve

The radial nerve provides sensation to the dorsum of forearm and hand (radial 3½ fingers). Its motor supply goes to the triceps before and after entering the radial groove. Then, it supplies brachioradialis, extensor carpi radialis longus (ECRL) and ECRB. Further, it enters the forearm via a tunnel under the supinator muscle. Thereafter it is called as *posterior interosseous nerve (PIN)* and supplies entire dorsal extensor compartment of the forearm.

(a) ***Sensory:*** Autonomous zone lies over the dorsum of first web space of the hand.

(b) ***Motor testing:*** The motor testing of radial nerve is discussed in Table 11.9.

Table 11.9: Motor testing of radial nerve.		
Muscle	**Action**	**How to test function**
Triceps	Elbow extension	Ask patient to extend his elbow (Fig. 11.10A)
Brachioradialis	Weak elbow flexor and forearm supinator	With forearm in midprone, ask the patient to flex the elbow against resistance. The brachioradialis stands up prominently on the radial border of the forearm (Fig. 11.10B).
ECRL	Wrist extensor and radial deviation	Ask the patient to extend his wrist and radially deviate against resistance (Fig. 11.11A)
Extensor digitorum	Finger extension at meta-carpophalangeal (MCP) joint	Check extension of fingers at the MCP joint against resistance. (Fig. 11.11B)
Extensor pollicis longus	Thumb extension at interphalangeal (IP) joint	Patient is asked to extend his thumb against resistance. (Fig. 11.11C)
Extensor carpi ulnaris	Wrist extension and ulnar deviation	Patient is asked to extend his wrist and ulnar deviate against resistance.

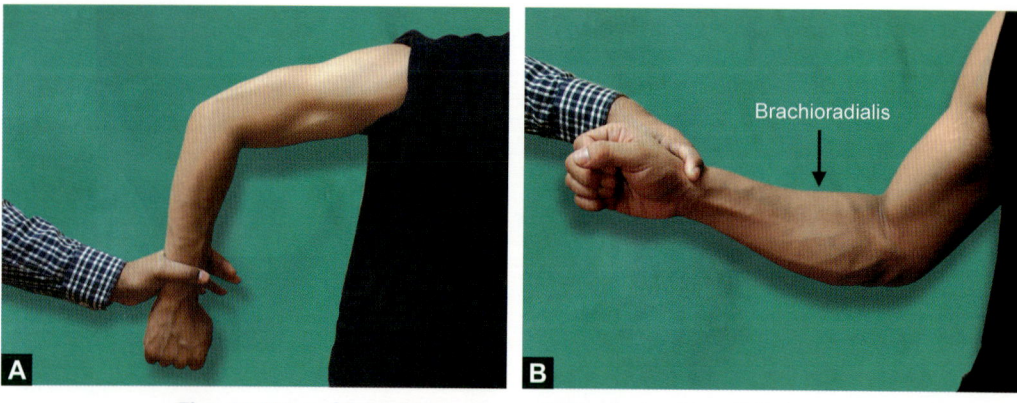

Figs. 11.10A and B: (A) Test for triceps. (B) Test for brachioradialis (arrow).

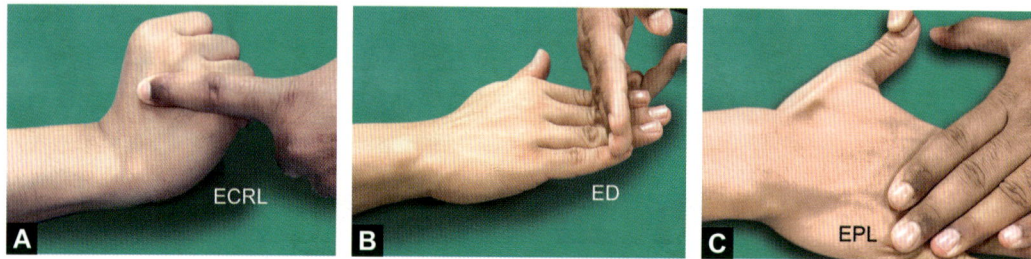

Figs. 11.11A to C: Test for wrist, finger, and the thumb extensors. (A) Extensor carpi radialis longus. (B) Extensor digitorum. (C) Extensor pollicis longus.

High radial nerve palsy (in the axilla): Loss of elbow extension, loss of wrist extension, and finger extension at MCP joint leading to "wrist, finger with thumb drop"
Low radial nerve paralysis (in the radial groove): "Wrist, finger with thumb drop"
Posterior interosseous nerve palsy: "Finger and thumb drop"
(*Note*: Patient will retain wrist extension and radial deviation due to intact ECRL and ECRB)

---

8. Median Nerve

The median nerve supplies lateral 3½ volar aspect of fingers and palm area for sensation. Its motor supply goes to **almost all flexors of the forearm** [*except flexor carpi ulnaris (FCU) and medial two tendons of flexor digitorum profundus (FDP), which are supplied by ulnar nerve],* ***all thenar muscles and lateral two lumbricals.***

  (a) *Sensory:* Autonomous zone lies over the volar tip of index finger.
  (b) *Motor:* The action and test for few muscles are mentioned in Table 11.10 while others are mentioned below in detail for better understanding.

Table 11.10: Motor testing of median nerve.

Muscle	Action	How to test function
Pronators	Forearm pronation	Ask patient to pronate forearm
Flexor carpi radialis	Flexion of the wrist, radial deviation	Ask patient to flex the wrist and radial deviate against resistance. (Fig. 11.12)
Flexor pollicis longus	Thumb flexion at IP joint	Ask patient to flex thumb IP joint against resistance.
Opponens pollicis	Opposition of thumb against all fingers	Opposition of thumb against all other fingers (Fig. 11.13)

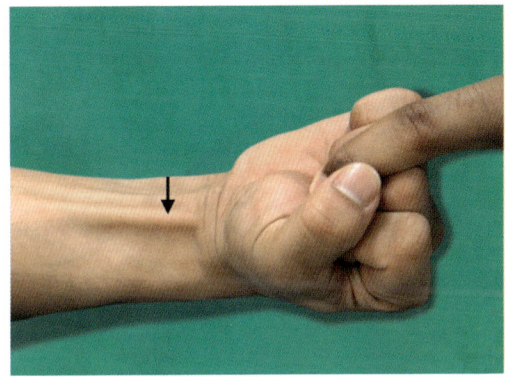

Fig. 11.12: Test for flexor carpi radialis (arrow).

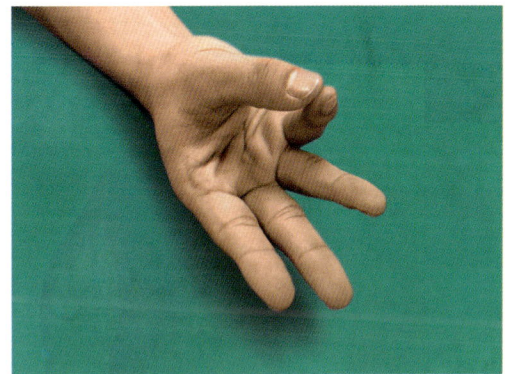

Fig. 11.13: Test for opponens pollicis.

- **Abductor pollicis brevis (APB):** *Thumb abduction " Pen test"*
Method: The patient is asked to lay his hand flat on a table. Then, a pen is brought above the thumb and patient is asked to touch the pen by abducting the thumb while APB muscle is palpated for contraction. If APB is paralyzed, the thumb will not be able to touch the pen (Fig. 11.14).

- ***Pointing index sign/Ochsner's clasping/Benediction test***

Method: The patient is asked to clasp both the hands. In a normal person, the patient will be able to clasp both hands together. In a patient with high Median nerve injury [affecting the all flexor digitorum superficialis (FDS) and lateral 2 flexor digitorum profundus (FDP)], the index finger fails to flex and remains as "pointing index finger" (Figs. 11.15A and B).

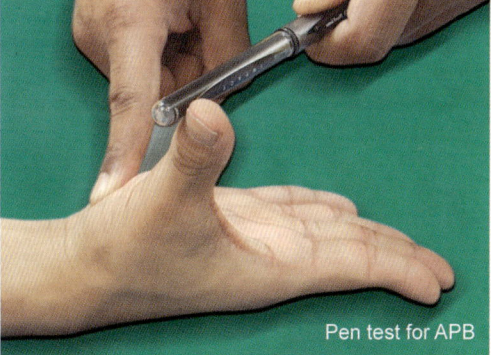

Pen test for APB

Fig. 11.14: Pen test for APB.

Even though FDP to both index and middle finger are paralyzed, only the index finger 'points' because FDP to index finger is independent, so its extension remains unopposed whereas FDP of middle finger remains flexed because its sheath is connected to FDP sheaths of ring and little finger (which are normal and flexed as it is supplied by ulnar nerve). Hence, FDP of middle finger remains flexed and 'doesn't point' despite being paralyzed.

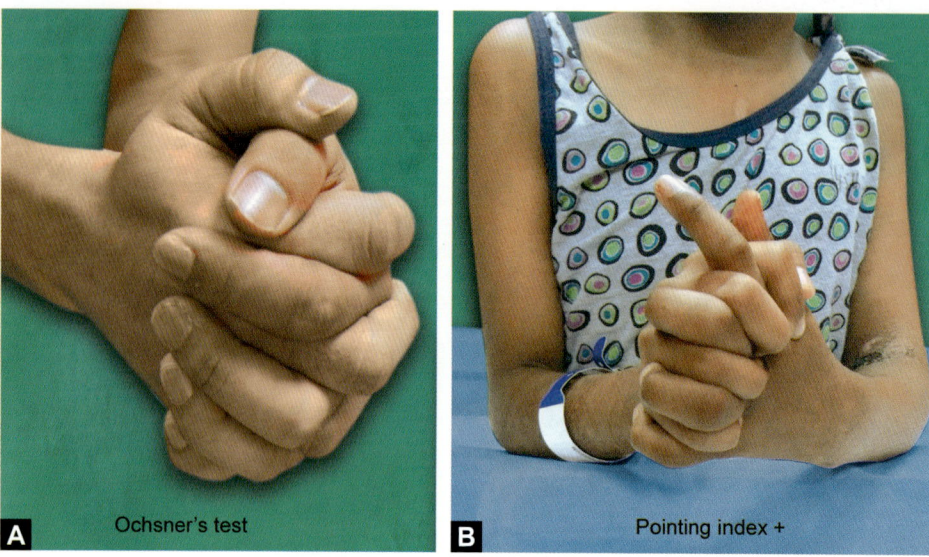

A Ochsner's test

B Pointing index +

Figs. 11.15A and B: (A) Ochsner test: Normal clasping. (B) Pointing index sign.

- **Flexor digitorum superficialis (FDS):** Proximal interphalangeal (PIP) joint flexion of four fingers

Method: The patient is asked to lay hand flat on the table. The examiner keeps his hand over other three fingers extended (to block FDP action) which are not to be tested, and 'finger to-be-tested' is left free. Then, the examiner asks the patient to flex his "free finger". The flexion happens only at proximal interphalangeal (PIP) joint of the free finger. The same action is repeated for all four fingers keeping others blocked (Fig. 11.16).

Anatomic basis of FDS test

FDS inserts over the base of middle phalanx and causes flexion at PIP joint. However, FDP while crossing PIP also causes PIP flexion. Hence, it will interfere in functional assessment of FDS. Nevertheless, due to a peculiar anatomic arrangement of FDP tendons (FDP tendons share common muscle belly), if one or more FDP tendons are not allowed to flex the fingers, other free FDP tendon cannot act in isolation. Hence, *to check the FDS function, the action of FDP has to be blocked by keeping fingers extended!*

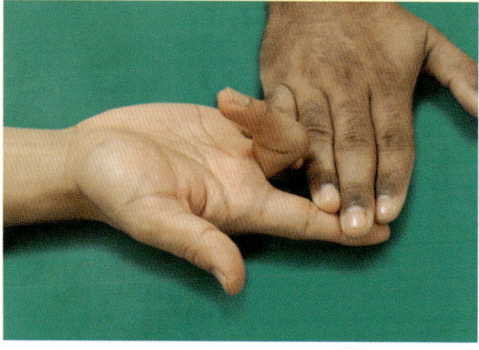

Fig. 11.16: Test for flexor digitorum superficialis.

- **Flexor digitorum profundus (FDP):** Distal interphalangeal joint (DIP) flexion (of lateral two fingers)

Method: The patient is asked to lay his hand flat on the table. The examiner stabilizes the middle phalanx of the finger whose DIP flexion has to be tested. Then, the patient is asked to flex his DIP and resistance is given by the examiner (Fig. 11.17).

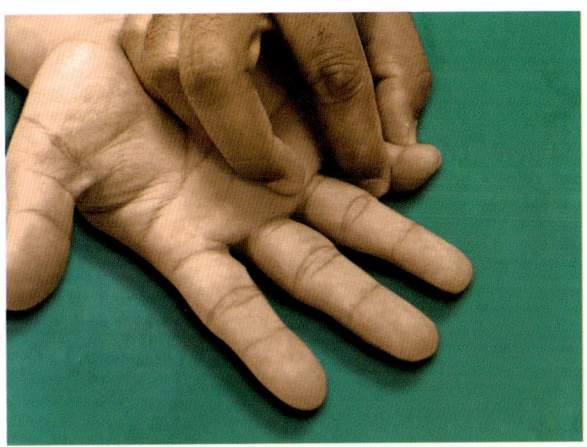

Fig. 11.17: Test for flexor digitorum profundus.

Median nerve palsy at elbow (high median nerve palsy): *Palsy of wrist flexors, long flexors of fingers, thenar muscles, and lateral two lumbrical*
Median nerve palsy at wrist (low median nerve palsy): *Spared wrist flexors and long flexors of fingers (FDS, lateral two FDP); ONLY palsy of thenar muscles (opponens, ADB), and lateral two lumbrical*
High/low, median nerve palsy leads to **"Ape thumb deformity/Simian hand"** wherein patient is unable to perform opposition due to palsy of opponens pollicis. The thumb lies in the plane of the palm unable to abduct and oppose to the tip of little finger tip.
(Note: Ape thumb deformity is a misleading term as monkeys have opposable thumb)

9. Ulnar Nerve

The ulnar nerve supplies sensation to medial 1½ fingers over dorsal and volar aspects. The motor supply goes to Flexor Carpi Ulnaris (FCU) and medial two heads of FDP in the forearm. Then it *crosses the wrist under Guyon's canal* and supplies the muscles of hypothenar eminence (abductor digiti minimi, opponens digiti minimi and flexor digiti minimi) followed by supply to all interossei (palmar and dorsal), medial two lumbricals and adductor pollicis.

(a) **Sensory:** Autonomous zone lies over the ulnar border of the little finger. Figure 11.22B shows the sensory innervation of the hand.

(b) **Motor:** The action and test for few muscles are mentioned in Table 11.11, while others are mentioned below in detail for better understanding.

Table 11.11: Motor testing of ulnar nerve.

Muscle	Action	How to test function
Flexor carpi ulnaris	Flexion of wrist, ulnar deviation	Ask the patient to flex his wrist and ulnar deviate against resistance. In case of ulnar nerve palsy, the hand deviates toward radial side (Fig. 11.18)
Abductor digiti minimi (ADM)	Abduction of little finger	The patient is asked to abduct his little finger against resistance (blue arrow) and taut ADM can be felt over the hypothenar eminence (white arrow) (Fig. 11.19)
Dorsal Interossei	Abduction of fingers	Ask the patient to abduct his index finger against resistance (blue arrow) and palpate the first dorsal Interosseous muscle between thumb and index finger (white arrow) (Fig. 11.20)
Palmar interossei	Adduction of fingers	*"Card test"*: Patient is given a card to hold between his fingers and examiner tries to pull it off with same fingers of his same hand. In case of ulnar nerve palsy, the patient fails to hold the card between fingers (Fig. 11.21)
Adductor pollicis	Adduction of thumb	*"Book test/Froment's sign"* The patient is asked to hold a book between his thumb and index finger and the examiner also holds it in the same way. In the case of adductor pollicis palsy, the patient uses his flexor pollicis longus (median nerve) to hold the book, and that leads to flexion of thumb (red arrow) (Fig. 11.22A).
FDP of medial two fingers	Flexion at DIP joint	Similar method as described in median nerve section

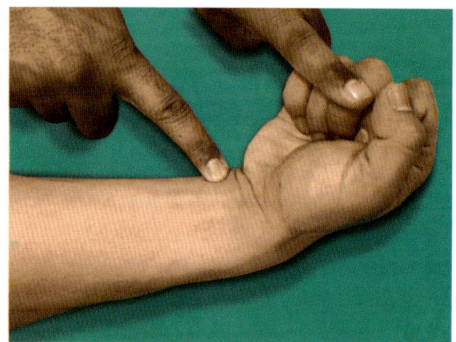

Fig. 11.18: Test for flexor carpi ulnaris.

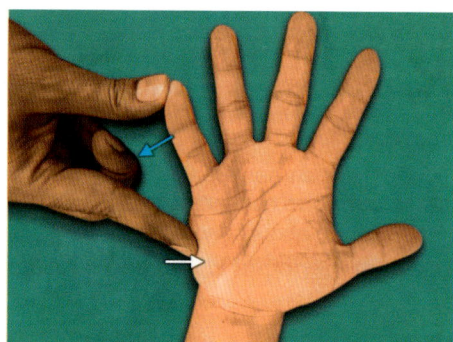

Fig. 11.19: Test for abductor digiti minimi.

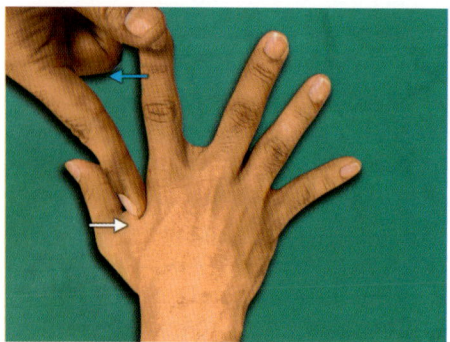

Fig. 11.20: Test for first dorsal interosseous muscle.

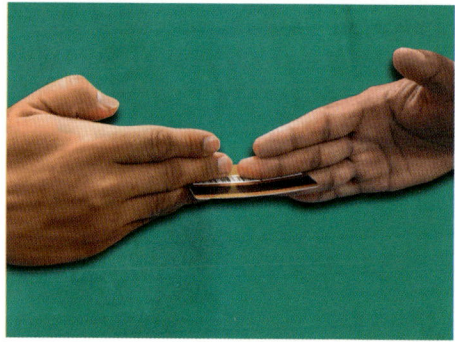

Fig. 11.21: Card test for palmar interosseous.

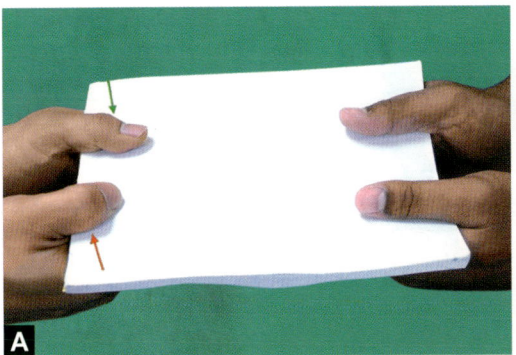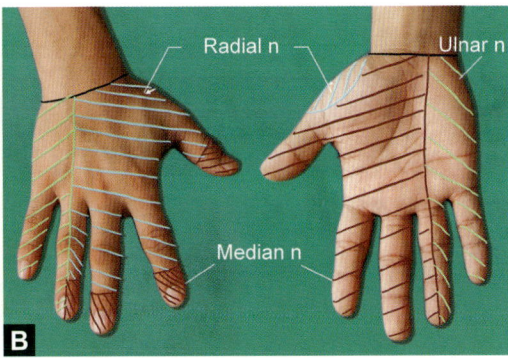

Figs. 11.22A and B: (A) Book test' for adductor pollicis. (B) Sensory innervation of hand. (n: Nerve)

Ulnar nerve palsy at elbow: Palsy of wrist flexors (FCU) and long flexors of fingers (medial two FDP), hypothenar muscles, medial two lumbrical, interossei, and adductor pollicis. Classic *ulnar paradox.*
Ulnar nerve palsy at wrist: *Spared FCU and medial two FDP;* Palsy of hypothenar muscles medial two lumbrical, interossei, and adductor pollicis. It leads to classic *"claw hand" deformity (intrinsic minus hand) wherein there is hyperextension at MCP and flexion at IP joints of little and ring finger.*

Ulnar paradox
Usually *higher the neurological lesion*, severe is the paralysis and consequently *more obvious deformity in extremity* is the rule! However, in case of ulnar nerve injury, there is a paradox!
- When ulnar nerve is paralyzed near the wrist (*lower lesion*), it leads to classic claw hand with MCP hyperextension and IP hyperflexion.
- Whereas when ulnar nerve is paralyzed near the elbow (*higher lesion*), it also paralyzes FDP to the fourth and fifth finger leading to no flexion at DIP joints. So, clawing is "not so prominent."
This is the paradox that in higher lesion of the ulnar nerve, the clawing is less prominent vis-à-vis lower lesion at the wrist.

Wartenberg's sign: Patient is asked to hold all fingers adducted with MCP and IPs extended. In case of ulnar nerve weakness, the little finger goes in abduction.
Jeanne's sign: Patient is asked to make a "key pinch." In case of ulnar nerve weakness, the thumb MCP goes in hyperextension.

Tardy ulnar nerve palsy
It is condition wherein there is delayed (Tardy) or gradual onset neuropathy of ulnar nerve. It is most commonly seen after non-union of lateral condyle fracture leading to gradual cubitus valgus deformity. Gradual cubitus valgus results in stretching and friction neuritis of ulnar nerve followed by peri- and intraneural fibrosis of the ulnar nerve affecting its sensory and motor function.

10. Femoral Nerve

(a) ***Sensory:*** Anteromedial aspect of the thigh and anteromedial aspect of the leg and foot (via saphenous nerve).
(b) ***Motor:*** It supplies knee extensors (quadriceps muscle) and few hip flexors (pectineus, iliacus, sartorius).
- **Quadriceps muscle:** Knee extension
Method: With the patient sitting on the couch, ask him to extend his knee against resistance (Fig. 11.23).

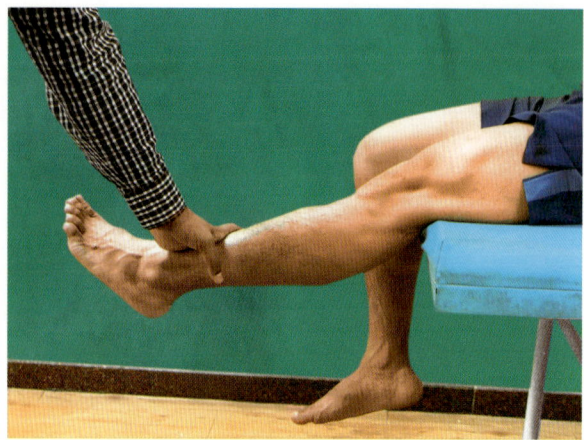

Fig. 11.23: Test for quadriceps femoris.

11. Obturator Nerve

(a) *Sensory:* Medial aspect of the thigh
(b) *Motor:* All adductors of the hip
  Method: Ask patient to adduct his thigh against resistance.

12. Sciatic Nerve

The sciatic nerve runs from the gluteal region to the back of thigh supplying hamstrings (knee extensors). So, to test the sciatic nerve proper, the patient is asked to flex his knee to check the strength of knee flexors (Fig. 11.24).

Further, while sciatic nerve crosses the superior part of the popliteal fossa, it divides into common peroneal and tibial division. Common peroneal further divides into superficial and deep peroneal nerve. Table 11.12 illustrates the muscle supplied and its action.

Table 11.12: Muscle supplied and its action.		
Nerve	*Muscle*	*Major action*
Superficial peroneal nerve	Peroneus longus and brevis	Eversion at subtalar joint and plantar flexion at the ankle joint.
Deep peroneal nerve	Tibialis anterior	Ankle dorsiflexion, inversion at subtalar joint
	Extensor hallucis longus	Extension of the great toe
	Extensor digitorum longus	Extension at lesser toes (2–5)
	Peroneus tertius	Dorsiflexion at ankle and evertor
Tibial nerve	Gastrocsoleus	Ankle plantar flexion, minor knee flexor
	Tibialis posterior	Ankle plantar flexion, inversion at subtalar joint
	Flexor hallucis longus	Flexion of great toe
	Flexor digitorum longus	Flexion of lesser toes (2–5)

Sensation over the foot is supplied by superficial and deep peroneal nerve, tibial nerve, saphenous, and sural nerve (Fig. 11.25):

- ***Tibial nerve:*** Plantar aspect of the foot. It divides into medial and lateral plantar nerve which supplies medial 3½ and lateral 1½ aspect of foot and toes.
- ***Superficial peroneal nerve:*** Dorsum of the foot except for first web space
- ***Deep peroneal nerve:*** First web space
- ***Saphenous nerve:*** Medial border of foot just upto ball of the great toe
- ***Sural nerve:*** Lateral border of foot.

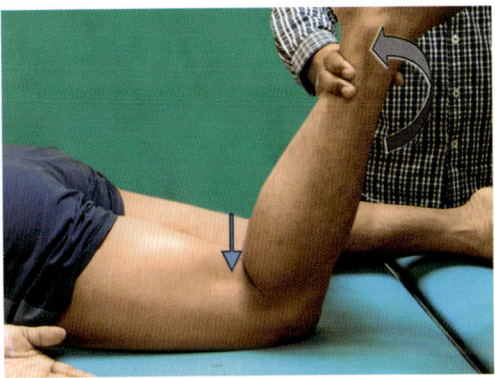

Fig. 11.24: Test for hamstrings.

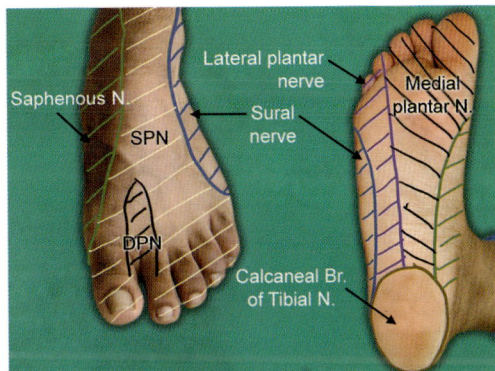

Fig. 11.25: Sensory innervation of foot. (SPN: Superficial peroneal nerve; DPN: Deep peroneal nerve)

▌METHOD TO TEST VARIOUS MUSCLES OF FOOT AND ANKLE

- **Peroneus longus and brevis:** Patient is sitting/supine. While the examiner holds the lower aspect of the leg, the ankle is kept in plantar flexion. Then, the patient is asked to evert the foot and the examiner gives resistance to the lateral border of the foot. Taut Peroneus longus is palpated behind lateral malleolus (Fig. 11.26).

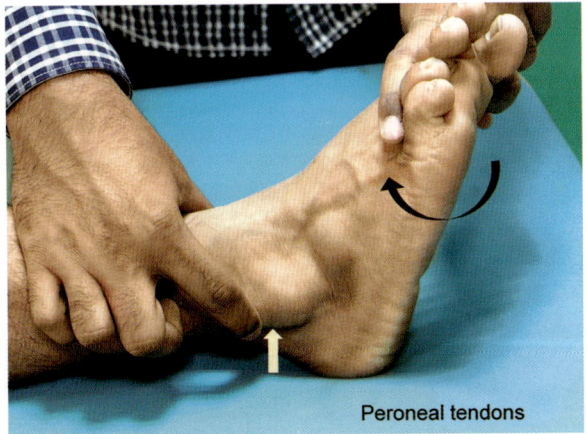

Peroneal tendons

Fig. 11.26: Test for peroneus longus and brevis.

- **Tibialis anterior (TA):** While patient is sitting/supine, he/she is asked to dorsiflex his ankle, invert at subtalar joint, and the examiner gives resistance to the medial border of the foot against inversion and feels for the taut TA tendon in front of the ankle (Fig. 11.27).
- **Tibialis posterior (TP):** While patient is sitting/supine, he/she is asked to plantarflex at ankle, invert at subtalar joint, and the examiner gives resistance to the medial border of the foot against inversion and feels for taut TP tendon behind the medial malleolus (Fig. 11.28).

> Both tibialis anterior (TA) and posterior (TP) are invertor at subtalar joint, the former is a dorsiflexor whereas latter is plantarflexor of the ankle joint. To test TA, the ankle is dorsiflexed which stretches the TP and nullifies TP's action. To test TP, the ankle is plantarflexed which stretches the TA and nullifies TA's action.

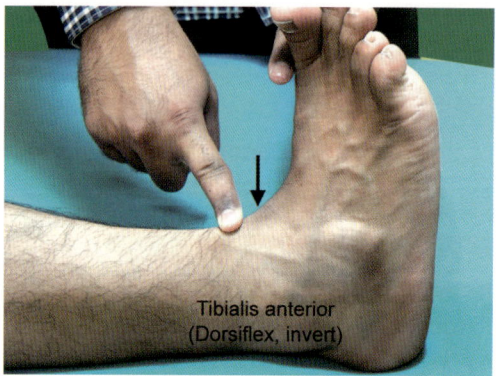

Fig. 11.27: Test for tibialis anterior (dorsiflex, invert).

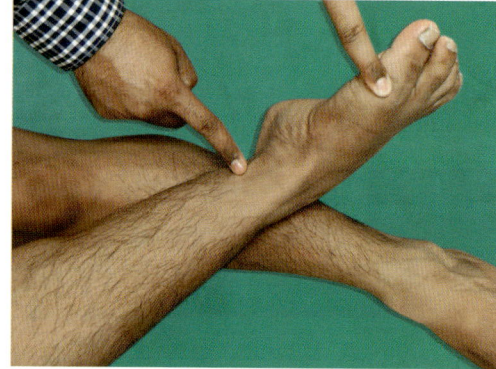

Fig. 11.28: Test for tibialis posterior (plantarflex, invert).

- **Extensor hallucis longus:** While patient is sitting/supine, the examiner holds the side of the proximal phalanx with his thumb and index fingers and patient is asked to dorsiflex his great toe. The examiner gives resistance to dorsiflexion with his index finger on the tip of the great toe (Fig. 11.29A).
- **Extensor digitorum longus:** While patient is sitting/supine, the ankle is held in slight plantar flexion and patient is asked to dorsiflex his second to fifth toe. The examiner gives resistance to dorsiflexion with his fingers on the tip of the toes (Fig. 11.29B).

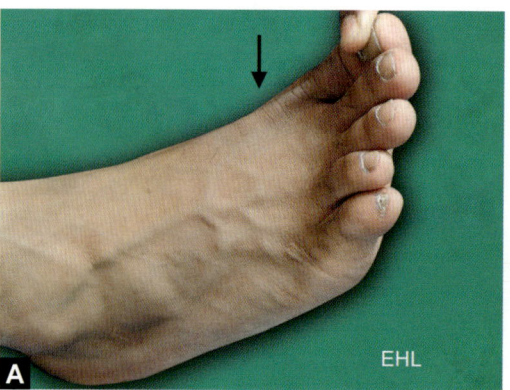

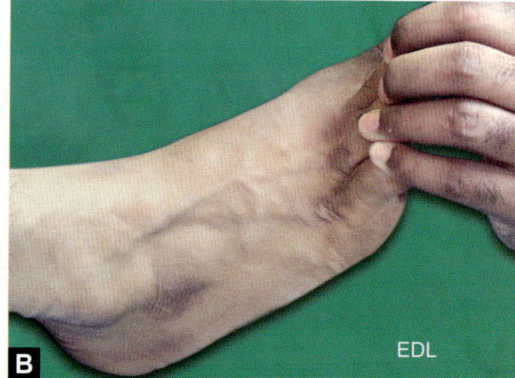

Figs. 11.29A and B: (A) Test for extensor hallucis longus (EHL). (B) Test for extensor digitorum longus (EDL).

- **Soleus:** The patient is asked to lie prone with knee flexed to 90° (this relaxes gastrocnemius and its action). The patient is asked to plantarflex his ankle and examiner provides resistance against plantar flexion (Fig. 11.30).
- **Gastrocnemius:** Patient is asked to stand on his forefoot by plantar flexing his ankle (Fig. 11.31).

> - *Sciatic nerve palsy at hip: Loss of knee flexion and flail foot*
> - *Common peroneal palsy: Loss of dorsiflexion at ankle and eversion of subtalar joint (foot drop).*
> - *Tibial nerve palsy: Gross weakness in ankle plantarflexion, weak inversion, and loss of toe flexion*

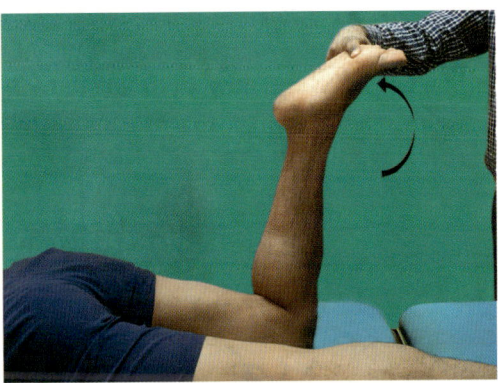
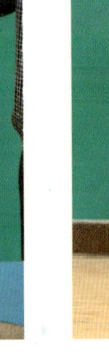
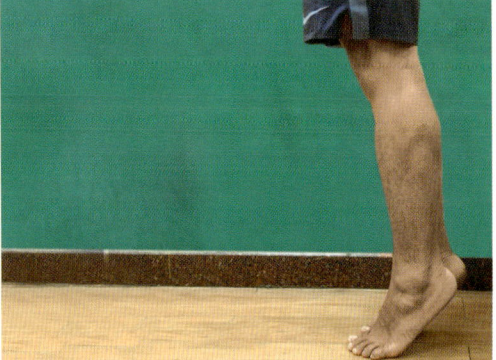

Fig. 11.30: Test for soleus muscle.   **Fig. 11.31:** Test for gastrocnemius muscle.

▌COMMON DEFORMITIES FOLLOWING SPECIFIC NERVE INJURIES

(1) Claw hand (Ulnar or combined median-ulnar palsy)
- Due to ulnar nerve or combined ulnar and median nerve palsy.
- Claw hand is characterized by hyperextension at MCP and hyperflexion at IP joints. Partial claw hand (involvement of ring and little finger) is due to Ulnar nerve injury, and total claw hand (all fingers are involved) is due to the Median and Ulnar nerve palsy.
- *Anatomical basis:* MCP flexion and IP joint extension occur due to the combined action of interossei and lumbricals which are supplied by Ulnar and Median nerve. Hence, its paralysis leads to MCP hyperextension and IP flexion giving a claw hand appearance.

(2) Wrist and finger drop
- Usually seen after injury to the radial nerve in fracture shaft humerus (radial nerve injured in radial groove) or fracture lower end humerus (Holstein–Lewis fracture).
- *Relevant anatomy:* The radial nerve after crossing the radial groove appears anteriorly after penetrating lateral intermuscular septum. Then, it supplies Brachioradialis, ECRL and ECRB. ECRL and ECRB cause wrist extension while in addition ECRL causes radial deviation. Further, radial nerve crosses elbow joint and enters supinator muscle while winding around the neck of the radius. From this point, the radial nerve continues as PIN. PIN supplies extensors of thumb, fingers and other dorsal compartment forearm muscles.
- *High radial nerve palsy/crutch palsy:* It occurs when radial nerve is injured in the axilla directly or due to the pressure from axillary crutch. It leads to triceps palsy (weakness of elbow extension), wrist, and finger drop.

- *Low radial nerve palsy:* It happens when the radial nerve is injured in the radial groove or near lower end of the Humerus (Holstein-Lewis fracture). This causes wrist, thumb and finger drop, but triceps is spared as most of the triceps fibers are supplied even before the nerve enters the radial groove.
- *Posterior interosseous nerve (PIN) injury:* It is commonly seen in Monteggia fracture-dislocation where it leads to loss of thumb and finger extension (no wrist drop). The wrist extensors (ECRL, ECRB) and brachioradialis are spared in PIN injury because it originates just above the elbow from the lateral intercondylar ridge and are supplied by the radial nerve and, hence no wrist drop.

(3) Foot drop
- It could be due to sciatic nerve injury (posterior hip dislocation, during posterior surgical approach) or common peroneal nerve injury (fracture neck fibula, posterolateral knee dislocation).
- *If sciatic nerve is injured* near the hip or at the upper end of posterior aspect of thigh, the patient loses knee flexion (hamstring), and there will be no foot and ankle movement (dorsiflexion, plantar flexion, inversion, and eversion) leading to *flail foot and ankle*. However, sciatic nerve injury just above the popliteal fossa spares the hamstrings but leads to foot drop (flail foot).
- *If common peroneal nerve alone is injured*, then dorsiflexion and eversion are lost (foot drop), but plantar flexion and inversion are possible due to spared tibial nerve. Further, there is sensory loss only over the dorsum of foot.
- *If tibial nerve alone is injured*, it leads to loss of plantar flexion at ankle and toes along with sensory loss over the plantar aspect of foot. Patient will be able to perform dorsiflexion and eversion (No foot drop). There is weakness in Tibialis posterior action too.

(4) Scapular winging (scapula alata): A condition where medial border becomes prominent due to weakness in scapular stabilizers.
- *Most common cause* is "Serratus anterior palsy" due to the involvement of *LTN*. It leads to *medial winging*.
- *Less common:* "Trapezius palsy" due to injury to the *spinal accessory nerve* (commonly injured during dissection of the posterior triangle of the neck [Fig. 11.32A]). It leads to *lateral winging*.
- *Rare causes:* Brachial plexus injury
  - *Serratus anterior palsy:* The serratus anchors the scapula against the rib cage during abduction or flexion of the shoulder like in boxing. When Serratus is paralysed, the medial scapular border becomes prominent as it is not anymore anchored to the rib cage.
    - Entire scapula displaced more medially and superior: "Medial winging," i.e. medial spine moves upward and medial due to over action of Trapezius, Levators and Rhomboids.
    - It is tested by asking the patient is asked to push against the wall with a hand
  - *Trapezius palsy:* Trapezius shrugs the shoulder and assists the mid abduction at the shoulder.
    - Its paralysis leads to discomfort or weakness in maintaining midarm abduction (*see* Fig. 11.6D).

- Superior angle of scapula displaced more laterally: "Lateral winging," i.e. medial spine moves more lateral and inferior (*see* Fig. 11.6C).
- *Positive triangle sign*: In the prone position, a normal person can forward flex his/her arm above the level of the head with ease. However, in case of trapezius palsy, the patient is unable to do that, and in that process, one lifts his shoulder and a part of the axilla. This makes a triangle (three sides of triangle by arm, chest wall, and couch) (Figs. 11.32B and C).

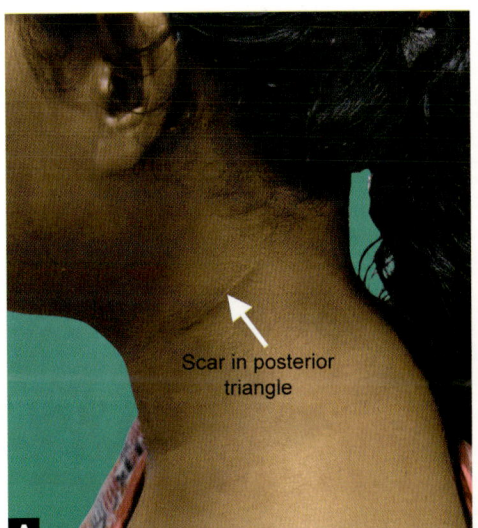

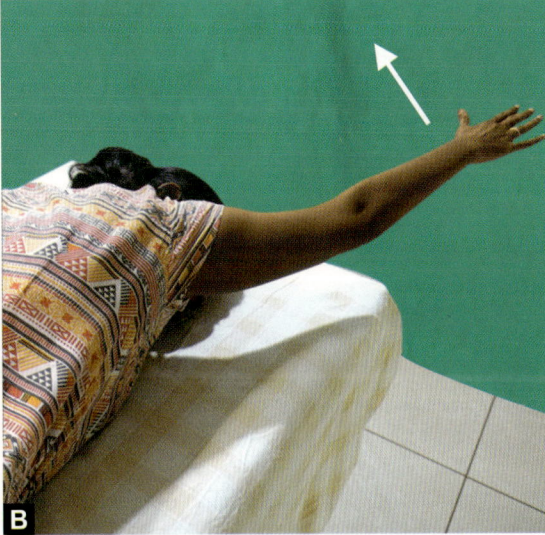

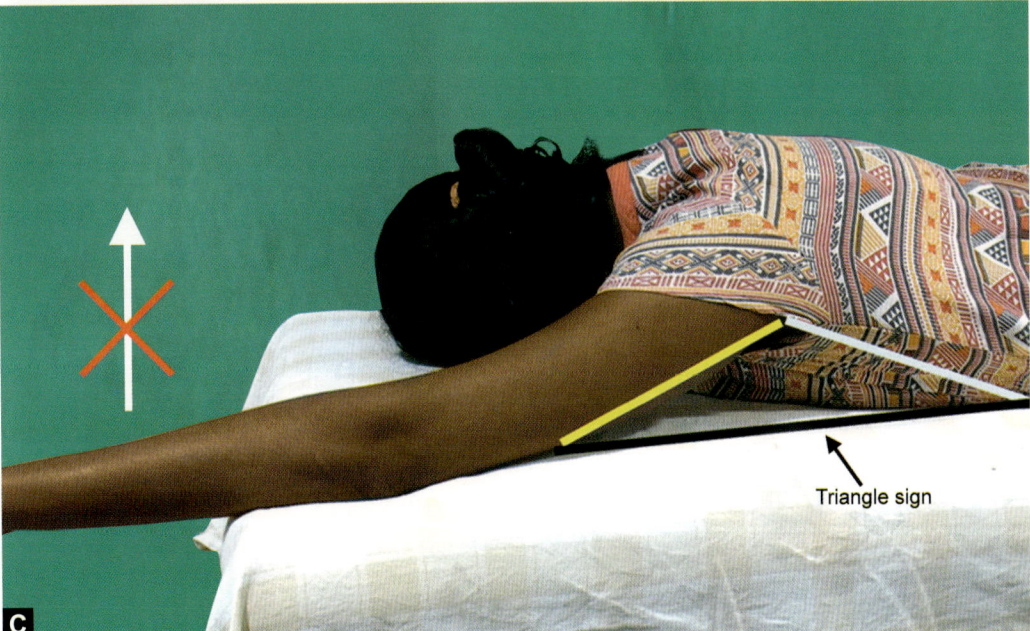

Figs. 11.32A to C: (A) Scar in posterior triangle (arrow). (B) Normal arm flexion in prone position (white arrow). (C) "Triangle sign": Poor or absent forward flexion of arm in prone position.

Peripheral nerve examination proforma

1. **Attitude, Gait**
2. **Inspection**
   - Deformity
   - Wasting of muscles
   - Scars
   - Skin and nail changes
3. **Palpation**
   - Temperature difference between two sides
   - Scar tenderness
   - Tenderness over the course of nerve: generalized/point tenderness
   - Palpation of any swelling, scar, bony irregularity or characteristics for the etiology responsible of nerve palsy.
4. **Movements:** Active and passive
   - Passive movement of paralyzed joints
   - Active movement of normal joints
5. **Measurements:** Limb length, muscle wasting
6. **Neurological examination**
   a) *Sensory examination*
   b) *Motor examination*: Bulk and nutrition, tone, power, reflexes (superficial and deep), coordination, abnormal movements
   c) *Individual nerve examination*
   d) *Nerve recovery pattern:* Tinel's sign, motor march
   e) *Autonomic system examination*
7. **Lymph node examination:** In case of infective/tumorous cause of nerve palsy

Notes

Clinical Evaluation of the Bone Tumors

CLASSIFICATION OF BONE TUMORS

Bone tumors can be classified into benign and malignant bone tumors and tumor-like lesions. The malignant bone tumors can be further classified as primary and secondary bone tumors. A clinical classification of bone tumor is shown in Flowchart 12.1. Table 12.1 illustrates the difference between a benign and malignant bone tumor.

Flowchart 12.1: Clinical classification of bone tumors.

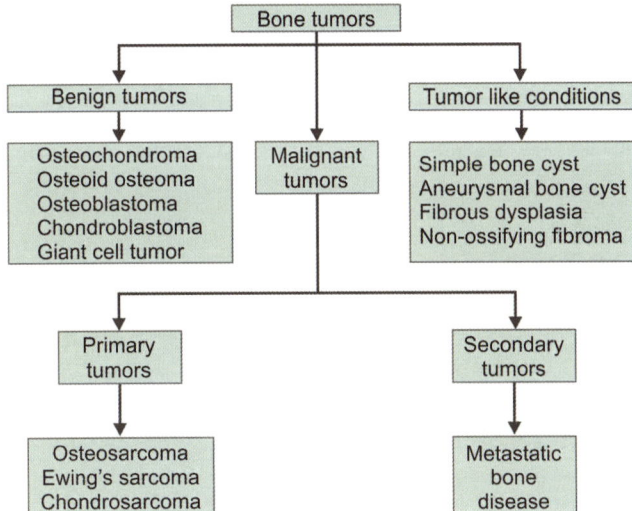

Table 12.1: Showing difference between benign and malignant bone tumors.

Characteristics	Benign	Malignant
Growth	Slow, may stop at maturity	Rapid
Duration	Long	Short
Pain and swelling appearance	Swelling followed by pain	Pain followed by swelling
Pain character	Localized, subsides with rest	Constant, present even on rest and night
Systemic features (weight and appetite loss, fever)	Rare	Common
Spread	Remains local	Infiltrate the adjacent bone/tissue
Swelling surface	Smooth	irregular
Local temperature	Normal	Raised
Consistency	Firm/hard	Variable
Metastasis	No	Yes
Radiograph	Limited 'geographic growth.'	'Moth eaten' or 'permeative' appearance
Encapsulated/well defined	Well encapsulated/defined	Non-encapsulated, Ill-defined margins
Histopathology	No features of malignancy	Numerous mitotic bodies Anisocytosis Anisonucleosis Hyperchromatism

Certain must know facts about the bone tumor during history assessment
1. Age of the patient
2. Site in the body
3. Location in bone
4. Single/multiple
5. Progression

HISTORY TAKING IN BONE TUMORS

A. Demographic data

1. **Age:** Certain benign and malignant tumors are common in specific age groups. The important bone tumors which are usually encountered in daily practice with its most common age group, are mentioned below:
   - *First and second decade of life:* Simple bone cyst, Aneurysmal bone cyst, Ewing's sarcoma, and osteosarcoma.
   - *After skeletal maturity (third and fourth decade of life):* Giant cell tumor (osteoclastoma) and malignant fibrous histiocytoma.
   - *After fifth decade of life:* Metastatic bone disease, multiple myeloma, secondary osteosarcoma, and chondrosarcoma.

2. **Sex:** Certain bone tumors have a predilection for males while some have a predilection for females.
   - *Osteosarcoma* is common in males in a ratio of 2:1.
   - *Ewing's tumor* has a slight male predilection with a ratio of 3:2.
   - *Giant cell tumor* of bone is common in females in a ratio of 2:3.

B. History of present illness
1. **Swelling:** Swelling is the most common symptom which the patient presents with, which may or may not be associated with pain.
   - *Onset*: Acute or insidious (an insidious onset swelling suggests a slow-growing tumor or probably a benign bone tumor).
   - *Duration*: In days, months, or years. Chronicity of the swelling favors a benign swelling (e.g. osteochondroma), whereas an acute onset may suggest malignant pathology.
   - *Progression*: Static or progressive. Slow-progressive tumor suggests a benign course of the tumor. A tumor which has a change to a rapid progression may indicate malignant transformation.
   - *Associated symptoms* (Pressure symptoms—numbness, claudication)
   - *Similar swellings elsewhere in the body*: Seen in multiple exostosis, metachronous osteosarcoma, and multiple enchondromatosis.
2. **Pain:** Pain is another symptom the patient presents with in bone tumors.
   - *Onset*: Insidious in benign tumors, whereas acute in the case of malignant tumors. Sudden onset pain may also be seen in case of pathological fractures.
   - *Duration*: Long duration in case of benign tumors, whereas relatively shorter duration in malignant tumors.
   - *Character*: Dull aching and boring pain in case of benign tumors, whereas sharp and throbbing and severe in malignant ones.
   - *Diurnal variation*: More in the night for specific tumors like osteoid osteoma. Malignant tumors may remain more painful in the night.
   - *Rest pain and night pain*: The presence of rest pain suggests a sinister pathology, probably a malignant bone tumor.

> **Benign tumor:** Swelling precedes the onset of pain.
> **Malignant tumor:** Pain precedes the onset of swelling.

   - *Pain relieved by nonsteroidal anti-inflammatory drugs (NSAIDs: Aspirin)*: It is characteristic of osteoid osteoma.
3. **Pressure symptoms:** A tumor may compress upon surrounding nerve or vascular structure (vein/artery) giving rise to several compression features such as distal swelling, claudication, sensory disturbance, or weakness in limb.
4. **Constitutional symptoms:** Symptoms of fever, weight loss, and loss of appetite are relevant in malignant bone tumors and would be absent in benign bone tumors.
5. **Symptoms suggestive of metastasis:**
   - Metastasis could be in the bones leading to bone pain in other areas or pathological fracture.
   - Metastasis could be in lungs, liver, abdomen and pelvis, brain, or other areas leading to area-specific symptoms such as a cough, hemoptysis, jaundice, hematuria, focal neurological deficit or epilepsy, etc.

6. **Activities of daily living:** Disabilities and limitation of activities of daily living have to be asked for in individuals with bone tumors irrespective of its benign or malignant nature. Individuals with bone lesions affecting the lower limb may find it difficult to walk, squat on the floor, and sit cross-legged. Individuals with pathology in the upper limb may find it difficult to carry out routine activities like combing his/her hair, lift weights.

C. Past history

D. Personal history

- History of loss of appetite/weight.
- *History of smoking:* Can lead to lung cancer with bony metastasis.

E. Treatment history

Detailed treatment history may suggest nature of tumor in question.

F. Family history

May be positive in tumors like multiple exostosis.

▌ EXAMINATION

General Examination

A detailed general and systemic examination is required in cases of bone tumors-especially if it is a case of malignant bone tumor. Several examples of importance of general examination are mentioned below.

1. *Pallor*: Patient may have pallor suggesting anemia in malignant bone tumors.
2. *Lymph node enlargement*: Bone tumors spread through hematogenous route. However, soft tissue infiltration and local spread of malignancy can be denoted by lymph node enlargement. Patients with metastasis to the liver may present with *icterus*.
3. *Edema*: Compression of the veins can cause bilateral or unilateral limb edema.

Systemic Examination

- A systemic examination should be undertaken to look for signs of metastasis in other major systems in the body.
- Likewise, a thorough systemic examination should be undertaken to locate the primary in case of the metastatic bone disease. The primaries which commonly cause bone metastasis are breast, lung, kidney, prostate, and thyroid.
- Per-rectal or per-vaginal examination may be required.
- Examination of other parts of skeletal system may be required in conditions where multiple bones may be involved like multiple exostosis, bony metastasis, etc.

Local Examination

Inspection

Swelling arising from the bone should be looked for the following specifics:

- **Size, shape, and location.** The location of bone tumor is the single most important inspection finding, and it can give a fair clue about the clinical diagnosis. There are tumors which occur specifically in epiphysis, metaphysis and diaphysis of long bones (Fig. 12.1).

- ***Extent:*** Extent to be described based on a landmark (joint line, tibial tubercle, anterior superior iliac spine, etc.)
- ***Overlying skin:***
  - Stretched and glistening suggest rapidly growing tumor
  - Puckered in case of skin infiltration
  - Dilated veins suggest an aggressive growth
- ***Any scars, sinuses*** overlying the swelling have to be highlighted upon. Surgical scars (of biopsy or other surgery) and drain site are an important part of tumor examination. *Note: Size, location, and extent to be described based on a fixed landmark. In this case, lateral joint line of the knee can be considered.*

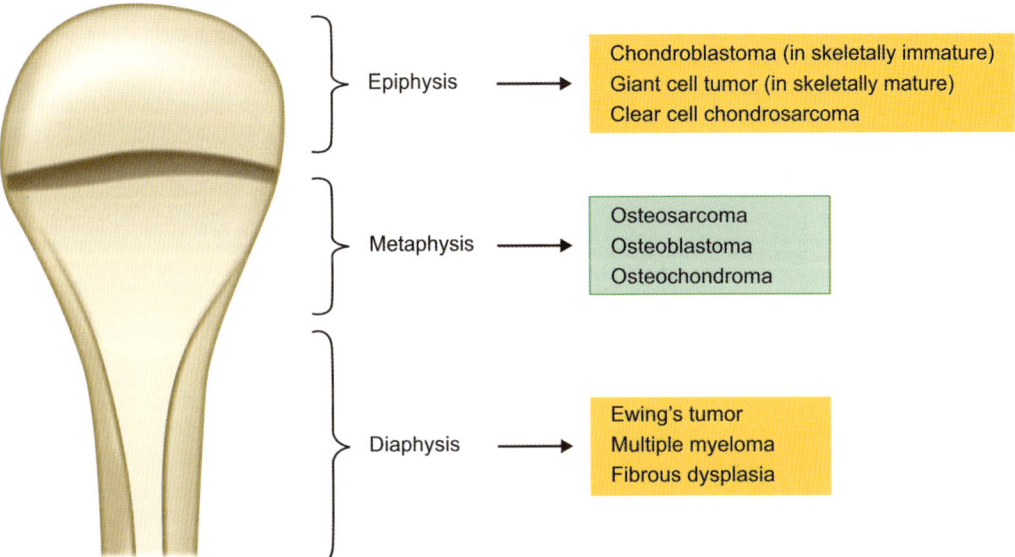

Fig. 12.1: Location of common tumors in bone.

Palpation

- ***Local rise of temperature*** over the swelling: Malignant tumors could have rise in local temperature.
- **Confirm site, size, shape and surface of the swelling:** (Fig. 12.2).
- ***Tenderness*** over the swelling (Fig. 12.3)
- ***Consistency:*** Variable consistencies from soft to firm in a centrifugal pattern may suggest malignant tumor as central necrosis may turn a tumor soft (Fig. 12.3). Hard consistency also suggests predominance of bony elements
  Firm consistency suggests predominance of cartilaginous elements
  Soft consistency suggests predominance of fibrous or vascular elements
- ***Surface: Smooth or bosselated:*** Smooth, regular surface may indicate benign tumor; whereas bosselated surface may be appreciated in malignant bone tumors (Fig. 12.3).
- ***Edge:*** An ill-defined edge may suggest a malignant bone tumor rather than a benign pathology (Fig. 12.4).

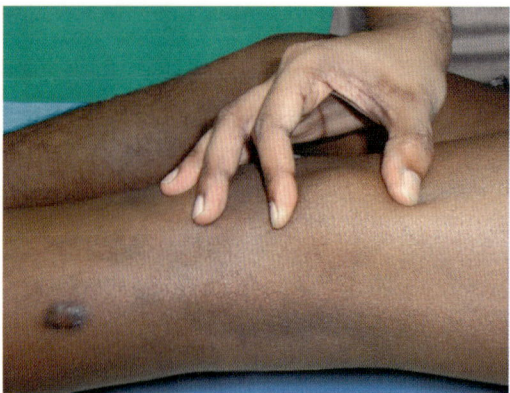

Fig. 12.2: *The site, size, shape* and extent of the swelling along with the mobility of the swelling should be assessed in palpation.

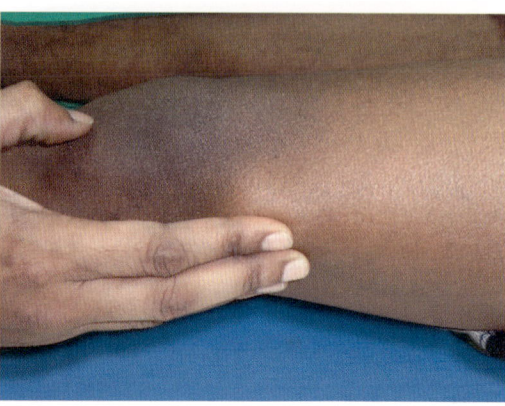

Fig. 12.3: Tenderness, surface and consistency of the swelling should be elicited as depicted in the figure.

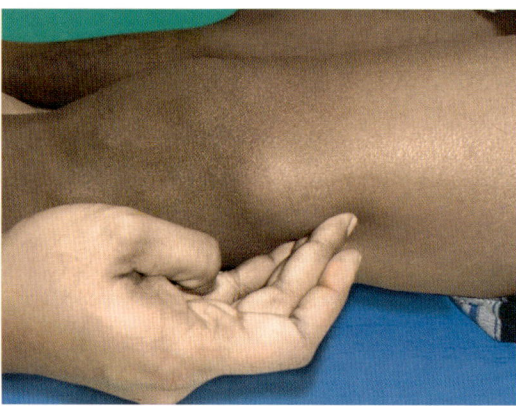

Fig. 12.4: The margin or edge is well defined when the tumor and the surrounding bone can be palpated as discrete entities as depicted in this figure.

- ***Plane of the swelling*** must be assessed (*Read chapter 15 for plane of swelling*)
- ***Skin pinchability:*** Inability to pinch the skin suggests infiltration of the skin—seen in malignant lesions.

Movements

Both active and passive range of movement (ROM) must be checked. In case of nerve palsy, the active ROM will be absent. *ROM may be restricted if*

- The ***lesion is in proximity with the adjacent joint, and may act as bony block*** in the movement. E.g., Osteochondroma arising from the posterior aspect of tibia restricting flexion of the knee. Similar restriction of supination and pronation movements may be appreciated in forearm suggesting a bone block caused due to the involvement of the radius or ulna.
- ***Intra-articular spread of tumor*** would restrict movement.
- ***Local muscle spasm*** due to infiltration into muscle and other soft tissues could result in restricted movement.

Measurements

- Pediatric bone tumors affecting the physis or in vicinity of physis are known to cause limb length discrepancies (shortening or lengthening).
- Adjacent muscle wasting may occur in long-standing bone tumors and has to be quantified.

Neurovascular Examination

Important to assess as tumors can have compressive features over the nerve, artery, and veins.

Lymph Node Assessment

The presence of enlarged adjacent draining lymph node is suggestive of soft tissue infiltration and spread of the bone tumor.

▉ IMPORTANT DIFFERENTIAL DIAGNOSIS

1. **Osteochondroma:**
   - *Affects*: Most common benign bone tumor affecting pediatric population.
   - *Site*: It usually affects the metaphyseal region of the bones and grows away from the joint.
   - *Clinically*:
     - Slow growing and painless exophytic swelling arising at the ends of long bones.
     - Usually asymptomatic and hence neglected by patients for a long time.
     - Solitary or multiple.
     - Multiple osteochondromas are associated with the autosomal dominant syndrome called as hereditary multiple exostosis (Diaphyseal Aclasis)
     - The growth of the tumor stops once skeletal maturity occurs. If it continues to grow or if there is sudden growth, it suggests a malignant transformation.
   - *Pathologically*: Cartilage tumor
   - *Diagnosis*: X-ray shows an excrescent growth with or without a pedicle (*sessile or pedunculated*), which may be disproportionate to the clinical picture. This is due to the cartilage cap which is not evident in the radiographs (Fig. 12.5).
   - *Treatment*: *Circumperiosteal resection* of symptomatic osteochondromas is recommended.
   - *Complications*: Bursa formation leading to bursitis (most common cause of pain), pathological fracture of the stalk, neurovascular compression, and malignant transformation into chondrosarcoma (rare, common in multiple exostosis).

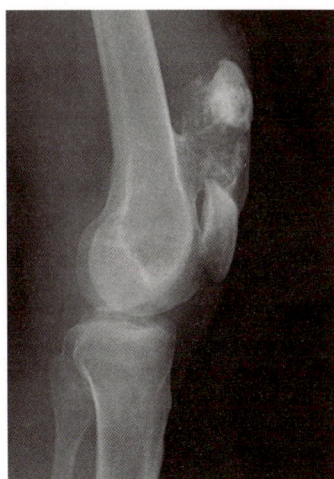

Fig. 12.5: Osteochondroma.

2. **Giant cell tumor (Osteoclastoma)**
   - *Affects:* Skeletally mature adults: 18–40 years, females are more likely to be affected.
   - *Site:* Epiphysis.
   - *Clinically:* Gradual swelling and dull aching pain.
   - *Pathologically:* A benign tumor but locally aggressive. Characterized by the neoplastic mononuclear stromal cells along with multinucleated giant cells. The incidence of malignant giant cell tumor (GCT) is around 1–6%, and lung is the most common site of metastasis.
   - *Diagnosis:* *X-ray* reveals a well-defined *eccentric, expansile geographic* lytic lesion at the epiphyseo-metaphyseal region of the bone. The "soap bubble appearance" on the radiograph is characteristic for GCT (Fig. 12.6).

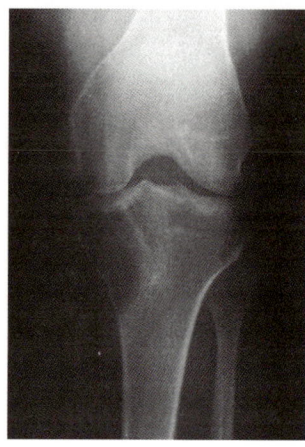

Fig. 12.6: Giant cell tumor.

   - *Treatment:* Extended curettage and reconstruction with graft/bone cement/combination.
     *Extended curettage means: Curettage followed treatment of cavity by mechanical (high speed burr)/chemical (phenol)/thermal means to kill the tumor cells in margin of tumor.
   - *Differential diagnosis:* Aneurysmal bone cyst—may be differentiated by internal septations and ballooning out of cortex.

3. **Osteosarcoma:** Most common primary bone malignancy
   - *Affects:* By far seen in the pediatric age group, it has a bimodal age distribution which is the second decade of life or seventh to eighth decade of life. It has a predilection toward males with a ratio of 2:1.
   - *Site:* Metaphyseal tumor. Commonly affects the growing end of bone-especially around the knee in 70% cases.
   - *Pathologically:* Large 'lacey' osteoid areas, Stromal cells show features of malignancy.
   - *Clinically:*
     - Vague, dull aching pain which may present or occur at rest.
     - Pain may precede a swelling associated with restricted mobility.

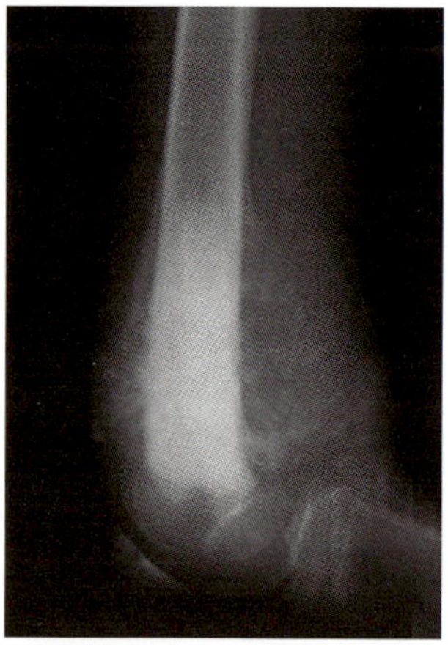

Fig. 12.7: Osteosarcoma of distal femur.

     - A pathological fracture may occur due to trivial injury.
     - Diffuse swelling along with tenderness and local rise of temperature.
     - Dilated veins may occur in the telangiectatic type of osteosarcoma or may suggest vascular impedance due to tumor infiltration.
     - Restriction of movements of the adjoining joint may be noted.
     - Neurovascular impairment may occur in case of infiltration of the tumor, clinically associated with swelling distal to the tumor with neurologic deficits.

- *Diagnosis:* Radiograph may show an Osteosclerotic and osteolytic lesion in the metaphyseal region of the bone. Characteristic radiographic findings of lesion are periosteal reaction in form of "Codman's triangle" and "sunburst appearance" (Fig. 12.7).
    - *A chest radiograph* is necessary to look for distant metastasis.
    - *Computed tomography (CT)* may better delineate the tumor
    - *Magnetic resonance imaging (MRI)* may help to stage the tumor, intramedullary spread (skip lesions) and to reveal the involvement of the neurovascular structures.
    - *Bone scan:* Three-phase Tc^{99} bone scan to detect metastasis.
- *Treatment:* Neoadjuvant chemotherapy followed by surgery followed by adjuvant chemotherapy. (chemo drugs: ifosfamide, methotrexate, and adriamycin).

4. **Ewing's sarcoma (Primitive neuroectodermal tumor group of malignancies)**
    - *Affects:* Second most common primary malignant bone tumor with a peak incidence in the second decade of life. It has a male predominance with a ratio of 1.5:1.
    - *Site:* Diaphysis; the most common site of occurrence is the lower extremity (most common—femur) with an incidence of 45%, followed by the pelvis, and the upper extremity.
    - *Clinically:*
        ○ Pain along with *swelling* (Fig. 12.8).
        ○ *Child may present with acute onset fever, associated pain and swelling (may be mistaken for acute or chronic osteomyelitis).*
        ○ *Metastasis is common in 10% of individuals at the time of presentation, and it commonly occurs in the lungs.*
    - *Diagnosis:* X-ray of the area concerned shows moth-eaten, permeative lucent lesion affecting the bone. Aggressive periosteal reaction characterized by "onion peel skin" is characteristically seen in a radiograph of Ewing's sarcoma (Fig. 12.8). Further, CT scan, MRI, and bone scan is required.
    - *Treatment:* Chemotherapy (Vincristine, doxorubicin, and ifosfamide) followed by surgery, radiation ±

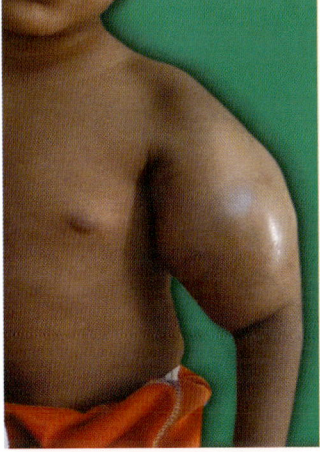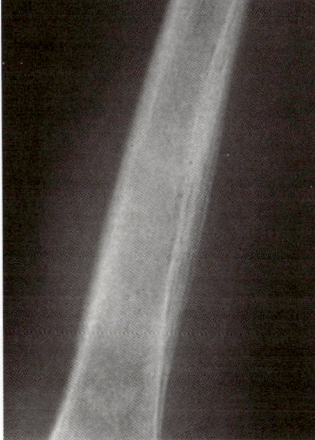

Fig. 12.8: Ewing's sarcoma of left humerus. X-ray shows Onion peel appearance.

Notes

Clinical Evaluation of the Amputation Stump

INTRODUCTION

Definition: Amputation is the intentional surgical removal of the limb by cutting through the bone or by disarticulating the joint.

The word amputation is derived from Latin word 'amputare' which implies 'to cut away'.

Amputation is a **constructive surgery** and not a destructive one, and is the first step towards return of comfortable and functional life.

CASE 1

- 64-year-old male
- Smoker
- Type 2 diabetic
- Claudication in his right lower limb
- Gradual blackening of the toes of his right foot
- Absent anterior tibial, posterior tibial, and dorsalis pedis pulsations to palpation
- Arterial Doppler shows critical stenosis with absent flow beneath the popliteal artery
- After obtaining informed consent, the patient underwent a below-knee amputation.

CASE 2

- 24-year-old male
- Working at a printing press
- Crush injury of the left hand with degloving of both palmar and dorsal aspects with fractures of metacarpals, carpals, and the distal end of radius and ulna, with contamination of the wound with the print ink.
- Disruption of the neurovascular bundles with the absence of sensation and capillary refill distally.
- After informed consent, patient underwent a below elbow amputation.

Here we see two patients of different age group, having undergone amputations for different reasons at different parts of the body. When such amputees come for their follow-up, one has to ask certain questions to know:

1. The cause of the amputation
2. The present state of the amputated limb
3. The functional disability of the limb in particular and the body, as a whole

4. The effectiveness of the prosthesis if already prescribed
5. The psycho-social aspect of leading a life with an amputated limb.

The history is thus important to obtain a general picture as to how the patient is dealing with an amputated limb.

INDICATIONS FOR AMPUTATION

Alan Apley highlighted the indications as "three Ds."

1. **Dead (or Dying):** It includes dry gangrene due to peripheral vascular disease and this is the commonest indication. Other examples of a dead limb are severely traumatized limb, burns and frostbite.
2. **Deadly:** It includes conditions which if not eradicated by amputation immediately might prove fatal. Examples include gas gangrene, severe sepsis, malignant tumors and crush injuries of limb which could lead to crush syndrome.
3. **Damned nuisance:** Retaining the limb may be worse than having no limb at all, because of
   • Pain
   • Gross malformation
   • Recurrent sepsis such as chronic osteomyelitis
   • Severe loss of function.

THE SCHEME OF HISTORY TAKING IN A PATIENT WITH AMPUTATION STUMP

1. **Demographic details:** It includes name, age, sex, occupation, and place of residence. If the upper limb is involved, then one must ascertain the dominant limb.
2. **Chief complaints:** The common complaints include:
   • Pain in the stump or the nearby joint
   • Swelling over the stump
   • Wound over the stump, with or without discharge
   • Deformities of the neighboring joints
   • Tingling/numbness/burning sensation while touching the stump or while donning the prosthesis.
3. **History of presenting complaint(s):** This part elaborates the presenting complaints and their not its associated problems.
   i. **It begins with the circumstances leading to the amputations.** The causes for the amputations can be broadly divided into traumatic and atraumatic.
      (A) Traumatic amputations are usually seen in young individuals following motor vehicle accidents and work-related injuries (the distal extremities of the upper limb, in particular).
      (B) Atraumatic amputations include those due to peripheral vascular disease (seen in older individuals) and those due to tumors.
   ii. **The present state of the limb:** Next, the focus should be on the present state of the limb and questions should be directed to know whether the patient is having any problems with the stump.
      (A) Pain at the stump may be due to a nonhealing wound, ill-fitting prosthesis, continual of claudication, recurrence of a tumor, and infection.

(B) *Phantom limb sensation* may also lead to pain at the stump, and the description is typical.

(C) *Tingling/numbness/burning sensation* while touching the stump or while donning the prosthesis.

(D) *Presence of any wound (sinus or ulcer)*: It may be due to persistent infection or an ill-fitting prosthesis

iii. **Fitting of the prosthesis:** Questions related to the fitting of the prosthesis should be asked. The ill-fitting prosthesis may be the reason for constant discomfort, pain, and nonhealing wound.

iv. **Present disability of the patient:** Further, the present disability of the patient should be discussed. The disability may stem from pain, weakness, deformity of the neighboring joint, and ill-fitting prosthesis.

4. **Past history:** This part elaborates the past medical and surgical histories. The medical history includes questions regarding diabetes mellitus, hypertension, and ischemic heart disease and is especially important in amputations secondary to peripheral vascular disease.

The past surgical history should include details on attempts at limb salvaging procedures such as vascular bypass surgeries, surgeries done for treatment of multiple non-healing wounds over an insensate limb with underlying osteomyelitis (In Charcot's arthropathy), etc.

5. **Personal history:** This includes the personal habits and daily routine of the patient. It is especially important to take a detailed history of tobacco consumption in any form (smoking, chewing) as there is a direct cause–effect relationship between smoking and peripheral vascular disease (Buerger's disease).

Alcohol history is equally important as the excess of alcohol promotes atherosclerosis.

6. **Family history:** Family history of peripheral vascular disease, musculoskeletal tumors, diabetes, etc., is important.

After these points mentioned above are asked, it is imperative to find out what are the patient's expectations, as the treatment should be planned to tailor to his/her needs.

Keeping these points in mind, let us now go through a general scheme of examination of a patient presenting with an amputation stump.

EXAMINATION

The General and Systemic Examinations

It is especially important in amputations secondary to the peripheral arterial occlusive disorder. The *general examination* includes a head to toe evaluation to look for signs of an underlying systemic condition(s).

The *systemic examination* includes a brief examination of the cardiovascular system, respiratory system, the central nervous system and the abdomen. The cardiovascular examination is especially important in peripheral vascular disease.

Local Examination

The examination of the affected limb (in case of lower limbs) begins with an assessment of following:

Gait

The patient is made to walk (as he normally does) and gait is observed from front, sides and behind. Mostly, gait is assisted with some orthosis or prosthesis (Fig. 13.1). However, the foot amputee may walk without a prosthesis (Syme's or Forefoot amputee).

Following the assessment of gait, the patient is then made to lie supine (position of rest) to comment upon other factors.

Attitude

The attitude of the limbs. It is described as the position assumed by each joint at rest.

Inspection of Stump

Inspection should include the following points (Fig. 13.2):

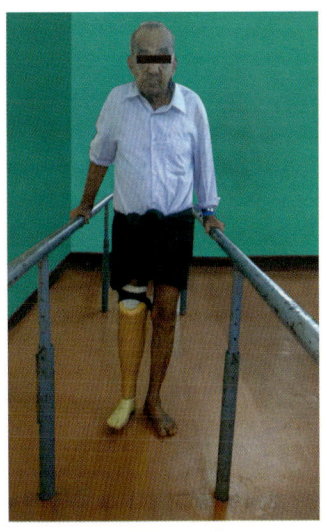

Fig. 13.1: Patient walking with below-knee prosthesis.

- The **shape** of the stump: Cylindrical, conical, bulbous or irregular.
- **Scar of the stump should be assessed with the following points is noted.**
    - State of the surgical incision: healed or the presence of gaping.
    - Whether scar has healed with the primary intention or secondary intention
    - Any hypertrophic scar/keloid formation
- **Swelling** of the stump.
- **Wasting** of the limb.
- Presence or absence of **sinus, discharge** from the wound, *excoriation, erythema, ulcer, or callosities*
- **Protruding or impinging bony ends.**

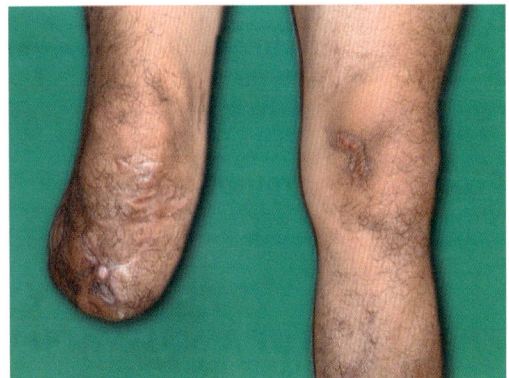

Fig. 13.2: Below-knee amputation stump shows badly scarred stump.

Palpation of Stump

Palpation should be gentle but informative and should confirm the findings obtained from inspection.

- *Local temperature*
- Presence/absence of **tenderness** *over the stump*, and site of tenderness should be noted.
- The bony stump is palpated to assess the *edge, the protruding prominence, and the soft tissue covering*.

- Whether **scar** is mobile or aderent to underlying tissues or bone.
- A detailed examination of **ulcer or sinus, if present,** should be done accordingly.
- The **joint proximal to the stump** should be palpated to assess the degenerative changes, such as joint line tenderness, synovial hypertrophy, joint effusion, bony deformities, and bony irregularities.

Movements of Neighboring Joints

- The ROM at the joint proximal to the stump should be assessed and compared to that of the normal limb.
- The presence of fixed deformities or contractures should be noted.
- Further, it is important to note the presence of pain during movement and joint crepitus, both of which may indicate degenerative changes.

Measurements

- The total length of the stump should be measured from a fixed proximal landmark or joint line.
- Next, the girth of the limb proximal to the stump should be measured and compared to the normal limb to assess muscle wasting.

Neurovascular Status

- Vascularity of the stump is assessed by skin temperature and the level of dependent rubor.
- The stump is then examined for the presence of neuroma (pain and localized paresthesia on percussion), sensory deficits, and paresthesia.

Prosthesis Examination

Once the amputated limb is examined, it is imperative to examine the prosthesis (if the patient is using one) to look for wear, loosening, breakage, etc.

▋ PRINCIPLES OF AMPUTATION

The following principles should be borne in mind while performing an amputation to create an ideal stump:

- The scar should be well healed and mobile, away from the subcutaneous bony edges.
- The skin should be as sensate as possible.
- The stump should have a cylindrical or conical shape at closure.
- Traumatized tissue must not be retained.
- Myoplastic techniques may be attempted in nonischemic limbs. (**Myoplasty**: suturing muscle-tendon to opposite group muscle. **Myodesis**: suturing muscle-tendon to the bone via a predrilled hole).
- Nerves should be gently sectioned and allowed to retract into proximal soft tissues to prevent neuroma formation in inappropriate places.
- The bone should be beveled to avoid sharp edges.

Ideal stump characteristics.
• Ideal length
• Ideal shape: Preferably conical or cylindrical
• Appropriately placed surgical scars healed with primary intention, non-adherent scars, No keloid or painful hypertrophic scars
• Bone ends well covered with muscles with no prominent/sharp bone ends
• Free from any soft tissue or bony Infection, no sinuses/ulcers
• No neuroma
• Full range of movement at the proximal joint, no fixed deformity
• Normal sensation at the stump
• Good muscle power.

TYPES OF AMPUTATIONS

1. **Provisional amputation:** It is performed when primary healing is unlikely. The limb is amputated as distal as the caudal condition will allow. Reamputation and closure of stump are performed when the local conditions are favorable, e.g. *Guillotine amputation*.

2. **Definitive end-bearing:** It is performed when pressure or weight is to be borne through the end of the stump. Hence, the scar must not be terminal, and the bone end must not be hollow, which means it must be cut through or near the joint, e.g. Syme's amputation (Fig. 13.3).

3. **Definitive non-end-bearing amputation:** It is performed when the weight is not taking at the end of the stump. This is the commonest variety, e.g. Below-knee amputation (Fig. 13.4).

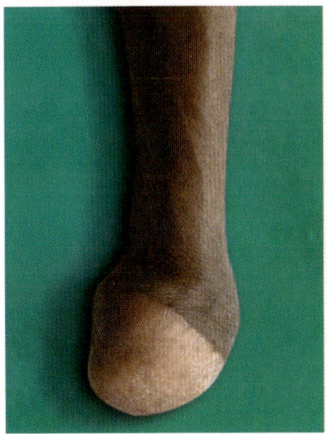 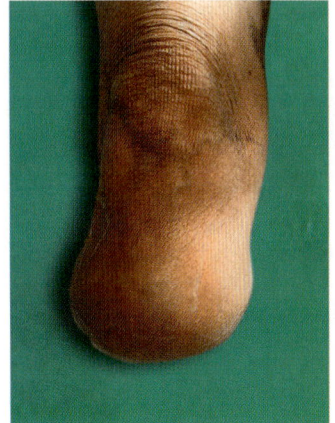

Fig. 13.3: Syme's amputation stump. **Fig. 13.4:** Below-knee amputation stump.

COMPLICATIONS OF AMPUTATION

The following are the common complications seen after amputation:
- Hematoma
- Infection
- Wound necrosis

- Pain
- Joint contractures
- Dermatological problems
- Phantom limb sensation: Mirror therapy should be done
- Neuroma formation
- Painful scars.

COMMON LEVELS OF AMPUTATION

The common level of amputation is explained in Figure 13.5.

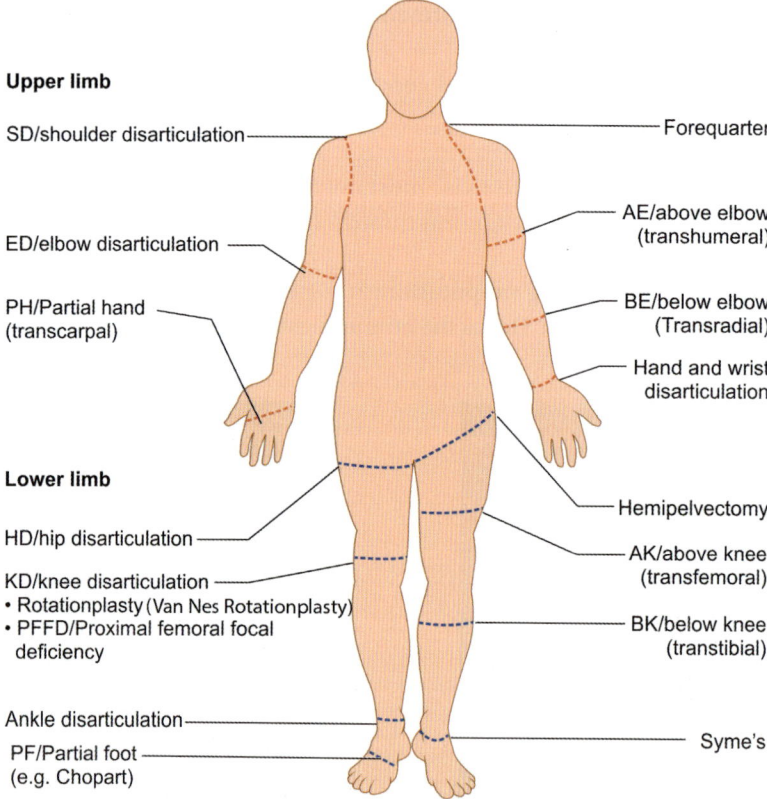

Upper limb

SD/shoulder disarticulation —————— Forequarter

ED/elbow disarticulation ———— AE/above elbow (transhumeral)

PH/Partial hand (transcarpal) — BE/below elbow (Transradial)

Hand and wrist disarticulation

Lower limb

HD/hip disarticulation ———— Hemipelvectomy

KD/knee disarticulation ———— AK/above knee (transfemoral)
- Rotationplasty (Van Nes Rotationplasty)
- PFFD/Proximal femoral focal deficiency — BK/below knee (transtibial)

Ankle disarticulation —————
PF/Partial foot — Syme's
(e.g. Chopart)

Fig. 13.5: Common levels of amputation and disarticulation.

THE OPTIMUM LEVEL OF VARIOUS AMPUTATION STUMPS

The optimal level of various stumps should be achieved to enable prosthesis fitting. However, in the era of modern prosthesis, the 'ideal' level of amputation is gradually becoming less important. The levels are listed in Table 13.1.

Table 13.1: Optimal level of various amputation stumps.			
Site of amputation	*Optimum level*	*Shortest level*	*Longest level*
Below elbow	Junction of proximal two-thirds and distal one-third of forearm	3 cm below to insertion of biceps brachii	5 cm above wrist joint
Above elbow	Middle-third of arm	4 cm below anterior axillary fold	10 cm above olecranon
Above knee	Middle-third of thigh	8 cm below pubic ramus	15 cm above medial joint line
Below knee	8 cm for every 1 m of height	7.5 cm below medial joint line	The level at which a myoplasty can be performed

▌ SPECIAL AMPUTATION STUMPS

1. ***Lisfranc's amputation:*** Foot amputation *through tarsometatarsal joint* while retaining the mid and hindfoot (calcaneus, talus, and heel pad) (Fig. 13.6).
2. ***Chopart's amputation:*** Foot amputation *through midtarsal joint* while retaining the hindfoot (calcaneus, talus, and heel pad).
3. ***Syme's amputation:*** Ankle disarticulation, removal of malleoli, *but* heel pad is retained. It works if there is patent posterior tibial artery. The retained heel pad gives excellent weight-bearing surface, and the patient can walk without a prosthesis (*see* Fig. 13.3).

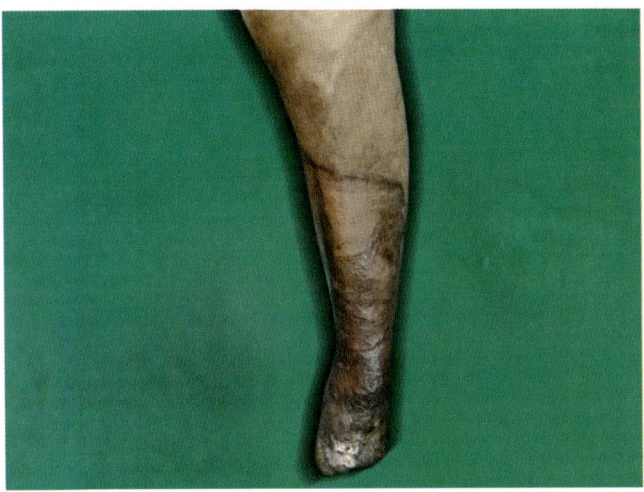

Fig. 13.6: Lisfranc amputation stump.

4. ***Pirogoff amputation:*** It is a Syme's variant wherein ankle disarticulation along with malleoli is removed; but along with heel pad, posterior part of calcaneum is retained.
5. ***Hindquarter amputation or external hemipelvectomy:*** Entire lower limb with the same side innominate bone is removed.

6. *Forequarter amputation*: Entire upper limb with scapula and clavicle is removed.

A note on disarticulation

Disarticulation: When amputation is done through the joint.

Advantages
- Long lever prevents contractures and allows consequently the better muscle and movement control due to longer lever arm
- Maintains muscle length and strength
- Preferred in children as it preserves the growth plates
- Candidates for end bearing prosthesis
- Better proprioception and distribution of pressure

Disadvantages
- Bulky prosthesis
- Poor cosmesis
- More demanding surgical procedure with the risk of increased wound complications

Notes

Gait Assessment and Various Patterns of Gait

INTRODUCTION

Gait analysis is an important part of an examination of the lower limb and spine evaluation as it indicates the way in which the pathological process has affected the main function of the lower limbs (bipedal mobility) and how the patient has compensated for it.

Definition: Gait is an energy-efficient, dynamic posture that allows bipedal mobility from one place to another. It involves neuromuscular coordination of the central nervous system, lumbar spine, pelvis, and the lower limbs.

PHASES OF GAIT

The gait cycle is divided into two phases—*stance and swing (Fig. 14.1).*

1. ***Stance phase:*** It is the time during which the limb is *in contact with the ground* and supporting the weight of the body. Stance phase occupies 60% of the gait cycle.
2. ***Swing phase:*** It is the time when the limb is advancing forward off the ground. During swing phase, the *advancing limb is not in contact with the ground* and body weight is supported by the contralateral limb. Swing phase occupies 40% of gait cycle.

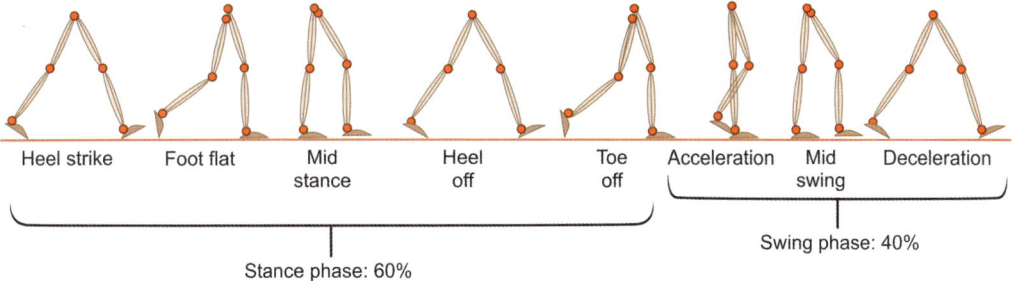

| Heel strike | Foot flat | Mid stance | Heel off | Toe off | Acceleration | Mid swing | Deceleration |

Stance phase: 60% Swing phase: 40%

Fig. 14.1: The role of stance phase and swing phase in gait cycle.

TEMPORAL PARAMETERS OF GAIT

These factors need to be understood while analyzing the gait. They are briefly described below.

- ***Step length:*** Distance between two feet during double-limb support.
- ***Stride length:*** Distance that one limb travels during stance and swing phases.
- ***Step time:*** Time needed to complete one step length.

- *Cadence*: Number of steps per minute.
- *Walking velocity*: Distance traveled per time (m/sec).

ASSESSMENT OF GAIT

It requires a systematic history taking and examination.
(A) History
(B) Examination

History

1. Gait analysis is mainly observational. However, the patient may present with certain complaints concerning his gait. The most common of these are:
   - Pain while walking
   - Stiffness
   - *Limp*: It may be painful or painless.
2. The onset, duration, and progression of the complaint (mainly, limp) have to be noted, and the disability resulting from an altered gait has to be analyzed. For example, a person with a stiff hip gait may complain of difficulty in getting into or out of a vehicle.
3. The history should also detail the use of a walking aid and the change of footwear.
4. Various neurological, systemic, and structural conditions influence the gait. The pertinent history detailing these disorders affecting the gait must be evaluated.
   - *Neuromuscular*: Cerebrovascular accident (CVA), cerebral palsy, poliomyelitis, Parkinson's disease, peripheral nerve injury or affection, and myopathy
   - *Structural*: Limb length discrepancy, developmental dysplasia of the hip (DDH), and congenital talipes equinovarus (CTEV).
   - *Due to congenital or acquired deformities*: Equinus, calcaneus, etc.

Examination

As mentioned before, gait analysis is observational. There are certain prerequisites that are to be followed while commenting on gait.

1. Gait should be observed from the front, behind, and sides.
2. The patient should be made to walk barefoot.
3. The lumbar spine, pelvis, and the lower limbs should be exposed with only the private parts being covered.
4. A walkway of sufficient length and width should be available.
5. The following structural and functional features should be observed while evaluating the gait.
   - Head position
   - Position of the shoulders
   - Arm swing
   - Trunk position
   - Pelvic tilt
   - The swing of the lower limbs

- Time spent in the stance and the swing phase
- Base (distance between the two feet).

For example, in a child with DDH on right side, the gait is described as, "a bipedal, unaided gait with the patient lurching to the right side and the pelvis dropping on the left side. The head is central in position, the arm swing is alternate and rhythmic, and the gait is painless. This is a description of a Trendelenburg gait on the right side."

■ COMMONLY ENCOUNTERED GAIT PATTERNS ARE BRIEFLY DESCRIBED BELOW

1. **Antalgic gait:** Seen in conditions causing *pain in any of the lower limb bones and joints.*
   - The patient walks with a shortened stance phase on the affected side.
   - Decreased swing of the normal side
   - Lurches on the affected side.
2. **Trendelenburg gait:** Seen in conditions causing *dysfunction of the abductor mechanism of the hip* (DDH, coxa vara, and perthes etc. *Read Hip examination chapter for details*).
   - The patient lurches on the affected side with normal stance phase, and the pelvis drops on the opposite (normal) side but lifts up due to lurch of trunk to the affected side. This causes rocking up and down of pelvis while walking.
   - A bilateral Trendelenburg's gait is called *Waddling gait.*
3. **High-stepping gait:** Seen in *foot drop.*
   - Because the patient is unable to actively dorsiflex the ankle during the swing phase, to avoid the dragging of foot, he/she lifts the affected limb higher (increased ipsilateral hip and knee flexion) and puts the forefoot to contact first during the stance phase.
4. **Extension lurch gait:** Seen in *paralysis of gluteus maximus* which is an extensor of the hip.
   - The patient lurches backward during walking. Patient's trunk moves forward and backward too much giving a rocking horse gait appearance (Fig. 14.2A).
5. **Stiff hip gait:** Seen in *ankylosis of the hip joint.*
   - The patient walks by moving his whole pelvis along with the affected side (swaying to the opposite side).
6. **Scissoring gait:** Due to *adductor contracture/spasm.* Classically seen in spastic cerebral palsy.
   - Here, the leg in swing phase crosses directly anteriorly over the leg in stance phase. (like a scissor, Fig. 14.2B)
7. **Festinant gait:** Seen in *Parkinson's disease.*
   - "Short, shuffling gait" where patient bends forward while taking short, quick steps with reduced arm swing and trembling of extremities. (Fig. 14.3A. (*The gait is something like, how a fast bowler bends forward in his initial run up with small steps!*)
8. **Hemiplegic gait:** Circumduction gait. Classically seen in *hemiplegia after cerebrovascular accident.*
   - Due to spasticity and hip in internal rotation, knee in extension, ankle in plantar flexion, and inversion; during swing phase, patient tries to *circumduct the hip* and clear the ground.

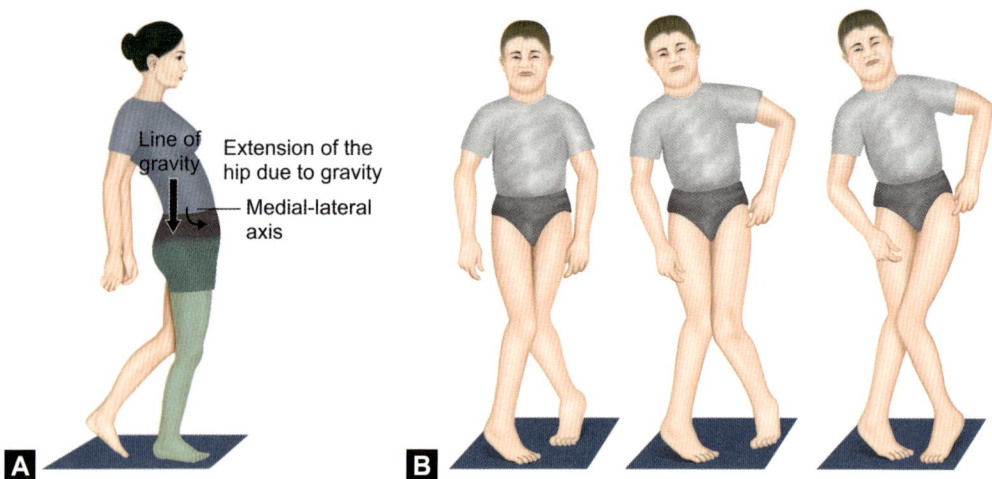

Figs. 14.2A and B: (A) Shows extension lurch gait. (B) Shows scissoring gait.

9. **Quadriceps weakness:** Classically described in *patients with Poliomyelitis affecting quadriceps muscle*. Here, patient bends forward to let the center of gravity fall in front of the knee to let the knee lock or knee goes in extension. In extreme quadriceps weakness, patient may adopt *hand to knee gait* wherein patient pushes the knee with his hand in order to extend and lock the knee to propel forward (Fig. 14. 3B).

10. **Ataxic gait:** Due to *cerebellar disorder*, the balance is impaired and the patient adopts wide base of support (BOS). This wide BOS creates large side—side swaying due to deviation of center of gravity.

11. **Stamping gait:** Seen in *posterior column disorder* where the patient has lost proprioceptive sensations from lower limb.
    - Here; patient raises his leg, jerks it forward to stamp the 'entire foot' on the ground. (c.f. foot drop where forefoot touches the ground first.)

12. **Knock knee gait:** Seen in *genu valgus deformity* wherein both knees knock with each other while walking (Fig. 14.3C).

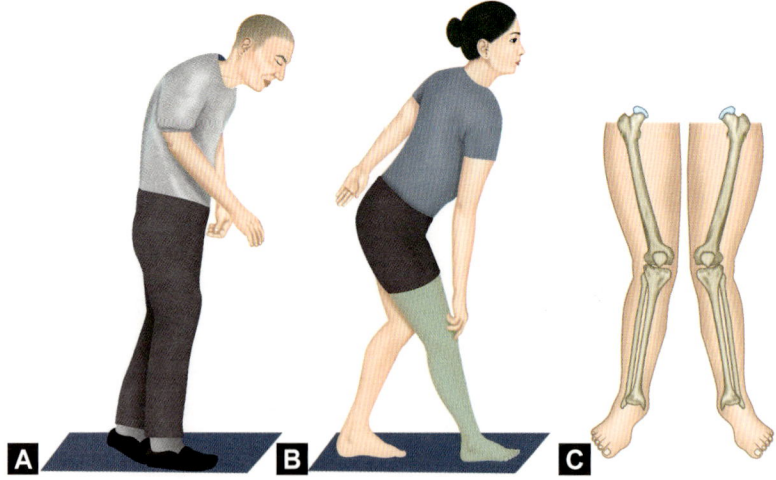

Figs. 14.3A to C: (A) Festinant gait. (B) Quadriceps weakness "hand to knee gait". (C) Knock knee gait.

Notes

Clinical Evaluation of the Swelling, Scar, Sinus, and Ulcer

▌HISTORY AND EXAMINATION OF A SWELLING

1. Onset

- *Acute onset:*
  - ○ *Following trauma:* Fractured displacement of bone, dislocation of joint, hematoma
  - ○ *Spontaneous:* Acute osteomyelitis, tumor (mostly malignant)
- *Insidious onset:* Tumor (mostly benign), inflammatory or chronic infective origin, ganglion, Baker's cyst

2. Painless/Painful

- *Painless:* Most tumors; initially ganglion, Baker's cyst
- *Painful:* Inflammatory (throbbing pain), later stages of tumors (dull aching pain)
  - ○ Pain followed by swelling: Inflammatory conditions, malignant tumors
  - ○ Initially painless swelling develops sudden pain: Malignant transformation, pathological fracture, hemorrhage, nerve entrapment/compression.

3. Duration

- *Since birth:* Congenital
- *Short duration (days to weeks):* Acute osteomyelitis, tumor (mostly malignant), inflammatory
- *Long duration (months to years):* Tumor (mostly benign), ganglion.

4. Progression

- *Growing slowly:* Benign swellings (Tumor, Ganglion, Baker's cyst)
- *Growing rapidly:* Malignant swellings
- *Suddenly increasing in size after remaining stationary for some time:* Malignant transformation of benign swellings
- *Fluctuation in size:* Inflammatory swellings.

5. Associated Sinus

- Mostly indicates chronic osteomyelitis.

6. Similar Swellings Elsewhere

- Multiple metaphyseal swellings: Diaphyseal Aclasis, Neurofibromatosis.

7. Exacerbating or Relieving Factors

- Vascular swellings may increase in size with dependency.

8. Other Associated Symptoms

- *Constitutional symptoms*: Tumor (mostly malignant), infection, inflammatory
- *Compressive symptoms*: Seen in tumors
  - *Nerve compression*: Pain, weakness, and paresthesia, distally.
  - *Vascular compression*: Venous congestion distally, edema
- *Growth disturbance/angular deformities:* Lesion damaging growth plate (Juxtaphyseal tumors like diaphyseal aclasis/osteomyelitis)
- *Functional disability*: Difficulty in using the limb
- Symptoms are suggestive of the location of the primary tumor in case of swelling due to secondaries in bone. E.g. Urinary complaints, breathing difficulty, neck swelling, breast lumps, etc.

9. Past History

- H/o infection elsewhere (must be asked in case of children and immunocompromised patients)*: Acute osteomyelitis.*

10. Family History

To rule out hereditary disorders like osteogenesis imperfecta, achondroplasia.

▍EXAMINATION

The general and systemic examination should be done in the standard fashion.

Local Examination of Swelling

Inspection

1. **Site:** Often a site may suggest the etiology of the swelling. E.g.
   - *Epiphysis*: Osteoclastoma, chondroblastoma
   - *Metaphysis*: Bone cyst, osteoid osteoma, osteosarcoma, acute pyogenic osteomyelitis
   - *Diaphysis*: Ewing's sarcoma, multiple myeloma, syphilitic osteomyelitis
   - *Small bones of the hand*: Enchondroma, spina ventosa (Tubercular dactylitis)

> *Note:*
> - Ganglions are very common over the dorsum of the wrist/around the wrist.
> - Rheumatoid nodules are seen over the extensor surface of the long bones, especially in the forearm.

2. **Size:** Approximate length and width of the swelling
3. **Shape:** Spherical/oval/irregular/other
4. **Number**
   - *Solitary:* Osteomyelitis, Ganglion, Most tumors
   - *Multiple*: Diaphyseal aclasis, Neurofibromatosis
5. **Extent:** Vertical and horizontal extent
6. **Surface**
   - *Smooth*: Usually benign tumors
   - *Irregular*: Malignant tumors, chronic infection
7. **Edge**
   - *Well defined*: Usually pedunculated swelling
   - *Indistinct*: Sessile swelling
8. **Skin overlying the swelling**
   - *Edematous and congested:* Acute osteomyelitis
   - *Stretched, shiny with dilated veins:* Malignant tumors
   - *Sinus*: Chronic osteomyelitis, tuberculosis
   - *Scar*: Chronic osteomyelitis, previous surgery
9. **Pressure effects** (limb distal to the swelling)
   - *Edema*: Venous compression
   - *Paresis/pain*: Nerve compression
10. **Muscle wasting**
11. **Shortening/Lengthening of bone:** Osteomyelitis, trauma, diaphyseal aclasis
12. **Neighboring joints**
   - Diffuse swelling seen in acute osteomyelitis over the adjacent joint is usually due to sympathetic effusion or when the pus breaks down into the joint cavity from the metaphysis leading to septic arthritis.
   - *Angular deformities:* Sequelae of osteomyelitis, diaphyseal aclasis.

Palpation

1. **Local temperature** (palpated by back of fingers)
   - Raised in acute inflammatory, infective, and malignant swelling
2. **Tenderness**
   - *Tender:* Inflammatory swellings, malignant tumors, infection, acute trauma
   - *Non-tender:* Chronic degenerative condition
3. **Swelling-specific characteristics**
   - *Site:* Same as inspection
   - *Size and Shape:* Same as inspection
   - *Surface*
     - *Smooth and lobulated:* Benign tumors
     - *Irregular*: Malignant tumors, chronic infection
   - *Edge*
     - *Well-defined*: New growth/benign (usually)
     - *Ill-defined*: Inflammatory/infective/malignant

- ○ *Initially well-defined and later rapidly progressing to ill-defined:* Benign turning malignant.
- **Consistency**
  - ○ Soft: Acute osteomyelitis with subcutaneous abscess (soft tissue over the swelling)
  - ○ *Variable (Hard to firm to soft):* Osteosarcoma
  - ○ *Bony hard*: Osteoma, osteoclastoma (egg shell crackling—must not be elicited), bone over chronic osteomyelitis area.
- **Pulsation:** Highly vascular tumors like telangiectatic osteosarcoma, aneurysmal bone cyst, highly vascular osteoclastoma and, rarely, highly vascular secondaries (from thyroid and renal adenocarcinoma) can be pulsatile.

> **Difference between pulsatile swelling and transmitted pulsation.**
> **Pulsatile swelling**: When a pair of fingers kept over the swelling move away from each other, it indicates a pulsatile swelling.
> **Transmitted pulsation**: when fingers move only vertically parallel to each other and not away from each other, it indicates transmitted pulsation.

- **Plane of the swelling:** It is extremely important to identify the plane of the swelling. Also, the swelling may possess some characteristic features when it arises from a particular structure.

> **Characteristic features of plane of the swelling.**
> - A **submuscular swelling** becomes less prominent when the muscle is contracted.
> - An **intramuscular swelling** remains the same when the muscle is contracted.
> - A **supramuscular swelling** becomes prominent when the muscle is contracted.
> - A **swelling arising from the tendon** does not move much along the axis of the tendon, but can be moved in the plane perpendicular to it, especially when the tendon is made to contract.
> - A **swelling arising from the nerve** may cause sensory motor symptoms. Also, when the swelling is percussed, it may cause shooting pains/tingling along the course of nerve.
> - An arterial swelling is pulsatile whereas venous is non-pulsatile.
> **With limb** in elevation, venous swelling decreases in size and fills slowly when emptied by milking it. Arterial swelling does not decrease in size with limb elevation and fill quickly after it emptied by milking.
> - Lipoma edges slip under the finger.
> - Bony swellings are hard, and often fixed to the bone if they arise from the same.

- **Fluctuation:** It should be tested in two planes, perpendicular to each other.
  - ○ Fix the swelling by placing the thumb and index finger of one hand at the opposite poles of the swelling. Now press the swelling at the summit with the index finger of the other hand and feel for the fluctuation with the index finger and thumb of other hand. Now, repeat the test by placing the fixing fingers on the plane perpendicular to the first ones. A positive fluctuation implies fluid or gas in the cavity.
- **Compressibility:**
  - ○ *Swelling of venous, lymphatic or capillary origin (varicose veins, saphenavarix, hemangioma, lymphangioma):* Reduces in size after elevation of limb, or by compressing it while it reappears after placing the limb at the level of heart or in a dependent position.

- ○ *Swelling of arterial origin (Aneurysm):* Reduces in size after compressing it directly or blocking the arterial feeder, and reappears when pressure is removed. However, the position of the limb may not have any effect on the size, unlike the swelling of venous origin.

> **Note: Compressible and reducible are different terms!**
> **Compressible** means that the swelling reduces in size when external pressure is applied over the swelling and gradually reappears once pressure is taken off.
> **Reducible** means that once the swelling is reduced with external pressure, it reappears only once intracavity (intra-abdominal) pressure is elevated, e.g. hernia

- *Transillumination:* In case of swellings with clear fluid, a torch light would pass through it and create a flare of light in the swelling.
- *Fixity* to the skin and underlying bone.
- *Auscultation:* Listen for arterial bruits and venous hums. An aneurysm or arterio-venous malformations could have bruits.

4. **Bony irregularity**
- It is felt in areas where the bone is relatively superficial and not covered by muscles. It is due to subperiosteal new bone formation classically seen in chronic osteomyelitis, Brodies abscess, united fracture

5. **Ulcer and sinus** (Read section on sinus examination)

6. **Presence of fracture**
- Abnormal mobility at the bone is suggestive of pathological fracture.

Movement

The adjacent joint movement should be assessed. It could be painful and decreased if the pathology involves the joint, muscle, and other local soft tissues.

Measurement

1. **Length of bone:** Limb length discrepancy (seen in osteomyelitis), tumors (diaphyseal aclasis)
- *Shortening*: Epiphyseal cartilage destruction
- *Lengthening*: Hyperemia of metaphysis and physis

2. **Circumference of limb:** Wasting of muscles.

Neighboring Joint Swelling and Movements

- Sympathetic effusion, septic arthritis.

Examination of Regional Lymph Nodes and Other Organs

- Important in case of infective and tumorous lesions. "If you are considering a possibility of a malignant swelling always visualize a possibility of a distant metastasis thus do not fail to examine possible organs where it might have metastasized."

Distal Neurovascular Assessment

HISTORY AND EXAMINATION OF A SCAR

Relevant History

1. **Etiology:** Trauma, history of infection or previous surgery, history of radiation or steroid exposure.
2. **The growth of scar:** The keloids can grow fast and irregularly, and then attain a plateau of growth.
3. **Associated symptoms:** Pain and itching.

Examination

1. **Site and extent:** The location of the scar may suggest the intention of surgical intervention or an approach to the region.
2. **Size**
3. **Color:** Normal color resembling the surrounding skin, hypo- or hyperpigmented.
4. **Shape and texture:** Suggestive of healing with primary or secondary intention.
   - *Linear scar with smooth margins:* Usually a surgical scar healed with primary intention (Fig. 15.1A).
   - *Linear scar with irregular margins:* Usually a surgical scar healed with secondary intention (Fig. 15.1B).
   - *Geographical/Irregular scar:* Usually a traumatic scar/post-infection scar healed with secondary intention (Fig. 15.1B).
   - *Exaggerated irregular scar:* Seen in keloid formation.

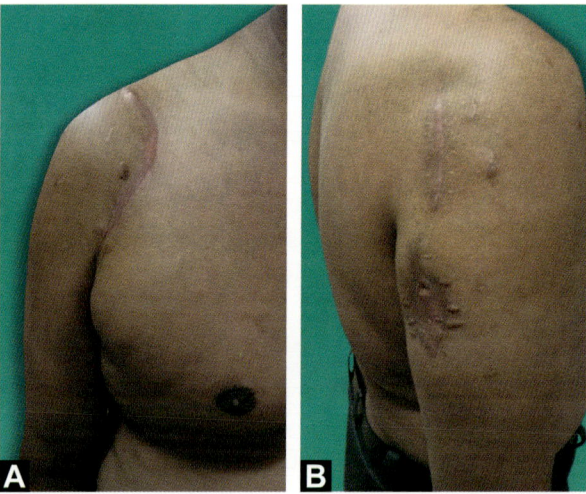

Figs. 15.1A and B: (A) Scar healed with primary intention. (B) Scar healed with secondary intention with sinus.

5. **Tethering and contracture:** Suggestive of the relationship of the scar to the surrounding structures.
6. **Tender:** Keloids and hypertrophic scars could be tender and pruritic.

■ HISTORY AND EXAMINATION OF A SINUS

Definition: The sinus is a blind track lined by granulation tissue which connects the surface to a cavity in the tissue.

Relevant History

1. **Onset and progression:** A patient with chronic osteomyelitis gives a typical history of the cyclical development of fever, swelling, and pain followed by the bursting of the abscess, resulting in the formation of a discharging sinus. There might be a history of extrusion of bone chip or pieces. Ask for any history of trauma, open fractures, past surgery etc. Often, there is periodical history of quiescence and exacerbation of sinus activity. Associated history of Diabetes and Tuberculosis are quite relevant.
2. **Pain:** It is suggestive of an inflammatory etiology or may be due to the blockage of the sinus, leading to increased intra-sinus or cavity (from where sinus is originating) pressure.

One has to remember that *presence of sinus in an orthopedic case does not always naturally mean osteomyelitis!* It implies that there is a dead tissue (sequestrum, other tissue)/dead material (foreign body, nonabsorbable suture material) inside the body, which harbors the infection. The infected material (pus) keeps coming out via the sinus and discharges over the surface. As long as the dead tissue survives, sinus will persist! Further, a weeping sinus may indicate an underlying malignancy.

Examination

Inspection

1. **Site:** It could be anywhere along the length of the bone, and the level of external opening might not correspond with the level of the cavity in the bone.
2. **Number**
3. **Margins**
   - Pouting granulation tissue at the margin of the sinus is suggestive of sequestrum (or a dead material) underneath (Fig. 15.2).
   - Undermined, the thin bluish margin is seen in the tubercular sinus.
4. **Discharge**
   - *Purulent discharge*: Pyogenic osteomyelitis
   - *Serosanguinous discharge:* Tuberculous osteomyelitis
   - *Sequestrum*: Hallmark of osteomyelitis
5. **Surrounding skin:** Scarring of the surrounding skin is usually seen in osteomyelitis.

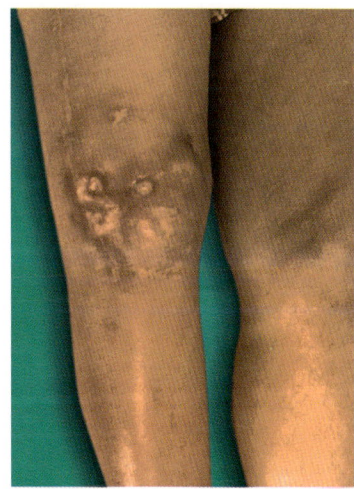

Fig. 15.2: Sinus along the granulation tissue.

Palpation

- *Tenderness* is usually a feature of sinus associated with chronic osteomyelitis.
- *Wall of the sinus* is thick due to fibrosis of surrounding tissue owing to chronic inflammation.
- *Fixity to the bone*: Hold the base of sinus and move it side-side. A sinus arising from bone (In chronic osteomyelitis) is always fixed to underlying bone whereas sinus arising from soft tissues retains its side-side mobility.

Standard Assessment of Movement at Neighboring Joint

Examination of Regional Draining Lymph Nodes

- Examination of regional draining lymph nodes should be done.

▌EXAMINATION OF ULCER

Definition: An ulcer is defined as a break in the continuity of the skin or mucous membrane with loss of surface tissue, disintegration and necrosis of the epithelial tissue with superadded infection.

The examination of the ulcer can be done under the following headings:

Inspection

1. **Site**
2. **Size**
3. **Shape**
4. **Floor:** Exposed surface of the ulcer *(the floor is seen while the base is felt!)*
   One can describe what is seen in the floor of the ulcer (granulation tissue, bone, muscle, dead tissue)
5. **Edge** (Fig. 15.3)
   - ***Sloping edge:*** Healing ulcer (with three zones from center to periphery; red in the center of the ulcer followed by a narrow blue zone due to a thin epithelium, followed by an outer white zone due to a fibrotic scar)
   - ***Punched out edge:*** Trophic ulcer (neuropathic ulcer, syphilis)
   - ***Undermined edge:*** Tuberculosis (Undermined edges because subcutaneous tissue is destroyed faster than skin)
   - ***Everted edge:*** Squamous cell carcinoma
   - ***Rolled-out edge:*** Basal cell carcinoma.

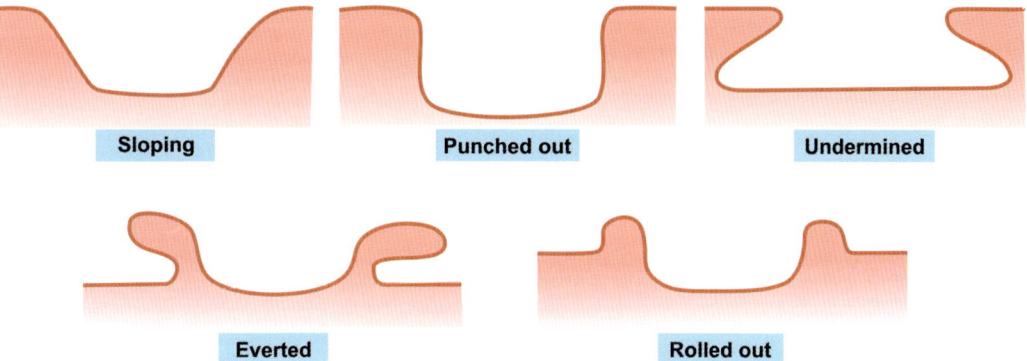

Fig. 15.3: Various types of ulcer edge.

6. **Discharge:** Serous or seropurulent or purulent
7. **Surrounding skin:**
   - Glossy red or edematous in acutely inflamed ulcers
   - Eczematous and pigmented in varicose ulcers.

Palpation

1. **Base:** It refers to the state of the tissue underneath the floor of ulcer. Induration and fixity to the underlying tissue is felt in inflammatory and malignant ulcers.
2. **Depth**
3. **Tenderness:** Acute ulcers may be tender
4. **Bleeding on touch:** Feature of a malignant ulcer
5. **Draining lymph node.**

Notes

Index

Page numbers followed by *f* refer to figure and *t* refer to table.